Pulmonary Pearls II

STEVEN A. SAHN, M.D.

Professor of Medicine
Director, Division of Pulmonary
    and Critical Care Medicine
Medical University of South Carolina
Charleston, South Carolina

JOHN E. HEFFNER, M.D.

Chairman, Academic Internal Medicine
St. Joseph's Hospital and Medical Center
Professor of Clinical Medicine
University of Arizona Health Sciences Center
Phoenix, Arizona

HANLEY & BELFUS, INC./Philadelphia
MOSBY/ST. Louis · Baltimore · Boston · Chicago · London
    Philadelphia · Sydney · Toronto

Publisher: HANLEY & BELFUS, INC.
Medical Publishers
210 S. 13th Street
Philadelphia, PA 19107
(215) 546-7293
FAX (215) 790-9330

North American and worldwide sales and distribution:

MOSBY
11830 Westline Industrial Drive
St. Louis, MO 63146

In Canada: Times Mirror Professional Publishing, Ltd.
130 Flaska Drive
Markham, Ontario L6G 1B8
Canada

Library of Congress Cataloging-in-Publication Data

Sahn, Steven A.
    Pulmonary pearls II / Steven A. Sahn, John E. Heffner.
        p.   cm.
    Includes bibliographical references and index.
    ISBN 1-56053-121-5
    1. Respiratory organs—Diseases—Case studies.   2.Chest—Diseases—Case studies.
    3. Chest—Radiography.   I. Heffner, John E.   II. Title.   III. Title: Pulmonary pearls 2.
    IV. Title: Pulmonary pearls two.
        [DNLM: 1. Lung Diseases—radiography—case studies.   WF 600 S131p 1994]
    RC732.S242   1994
    616.2—dc20
    DNLM/DLC   94-23207
    for Library of Congress   CIP

PULMONARY PEARLS II   ISBN 1-56053-121-5

Library of Congress catalog card number 94-23207

Last digit is the print number: 9 8 7 6 5 4 3 2 1

DEDICATION

To Ellie for always being there with love and understanding

— SAS

To Ann for her never-ending love and support

— JEH

THE PEARLS SERIES

Series Editors

Steven A. Sahn, M.D.
Professor of Medicine
Director, Division of Pulmonary
and Critical Care Medicine
Medical University of South
Carolina
Charleston, South Carolina

John E. Heffner, M.D.
Chairman, Academic Internal Medicine
St. Joseph's Hospital and Medical Center
Professor of Clinical Medicine
University of Arizona Health Sciences
Center
Phoenix, Arizona

The books in the Pearls Series contain 100 case presentations that provide valuable information that is not readily available in standard textbooks. The problem-oriented approach is ideal for self-study and for board review. A brief clinical vignette is presented, including physical examination and laboratory findings, accompanied by a radiograph, EKG, or other pertinent illustration. The reader is encouraged to consider a differential diagnosis and formulate a plan for diagnosis and treatment. The subsequent page discloses the diagnosis, followed by a discussion of the case, clinical pearls, and key references.

CARDIOLOGY PEARLS

Blase A. Carabello, MD, **William L. Ballard, MD**, and **Peter C. Gazes, MD**, Medical University of South Carolina, Charleston, South Carolina
1994/223 pages/illustrated/ISBN 0-932883-96-6

CRITICAL CARE PEARLS

Steven A. Sahn, MD, Medical University of South Carolina, Charleston, South Carolina, and **John E. Heffner, MD**, St. Joseph's Hospital and Medical Center, Phoenix, Arizona
1989/300 pages/illustrated/ISBN 0-932883-24-9

INTERNAL MEDICINE PEARLS

Clay B. Marsh, MD, and **Ernest L. Mazzaferri, MD**, The Ohio State University College of Medicine, Columbus, Ohio
1992/300 pages/90 illustrations/ISBN 1-56053-024-3

PULMONARY PEARLS I

Steven A. Sahn, MD, Medical University of South Carolina, Charleston, South Carolina, and **John E. Heffner, MD**, St. Joseph's Hospital and Medical Center, Phoenix, Arizona
1988/250 pages/illustrated/ISBN 0-932883-16-8

PULMONARY PEARLS II

Steven A. Sahn, MD, Medical University of South Carolina, Charleston, South Carolina, and **John E. Heffner, MD**, St. Joseph's Hospital and Medical Center, Phoenix, Arizona
1995/300 pages/illustrated/ISBN 1-56053-121-5

CONTENTS

FOREWORD

The diagnosis and management of patients with pulmonary problems are fun. This is as it should be. The modern pulmonologist encounters a wide array of diagnoses and treatment problems that embrace all age groups, and the field intertwines with all of medicine itself. The acquisition of extensive experience takes a lifetime, and disciplined clinicians continue to add to their armamentarium of mental and intuitive resources that allow the pursuit of a systematic approach to problem solving. Yet no one clinician has seen it all.

Pulmonary Pearls II presents 100 new clinical vignettes and the associated "pearls" of wisdom that derive therefrom. Two astute clinicians have presented a most delightful format, as they did with their previous book, *Pulmonary Pearls*, and with other books in the Pearls Series, which they edit.

This new book is as challenging and instructive as the first, and, of course, complements it. My hat is off to two former fellows of the Colorado program. These exciting and energetic individuals are not only excellent clinicians, but two of the most seasoned journalists in our field.

Thomas L. Petty, M.D.
Director of Academic Affairs
Presbyterian-St. Luke's Medical Center
Denver, Colorado

ACKNOWLEDGMENTS

The authors wish to thank Celia Barbieri, Louisa Cory, and Ruth DeHaven for their tireless and invaluable efforts in assisting us with manuscript preparations. We also acknowledge the contributions of the internal medicine residents from St. Joseph's Hospital and Medical Center and the following pulmonary and critical care fellows from the Medical University of South Carolina: Dalton E. Dove, M.D., Scott R. Dryzer, M.D., Mikell J. Jarratt, M.D., Jose Joseph, M.D., Lisa Kennedy, M.D., Timothy C. Keys, M.D., Sola Kim, M.D., Gregory P. LeMense, M.D., Lalaine E. Mattison, M.D., and Philip P. Retalis, M.D. We thank our colleague Lee K. Brown, M.D. for providing a resonant sounding board for validating concepts and ideas.

Our greatest debt is to our publisher, Linda Belfus, who continues to provide us with guidance, patience, and good will.

The authors gratefully acknowledge that several cases were adapted or reprinted with permission from material that appeared previously in the following journals:

Case 6: J Respir Dis 1990;11:1007–1010
Case 8: J Respir Dis 1991;12:586–589
Case 10: J Respir Dis 1990;11:819–822
Case 12: J Crit Illness 1991;6:131–137
Case 25: J Crit Illness 1991;6:670–676
Case 30: J Crit Illness 1990;5:932–936
Case 31: J Respir Dis 1990;12:81–84
Case 33: J Crit Illness 1993;8:414–421
Case 37: J Respir Dis 1992;13:603–606
Case 51: J Respir Dis 1993;14:283–286
Case 61: J Respir Dis 1993;14:125–129

Case 63: J Crit Illness 1992;7:200–204
Case 65: J Respir Dis 1992;13:193–197
Case 67: J Respir Dis 1990;11:399–401
Case 69: J Respir Dis 1991;12:943–948
Case 71: J Crit Illness 1992;7:1436–1444
Case 73: J Respir Dis 1993;14:827–831
Case 75: J Respir Dis 1993;8:693–696
Case 77: J Crit Illness 1993;8:995–998
Case 79: J Respir Dis 1993;14:1343–1351
Case 83: J Crit Illness 1992;7:691–697

PREFACE

When chest physicians distill their interests in pulmonary medicine down to a fundamental essence, many of us speak of our fascination for facing difficult diagnostic challenges armed with a broad-based fund of medical knowledge. In that regard, we have been gratified with the reception during the last four years of *Pulmonary Pearls*, the first book in the Pearls Series. The Pearls Series challenges the reader with a brief clinical vignette to formulate a differential diagnosis and evaluative plan. In the pages that follow the case summary, a patient's primary disorder is discussed in a manner that provides both fundamental knowledge along with recent advances in understanding of the disease processes. The content is structured to supplement the learning of both medical student and master clinician alike. The more salient points are classified at the end of the discussion as "pearls"—those "difficult-to-find" and clinically valuable concepts that provide insight into differential diagnosis and patient care.

The publication of *Pulmonary Pearls II* marks several milestones for the authors. It is the first book published in the Pearls Series that builds upon a predecessor—*Pulmonary Pearls*. We have retained the original format that has assisted physicians in practice, young clinicians learning pulmonary medicine, and pulmonologists preparing for their board examinations. But the book contains entirely new material. Case presentations of 100 patients challenge the reader with clinical conditions that rarely overlap with those discussed in its companion volume, *Pulmonary Pearls*. But perhaps the most meaningful milestone for us is that this book marks the 20th anniversary of the authors' professional collaboration and shared fascination with pulmonary medicine and ongoing efforts to hone our differential diagnosis skills.

Steven A. Sahn, M.D.
Charleston, South Carolina
John E. Heffner, M.D.
Phoenix, Arizona

PATIENT 1

A 68-year-old woman with a dry cough, myalgias, and respiratory failure

A 68-year-old woman with chronic lymphocytic leukemia treated with prednisone noted in early January a 2-day history of fever, headache, and myalgias, followed by a dry nonproductive cough. She presented for evaluation when dyspnea developed that rapidly progressed to severe shortness of breath. Several members of her family had similar symptoms, except for the shortness of breath, and ascribed their illnesses to the flu. The patient had not received an influenza vaccination.

Physical Examination: Temperature 103°; respirations 28; pulse 120; blood pressure 110/80. General: severe dyspnea. Skin: normal except for peripheral cyanosis. Chest: diffuse crackles. Cardiac: normal heart sounds. Abdomen: no organomegaly.

Laboratory Findings: Hct 39%; WBC 27,500 μl with 60% lymphocytes. Electrolytes and renal indices: normal. CPK 650 IU/L. ABG (4 L nasal cannula): PO_2 49 mmHg; PCO_2 29 mmHg; pH 7.48.

Hospital Course: The patient was intubated in the emergency department because of severe dyspnea. The postintubation chest radiograph is shown below.

Question: What is the likely diagnosis? What specific therapy is available?

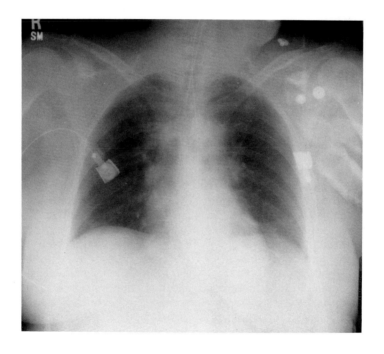

Diagnosis: Influenza with influenza pneumonia.

Discussion: Despite the availability of effective influenza vaccines and widespread recommendations for their use in older persons, influenza remains a major cause of lower respiratory tract infections and a leading cause of annual excess mortality. During serious epidemics that occur every 1–3 years, influenza accounts for 10,000 deaths per year in the United States.

The major complications of influenza infection include primary viral pneumonia, which can be followed by secondary bacterial pneumonias, exacerbation of chronic pulmonary conditions, rhabdomyolysis with myoglobinuric renal failure, encephalitis, pericarditis, transverse myelitis, and Reye's syndrome in children. Although most patients with influenza experience spontaneous recovery, elderly patients or patients with chronic comorbid conditions may have a complicated course. The potential for serious complications prompts the recommendations for annual vaccination in patient groups considered at risk for severe influenza and warrants consideration of antiviral medications in certain clinical situations. It has been stated that antiviral drugs are presently underutilized both in prophylaxis against infection and in the management of patients with early established disease.

Agents with activity against influenza include amantadine, rimantadine, ribavarin, isoprinosine, and interferon. These drugs have specificity to viral type in that amantadine and rimantadine are active only against influenza A, ribavarin is active against types A and B, and no agents have been reported to have definite activity against influenza C.

The role of antiviral agents in preventing and managing influenza is based on less than complete data. Amantadine was the first drug to receive release for therapy of influenza. When used for prophylaxis, amantadine is 70–90% effective in preventing disease, which is similar to the success of influenza vaccines. Most of the studies showing efficacy, however, were performed in healthy young adults and limited data are available from elderly patients with chronic medical problems. Nevertheless, because of its low rate of serious adverse reactions and demonstrated efficacy, amantadine at a dose of 100 mg twice a day is recommended for high-risk unvaccinated adults during outbreaks of influenza. Also, family members of patients with influenza A, hospital workers, residents of long-term care facilities, or other closed populations should receive amantadine prophylaxis during epidemics if contraindications for vaccination exist. Amantadine can also be administered during an outbreak for 2 weeks after vaccination until immunity develops.

Amantadine can also play a role in patients who have already developed active disease. Double-blind, placebo-controlled studies have demonstrated a more rapid rate of clinical improvement and resolution of influenza symptoms, including fever, in patients treated with amantadine. Furthermore, peripheral airway abnormalities due to influenza infection return to normal more rapidly in amantadine-treated patients. Although general recommendations are to prescribe amantadine in a dose of 200 mg/day for 5–10 days, 100 mg/day may be equally as effective. The lower dose should be used in the presence of renal failure, and patients older than 65 years of age should be observed for neurologic complications. To have an impact on the clinical course, however, amantadine must be initiated within the first 48 hours of symptom onset. Since it takes several days for infected patients to shed virus particles and allow laboratory diagnosis, patients at high risk for complications from influenza and patients severely ill from influenza should receive amantadine promptly on the basis of a clinical diagnosis. A potential concern with regard to therapy is the resistance that can develop in viruses shed within a household by amantadine-treated patients. The clinical significance of this observation is uncertain.

Rimantadine, a recently released derivative of amantadine with antiviral properties, is considered superior to amantadine and has fewer side effects. It is effective both as a prophylactic agent and in patients with active disease when given at a dose of 200 mg/day.

Ribavarin is a nucleoside analogue that has activity against a wide variety of DNA and RNA viruses, including influenza A and B. Although its mechanisms of antiviral actions are not clearly defined, ribavarin probably interferes with viral replication at several different points. In contrast to the oral route required for amantadine and rimantadine, ribavarin can be administered intravenously, orally, or by aerosolization. Delivery by aerosol is the most common mode of drug delivery and is generally well tolerated except for occasional occurrences of bronchospasm, rash, and skin irritation.

Orally administered ribavarin has been investigated as a method for preventing influenza in high-risk patients. To date, the results of clinical trials are conflicting and ribavarin has not yet gained a role in influenza prophylaxis. Aerosolized ribavarin had gained attention for the management of patients with established influenza infection. Most but not all reports indicate that treated patients have reduced signs and symptoms of infection and that viral resistance does not occur. Anecdotal reports suggest a beneficial role in patients with severe respiratory complications such as influenza pneumonia.

Although more data are required to define fully the role of ribavarin in influenza infections, its use with amantadine or rimantadine should be considered for patients with influenza pneumonia or in immunocompromised patients with severe influenza infections. Some viral experts reserve its use for patients with severe influenza B infections only. Because ribavarin is teratogenic and embryotoxic in small mammals, it should not be used in pregnant patients or aerosolized in the vicinity of pregnant health workers. Limited experience exists with the use of isoprinosine and interferon in patients with severe influenza infections.

The present patient appeared on the basis of her history and her family's recent illnesses to have severe influenza with influenza pneumonia and respiratory failure. The postintubation chest radiograph showed a fine interstitial diffuse infiltrate that progressed during the subsequent 24 hours. Because of the severity of her symptoms and her underlying immunocompromised state, she was treated with aerosolized ribavarin in addition to rimantadine. She recovered 2 weeks later and underwent successful extubation. Her rhabdomyolysis did not progress to myoglobinuric renal failure.

Clinical Pearls

1. Amantadine and rimantadine are the two agents with clearly demonstrated efficacy against influenza A. On the basis of available data, rimantadine appears to be more effective and better tolerated than amantadine.

2. Amantadine and rimantadine accelerate clinical recovery in patients with established influenza if started within 48 hours of onset of symptoms.

3. Aerosolized ribavarin reduces the signs and symptoms of influenza infections and should be considered in patients with severe manifestations of infection or influenza pneumonia.

4. Some viral experts reserve the use of aerosolized ribavarin for patients with severe infections with influenza B, treating influenza A with amantadine or rimantadine.

REFERENCES

1. McChung HW, Knight V, Gilbert BE, et al. Ribavarin aerosol treatment influenza B virus infection. JAMA 1983;249:2671–2674.
2. Hayden FG. Clinical applications of antiviral agents for chemoprophylaxis and therapy of respiratory viral infections. Antiviral Res 1985;Suppl 1:229–239.
3. Douglas RG. Prophylaxis and treatment of influenza. N Engl J Med 1990;322:443–450.
4. Gilbert BE, Wyde PR, Ambrose MW, et al. Further studies with short duration ribavarin aerosol for the treatment of influenza virus infection in mice and respiratory syncytial virus infection in cotton rats. Antiviral Res 1992;17:33–42.
5. Van Voris LP, Newell PM. Antivirals for the chemoprophylaxis and treatment of influenza. Semin Respir Infect 1992;7:61–70.

PATIENT 2

**A 20-year-old man with end-stage renal disease, painful skin lesions,
diffuse pulmonary infiltrates, and respiratory failure**

A 20-year-old man with end-stage renal disease and a painful, violaceous, plaque-like skin eruption over the lower extremities was admitted to the hospital. His past medical history was remarkable for a rapidly progressive glomerulonephritis, an unsuccessful cadaveric renal transplant, and poorly controlled hypertension. Shortly after admission, he developed respiratory distress requiring mechanical ventilation. Over the next few weeks, his skin lesions spread to the abdomen and back and became ulcerative and necrotic, forming eschars. The patient eventually required a tracheotomy for chronic ventilator support.

Physical Examination: Afebrile; respirations 24 on the ventilator; blood pressure 100/90. General: chronically ill appearing. Chest: scattered rhonchi. Cardiac examination: II/VI systolic ejection murmur at the left sternal border. Skin: multiple plaque-like lesions with areas of necrosis, ulceration, and eschars.

Laboratory Examination: Hct 19.7%; WBC 14,500 μl. Na^+ 125 mEq/L; K^+ 3.6 mEq/L; Cl^- 89 mEq/L; HCO_3^- 16 mEq/L; BUN 95 mg/dl; creatinine 10.3 mg/dl; phosphate 6.5 mg/dl; calcium 7.2 mg/dl. Chest radiograph (shown below left): diffuse infiltrates. Right heart catheterization: PAOP 12 mmHg; CI 3.7 L/min/m²; SVR 1170 dyne sec cm⁻⁵.

Hospital Course: Later in the hospitalization, the serum calcium increased to 14 mg/dl, and a serum mid-chain parathyroid hormone level was increased at 246 pg/ml. A skin biopsy revealed diffuse subcutaneous and vascular calcification with in situ thrombosis. A bone scan is shown below right.

Question: What is the cause of the patient's respiratory failure?

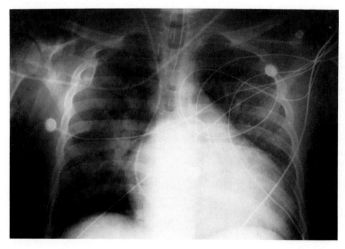
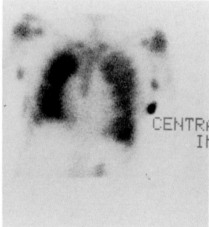

Diagnosis: Pulmonary calcinosis and calciphylaxis from secondary and tertiary hyperparathyroidism. The patient's respiratory failure was caused by severe pulmonary calcinosis.

Discussion: Diffuse tissue calcification occurs in two distinct clinical presentations: calciphylaxis and systemic calcinosis. In 1962, Seyle coined the term calciphylaxis to describe a process of soft tissue calcification and necrosis produced in laboratory animals when an appropriate biochemical milieu was present with "sensitizing" and "precipitating" influences. Sensitizing factors, which include azotemia, elevated parathyroid hormone, increased calcium and phosphate product, and vitamin D compounds, create an environment for tissue calcification. Precipitating influences are throught to initiate the process and include elevated parathyroid hormone, ionized calcium, intravenous albumin, warfarin, corticosteroids, and immunosuppressants.

Calcification occurs in subcutaneous connective tissue, including small and intermediate blood vessels. Subsequent tissue ischemia occurs, and patients develop painful, violaceous mottling of the skin (livedo reticularis) that can progress to well-demarcated plaques, ulcers, and eschar formation. Mortality is high, with uncontrollable sepsis being the usual lethal event. Systemic calcinosis refers to deposition of calcium in the connective tissue of various organs, including the lungs, kidney, stomach, heart, and skin.

In contrast to calciphylaxis, patients with systemic calcinosis are usually asymptomatic. The lack of an inflammatory reaction to calcium deposition may be in part due to its smaller crystal composition when compared to calcification in calciphylaxis. Pulmonary calcinosis, at least on a microscopic level, appears common in chronic renal failure. Calcification occurs in the alveolar septa, alveolar wall, bronchial submucosa, and the pulmonary arterioles. Most cases are clinically silent, with patients being asymptomatic and having normal chest radiographs. With extensive calcification, the chest radiograph may show a persistent, dense alveolar infiltrate. Pulmonary function may be reduced, and symptoms may progress from long periods of relative quiescence to respiratory failure.

The differential diagnosis of pulmonary calcinosis includes pulmonary alveolar microlithiasis, granulomatous disease, mitral stenosis, ectopic parathyroid hormone-producing tumors, bone-destroying tumors, and other conditions associated with hypercalcemia (milk-alkali, vitamin D intoxication, and primary, secondary, and tertiary hyperparathyroidism). Computerized tomography, gallium scan, and technetium 99m methylene diphosphonate bone scan have been used to screen patients in whom systemic calcinosis is suspected. Lung biopsy may be required for a definitive diagnosis. Elimination of any known precipitating or sensitizing influences is the cornerstone of therapy for calciphylaxis and systemic calcinosis.

The present patient had clinical and laboratory features of pulmonary calcinosis and calciphylaxis from secondary and tertiary hyperparathyroidism. After parathyroidectomy, the patient's calcium and phosphate product was lowered, and he underwent successful weaning from the ventilator.

Clinical Pearls

1. Calciphylaxis, an uncommon but severe complication of secondary and tertiary hyperparathyroidism in patients with chronic renal failure, presents with painful, necrotic skin lesions. The condition is associated with high morbidity and mortality, usually due to sepsis.

2. Pulmonary calcinosis, a subtype of systemic calcinosis, is usually clinically silent but can progress to respiratory failure.

3. Treatment of both systemic calcinosis and calciphylaxis consists of eliminating known sensitizing or precipitating factors. These efforts include lowering the calcium and phosphate product and parathyroidectomy when appropriate.

REFERENCES
1. Conger JD, Hammond WS, Alfrey AC, et al. Pulmonary calcification in chronic dialysis patients: clinical and pathologic studies. Ann Intern Med 1975;83:330–336.
2. Khafif RA, DeLima C, Silverberg A, et al. Calciphylaxis and systemic calcinosis: collective review. Arch Intern Med 1990;150:956–969.
3. Duh QY, Lim RC, Clark OH. Calciphylaxis in secondary hyperparathyroidism. Arch Surg 1991;126:1213–1219.

PATIENT 3

A 56-year-old man with cough, hemoptysis, and syncope

A 56-year-old man with a long smoking history noted a cough and mild dyspnea that persisted for 3 months. He presented for evaluation when his sputum became blood streaked and his shortness of breath worsened.

Physical Examination: Temperature 98.4°; respirations 22; pulse 140; blood pressure 90/53. Neck: no lymphadenopathy; normal neck veins. Chest: dullness at the left base with decreased breath sounds. Cardiac: normal heart sounds.

Laboratory Findings: Hct 39%; WBC 7,800/μl; platelets normal. Prothrombin time normal; partial thromboplastin time normal. Sputum: clear sputum with blood streaks. Chest radiograph (below left): left lower lobe atelectasis.

Clinical Course: The patient was scheduled for outpatient bronchoscopy but 2 days later experienced the sudden onset of left-sided chest pain and worsening dyspnea. On the way to the hospital, he transiently lost consciousness. In the emergency department, his Hct was 31%. A chest radiograph is shown below right.

Question: What intrathoracic disorder requires immediate detection and management?

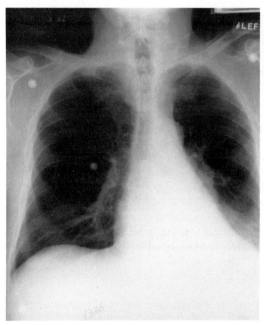 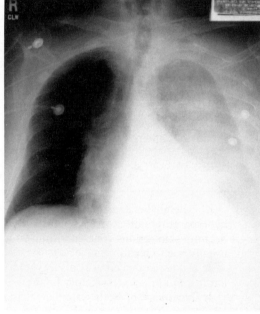

Diagnosis: Spontaneous hemothorax from a primary lung cancer.

Discussion: A spontaneous hemothorax is defined as a nontraumatic collection of bloody pleural fluid with a hematocrit $\geq$ 50% of the venous blood value. Although spontaneous hemothorax is rare, its lethal potential warrants its immediate exclusion in patients presenting with rapidly developing pleural effusions and symptoms of chest pain, hemoptysis, dyspnea, syncope, or hemodynamic instability.

Of the disparate disorders that can result in spontaneous hemothorax, the most common etiology is bleeding from pleural tears or adhesions in patients with a pneumothorax. Considered the other way, however, only 5% of patients with pneumothoraces experience the formation of a true hemothorax. In this setting, the pleural blood collection is usually small or moderate in size and resolves during chest tube drainage instituted for management of the pneumothorax.

Seventy percent of pleural effusions in patients with pulmonary emboli are hemorrhagic in nature. It is interesting, therefore, that a true hemothorax is a rare event in patients undergoing heparin or coumadin anticoagulation for thromboembolic disease. Most patients with this complication have an underlying hemorrhagic pulmonary infarction and present with pleural bleeding within 1 week of anticoagulation initiation. Most reported patients with spontaneous hemothorax have been anticoagulated within the therapeutic range. Underlying blood dyscrasias with autoanticoagulation are additional causes of spontaneous hemothorax that are extremely rare.

Microbial etiologies of hemothorax include pulmonary infections with *Mycobacterium tuberculosis*, necrotizing bacteria, and fungi. Tuberculosis commonly causes hemorrhagic pleural effusions, but frank hemothorax is exceedingly rare. Bacterial pneumonias associated with hemothorax are necrotizing and have usually proceeded to pulmonary gangrene and disruption of medium- or large-sized pulmonary arteries. Cavitary mucormycosis and aspergillosis are the leading fungal causes of hemothorax formation. These pathogens invade muscular arteries, causing pulmonary necrosis and formation of lung cavities that can rupture and hemorrhage into the pleural space. Pulmonary mucormycosis and aspergillosis can also erode into the chest wall and intercostal arteries, causing hemothorax and hemoptysis from the systemic circulation.

Subdiaphragmatic endometriosis represents a rare cause of hemothorax that nearly always results in right-sided rather than left-sided pleural blood collections. All patients with hemothorax have extensive pelvic endometriosis and many have coexisting bloody ascites. Hemothorax occurs in this condition either from passage of bloody ascites across the diaphragm into the pleural space or bleeding from transplanted endometrial tissue attached to the pleural surface. Hemothorax can also occur in patients with other causes of intra-abdominal bleeding that communicate with the pleural space.

Spontaneous bleeding from major intrathoracic vasculature can also result in hemothorax formation. Aortic dissection with rupture into the pleural space is the most common systemic vascular event causing hemothorax. Bleeding is four times more likely to occur into the left compared to the right pleural space. Patient survival depends on rapid diagnosis and immediate surgical repair. Intrapleural bleeding from pulmonary vessels most commonly occurs in patients with vascular malformations with or without accompanying hereditary hemorrhagic telangiectasia. Hemoptysis due to intrabronchial bleeding is a frequent associated manifestation. Early thoracotomy appears to enhance survival, although some patients may be managed by embolization of the feeding vessels to the vascular malformations.

Primary pulmonary malignancies are very rare causes of hemothorax, even though they are the most common etiology of hemorrhagic pleural effusions. Most patients have direct pleural tumor invasion as a cause of intrapleural hemorrhage, although neoplastic disruption of intrapulmonary blood vessels can also occur. Scattered reports exist of hemothorax due to diffuse mesothelioma. Choriocarcinoma and neurofibromatosis are unusual causes of hemothorax.

Patients with suspected hemothoraces should undergo immediate thoracentesis and determination of the pleural fluid hematocrit. Although a pleural fluid hematocrit of $\geq$ 50% of the venous value defines the presence of a hemothorax, dilution of the pleural blood and lysis of red blood cells can lower the pleural fluid hematocrit within several hours. The pleural fluid hematocrit will decrease to one-fifth of its initial value within 3 days after the control of bleeding.

After diagnosis, the patient is treated in a manner similar to patients with traumatic hemothoraces. A chest tube is placed to remove blood and monitor the rate of continued bleeding. Reexpansion of the lung to the chest wall can also serve to tamponade a pleural site of bleeding. Thoracotomy is considered when the patient is hemodynamically unstable or the chest tube is draining more than 150–500 ml of blood each hour.

The present patient underwent a thoracentesis after initial intravascular volume expansion. The pleural fluid was bloody, with a hematocrit that was 70% of the venous blood value. A chest tube was placed and the patient taken to surgery when bleeding continued unabated. The left lower lobe was removed and a large adenocarcinoma was found to be invading a major pulmonary artery, which was the source of bleeding. The patient recovered from surgery and underwent oncologic evaluation.

Clinical Pearls

1. Hemothorax is defined by a pleural fluid hematocrit that is $\geq 50\%$ of the pleural fluid value.

2. Although tearing of pleural adhesions in patients with pneumothoraces is the most common cause of spontaneous hemothorax, pleural bleeding is rarely severe or continues unabated in this condition.

3. Aortic dissection is the most common condition associated with major intrathoracic vasculature to cause spontaneous hemothorax. Pleural blood most often collects in the left hemothorax.

4. A chest tube is required in patients with spontaneous hemothorax to drain intrapleural blood, monitor the rate of bleeding, and tamponade pleural bleeding sites. Patients with continued bleeding of 150–500 ml should be considered for thoracotomy.

REFERENCES

1. Conlan AA. The management of complicated haemothorax. S Afr J Surg 1981;19:165–169.
2. Burke CM, Safai C, Nelson DP, Raffin TA. Pulmonary arteriovenous malformations: a critical update. Am Rev Respir Dis 1986;134:334–339.
3. Martinez FJ, Villanueva AG, Pickering R, et al. Spontaneous hemothorax: report of 6 cases and review of the literature. Medicine 1992;71:354–368.
4. Chou S-H, Cheng Y-J, Kao E-L, Chai C-Y. Spontaneous haemothorax: an unusual presentation of primary lung cancer. Thorax 1993;48:1185–1186.

PATIENT 4

A 28-year-old man with AIDS-related Kaposi's sarcoma and bilateral pleural effusions

A 28-year-old man with HIV infection was admitted to the hospital with dyspnea on exertion and fever. Fourteen months earlier, skin and rectal lesions appeared that were diagnosed as Kaposi's sarcoma. An episode of respiratory failure occurred 12 months prior from *Pneumocystis carinii* pneumonia. Pleural effusions were noted 4 months before admission.

Physical Examination: Temperature 101.4°; pulse 120; respirations 28; blood pressure 108/68. General: thin, minimal respiratory distress. Skin: diffuse lesions of Kaposi's sarcoma. Chest: dullness and decreased fremitus over both lower lung zones. Cardiac: normal heart sounds; no murmurs or gallops.

Laboratory Findings: Hct 28%; WBC 6300/μl with 86% PMNs, 7% lymphocytes, 7% monocytes. Electrolytes and renal indices: normal. ABG (room air): pH 7.49; PCO_2 30 mmHg; PO_2 63 mmHg. Chest radiograph: shown below left. Pleural fluid analysis: shown below right. Pleural biopsy: nonspecific inflammation.

Question: What is the most likely cause of the pleural effusions?

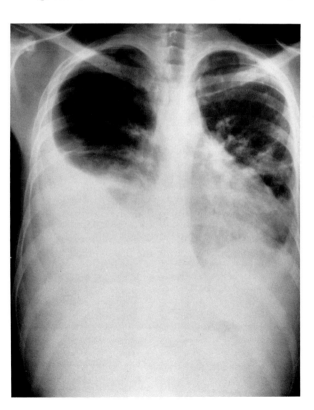

Pleural Fluid Analysis

Appearance: bloody

Nucleated cells: 1254/μl

Differential:
  11% PMNs
  68% lymphocytes
  21% mononuclear cells

RBC: 88,000/μl

Protein: 4.8 g/dl (serum 6.8 gm/dl)

LDH: 134 IU/L (serum 200 IU/L)

Glucose: 80 mg/dl

Cytology: negative

pH: 7.37

Smears: Gram, AFB, and KOH: negative

Cultures: negative

Diagnosis: Kaposi's sarcoma (KS).

Discussion: Kaposi's sarcoma is a multicentric disease that affects lymphatic endothelium and commonly presents at external sites, such as the skin and oral cavity. In the variant of the condition associated with AIDS, visceral involvement frequently occurs, with the lung being the most clinically important site. Dyspnea and a nonproductive cough are the most common symptoms of pulmonary disease, with wheezing, hemoptysis, pleuritic pain and stridor less frequently observed. The presence of the latter findings in patients with AIDS, however, suggests the diagnosis of KS because these signs and symptoms occur less commonly with opportunistic lung infections.

The chest radiographic findings of KS vary depending on the extent of the disease and the presence of concomitant pulmonary disorders. Ill-defined nodules, reticular infiltrates, homogenous infiltrates, and pleural effusions are commonly observed. Some affected patients, however, may have a normal chest radiograph.

Pleural effusions develop in 50–70% of patients with pulmonary KS at some time during the course of their disease. Effusions are usually bilateral and moderate to large in volume (reported range 200–2000 ml) but can be unilateral and small. The effusions tend to develop rapidly over 1–2 weeks. Other diagnoses associated with large effusions in AIDS are lymphoma, tuberculosis, and empyema. Nearly all patients with pleural effusions have accompanying parenchymal lesions, although the pleural fluid may obscure radiographic detection of the parenchymal abnormalities.

The pathogenesis of pleural effusions in KS appears related to subpleural and pleural vessel infiltration of tumor. Tumor deposits result in capillary leakage of fluid that crosses the mesothelium due to a pressure gradient and/or alteration of mesothelial cell junctions. Lung lymphatic drainage may also be impaired and contribute to increased extravascular lung water.

Pleural KS should be suspected when patients with AIDS present with bilateral pleural effusions and any combination of the following features: skin lesions, dyspnea, cough, wheezing, hemoptysis, pleuritic pain, or radiographic findings of ill-defined nodules or interstitial infiltrates. Pleural fluid analysis demonstrates a serous or serosanguinous exudate with a small number of mononuclear cells. Pleural fluid acidosis and low pleural fluid glucose have not been reported. Cytologic examination usually does not reveal malignant cells probably because the pleura usually remains intact over the visceral lesions. Percutaneous pleural biopsy is seldom diagnostic because KS involves the visceral rather than the parietal pleura.

Bronchoscopy with BAL is helpful in excluding opportunistic infections in patients with pleural effusions from KS. In the proper clinical setting, visualization of characteristic oval or circular raised cherry-red lesions on the tracheobronchial mucosa confirms the diagnosis. It is difficult to establish a histologic diagnosis by endobronchial biopsy of these lesions because adequate tissue can seldom be obtained. The highest yield appears to be from lesions at carinae of distal airways. In some centers, transbronchial biopsy of parenchymal lesions has had a low diagnostic yield due to the focal nature of the disease. Other reports indicate that transbronchial biopsy can establish the diagnosis even in early disease. In some patients, KS may even be missed at open lung biopsy.

The prognosis for patients with pulmonary KS is exceedingly poor; chemotherapy and radiation therapy have not been proved to prolong survival. Therapeutic thoracentesis and pleurodesis may relieve dyspnea in selected patients.

The present patient was treated with alpha interferon and VP-16 without clinical response and died 6 months after the discovery of the pleural effusions.

Clinical Pearls

1. Pleural effusions occur in 50–70% of patients with KS of the lung.

2. Bilateral pleural effusions in a patient with AIDS and KS of the skin with nodular radiographic densities are invariably due to KS of the lungs and pleura. The diagnosis can be substantiated by noting raised cherry-red lesions at bronchoscopy.

3. KS pleural effusions are serous or serosanguinous exudates with a small number of lymphocytes and mononuclear cells. Pleural fluid acidosis and low glucose values have not been demonstrated.

4. Pleural fluid cytology and percutaneous pleural biopsy are usually negative because the visceral pleura tends to remain intact and the parietal pleura is not involved.

REFERENCES

1. Meduri GU, Stover DE, Lee M, et al. Pulmonary Kaposi's sarcoma in the acquired immunodeficiency syndrome. Am J Med 1986;81:11–18.
2. Purdy LJ, Colby TV, Yousem SA, et al. Pulmonary Kaposi's sarcoma: premortem histologic diagnosis. Am J Surg Pathol 1986;10:301–311.
3. Davis SD, Henschke CI, Chamides BK, et al. Intrathoracic Kaposi's sarcoma in AIDS patients: radiographic-pathologic correlation. Radiology 1987;163:4495–4500.
4. Garay SM, Belenko M, Fazzini E, et al. Pulmonary manifestations of Kaposi's sarcoma. Chest 1987;91:39–43.
5. Judson MA, Sahn SA. Endobronchial lesions in HIV-infected individuals. Chest 1994:105:1314–1323.

PATIENT 5

A 27-year-old woman with hemoptysis, dyspnea, and lower extremity swelling

A 27-year-old woman noted 3 months before admission the gradual onset of painless ankle swelling and mild dyspnea during exertion. A chest radiograph was normal, and the patient was managed with a thiazide diuretic. The symptoms progressed to include bilateral leg swelling to both knees and dyspnea while at rest. After expectorating 30 ml of blood, the patient was admitted for evaluation. She denied previous illnesses, illicit drug use, or a smoking history.

Physical Examination: Temperature 98.5°; respirations 22; pulse 120; blood pressure 113/87 (no paradox). General: moderate dyspnea with frequent coughing of blood-streaked sputum. Neck: elevated neck veins. Chest: bilateral crackles and tubular breath sounds. Cardiac: right ventricular heave; right-sided S3; systolic ejection murmur over the second intercostal space left of the sternum. Abdomen: no organomegaly. Extremities: moderate edema below both knees.

Laboratory Findings: Hct 24%; WBC 7900/µl. Electrolytes and renal indices: normal. EKG: right axis deviation. Chest radiographs: shown below.

Question: What rare neoplasm should be included in the differential diagnosis?

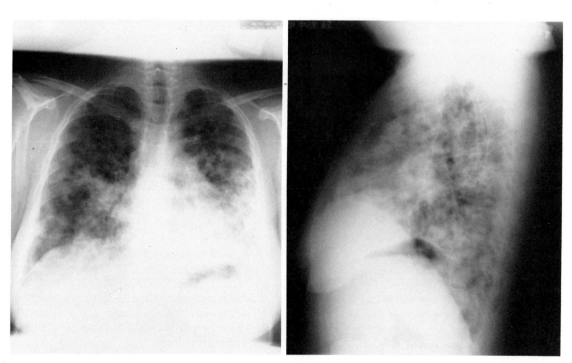

Diagnosis: Angiosarcoma of the main pulmonary artery with pulmonary metastases.

Discussion: Angiosarcomas are rare vascular malignancies that represent only 2% of all sarcomas. Most widely recognized as hepatic tumors associated with exposure to vinyl chloride, phenylethyl hydrazine, and thorotrast, primary angiosarcomas have been reported to develop in nearly every organ system. Within the thorax, primary angiosarcomas most commonly affect the heart and originate in the right atrium, right ventricle, or mainstem pulmonary arteries. Patients typically present with right ventricular flow obstruction or a restrictive cardiomyopathy that creates clinical manifestations of right-sided congestive heart failure.

Primary pulmonry angiosarcomas are extremely rare, with only a few bonafide reports existing in the literature. Most patients with lung involvement have metastatic disease from a cardiac or extrathoracic primary site. Cardiac and cutaneous angiosarcomas account for over 80% of pulmonary metastases. Cardiac angiosarcomas tend to involve the lungs by local extension from the mediastinum or through vascular embolization. Of interest, most patients with cutaneous angiosarcomas with pulmonary metastases have a primary tumor originating on the scalp.

Although the clinical manifestations of primary and metastatic pulmonary angiosarcomas vary in the existing clinical reports, common features include chest pain, progressive dyspnea, low-grade fever, persistent cough, and malaise. The tumor tends to grow slowly with the subtle onset and progression of symptoms, so that patients present relatively late in their disease with extensive pulmonary tumor deposits. After diagnosis, however, symptoms progress rapidly and acute complications occur. Because of the vascular nature of these tumors, hemoptysis with pulmonary parenchymal hemorrhage and hemothoraces are classic complications of far advanced disease. A proclivity for tumor necrosis, cavitation, and extension to the pleura results in pneumothoraces, which are unusual occurrences in other forms of lung cancer. Patients with primary tumors located on the scalp appear to be especially predisposed to hemothoraces and pneumothoraces.

The chest radiograph in patients with pulmonary angiosarcomas ranges from a normal appearance to multiple nodular densities with or without associated pleural effusions. Localized or diffuse alveolar infiltrates may occur in regions of parenchymal hemorrhage. Metastatic nodules can rapidly progress to thin-walled cavities, suggesting an infectious pulmonary disorder.

The diagnosis of pulmonary angiosarcoma is commonly delayed because of the indolent progression of symptoms until the late stages of the disease. The radiographic or chest CT appearance of the pulmonary nodules is nonspecific; an MRI scan may suggest the vascular nature of the disease. In the absence of a clinically apparent primary lesion, most patients require fiberoptic bronchoscopy with transbronchial biopsy, transthoracic needle biopsy, or open lung biopsy/thoracoscopy to obtain tissue for diagnosis. The pathologic diagnosis, however, is complicated because multicentric hemangiomas, chemodectomas, congenital malformations, vasoproliferative lesions, bronchoalveolar cell tumors with vascular invasion, and Kaposi's sarcomas may have similar or identical histologic appearances. Electron microscopy and immunohistochemistry techniques may be required to confirm the diagnosis.

No curative therapy exists for patients with pulmonary angiosarcoma. Clear benefit from surgery or chemotherapy has not been demonstrated probably because of the highly resistant nature of these tumors and the late stages in which they present. Palliative pulmonary resections may improve symptoms in patients with persistent pneumothoraces or pulmonary hemorrhages but do not appear to enhance survival. Well-differentiated angiosarcomas may follow a slower course and offer a better prognosis compared to undifferentiated forms.

The present patient underwent an echocardiogram and chest CT that demonstrated right atrial and ventricular dilatation and a large mass that enveloped and constricted the main pulmonary artery. A transbronchial lung biopsy obtained by fiberoptic bronchoscopy demonstrated pathologic and immunohistologic features of metastatic angiosarcoma, which was presumed to be from a pulmonary artery primary site. The patient underwent chemotherapy but rapidly deteriorated with worsening manifestations of cor pulmonale and died several weeks later.

Clinical Pearls

1. Angiosarcomas can originate in any organ system. Cardiac angiosarcoma, however, is the most common primary intrathoracic form of the disease.

2. Patients with cardiac angiosarcomas most commonly present with manifestations of right ventricular failure due to right atrial, right ventricular, or pulmonary artery neoplastic invasion.

3. Primary pulmonary angiosarcoma is extremely rare. Metastatic pulmonary involvement is common, however, in patients with cardiac or extrathoracic sites of primary disease.

4. Pulmonary parenchymal hemorrhage, hemothorax, and pneumothorax are classic manifestations of pulmonary angiosarcomas.

5. More than 80% of patients with metastatic pulmonary angiosarcomas have primary tumors of the heart or skin. Most patients with cutaneous tumors metastatic to the lung have a primary lesion located on the scalp.

REFERENCES

1. Kitagawa M, Tanaka I, Takemura T, et al. Angiosarcoma of the scalp: report of two cases with fatal pulmonary complications and a review of Japanese autopsy registry data. Virchows Archiv 1987;412:83–87.
2. Ott RA, Eugene J, Kollin J, et al. Primary pulmonary angiosarcoma associated with multiple synchronous neoplasms. J Surg Oncol 1987;35:269–276.
3. Palvio DHB, Paulsen SM, Henneberg EW. Primary angiosarcoma of the lung presenting as intractable hemoptysis. Thorac Cardiovasc Surgeon 1987;35:105–107.
4. Aronchick JM, Palevsky HI, Miller WT. Cavitary pulmonary metastases in angiosarcoma: diagnosis by transthoracic needle aspiration. Am Rev Respir Dis 1989;139:252–253.
5. Ashokakumar M, Patel MD, Ryu JH. Angiosarcoma in the lung. Chest 1993;103:1531–1535.

PATIENT 6

A 29-year-old woman with chest pain and pulmonary nodules

A 29-year-old woman presented with chest pain and dyspnea of several days' duration. She denied cough, hemoptysis, edema, or leg pain. Before the onset of the present illness, she was healthy. She was gravida 2, para 1, AB1.

Physical Examination: Temperature 100.3° F; respirations 30; pulse 100; blood pressure 100/60 mmHg. General: moderate chest discomfort and slight respiratory distress. Chest: decreased bilateral expansion; no adventitious sounds. Cardiac: regular tachycardia; no jugular venous distention; heart sounds normal without gallops. Abdomen: nontender without organomegaly. Extremities: no cyanosis, clubbing, or edema.

Laboratory Findings: Hct 35%; WBC 14,200/μl with 90% PMNs. Electrolytes and liver function test: normal. ABG (2 L nasal oxygen): pH 7.48; PCO_2 34 mmHg; PO_2 75 mmHg. Chest radiographs: shown below.

Question: What is the diagnosis? What test will confirm the diagnosis?

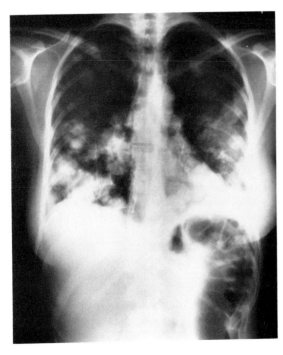 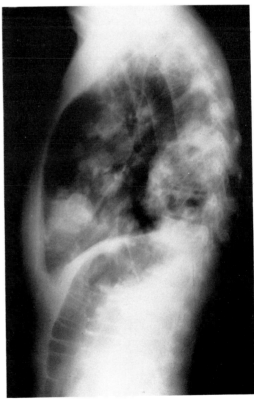

Diagnosis: Choriocarcinoma metastatic to the lung. A serum βHCG level was markedly elevated, and pregnancy was excluded by physical examination and ultrasound.

Discussion: Choriocarcinoma is a form of gestational trophoblastic disease that commonly metastasizes. The other types of trophoblastic disease include hydatidiform mole, which is limited to the uterus, and invasive mole (chorioadenoma destruens), which invades the uterus but rarely metastasizes.

The lung is the organ most often involved with metastases from choriocarcinoma because of the propensity of trophoblastic tissue to disseminate hematogenously. Other sites of metastasis include the vagina, uterus, and brain. Metastasis to the brain is particularly ominous because of the inclination for metastatic choriocarcinoma to bleed and cause massive cerebral hemorrhage. This hemorrhagic potential can be disastrous if patients with metastatic choriocarcinoma undergo anticoagulant therapy.

Most patients with choriocarcinoma are multiparous and have had a preceding molar pregnancy. Fewer than 5% of patients experienced a normal term pregnancy or underwent an abortion immediately preceding onset of the tumor. Pulmonary symptoms are commonly absent but may include: (1) acute dyspnea and chest pain secondary to tumor emboli and pulmonary infarction; (2) cough and hemoptysis resulting from either bronchial or parenchymal involvement; (3) insidious dyspnea secondary to pulmonary parenchymal metastases or emboli; and (4) pleurisy resulting from pleural metastases. Pleural effusions may be caused by metastatic disease to the pleura or the subpleural parenchyma, or by pulmonary infarction. Pleural fluid is usually hemorrhagic; severe bleeding into the pleural space can in some instances cause patient exsanguination.

The chest radiograph may demonstrate multiple nodules or a diffuse, miliary pattern. Pleural effusions may be apparent. Patients with tumor emboli may have a normal chest radiograph. In patients with metastatic disease who are asymptomatic, the disease may be "discovered" on a routine chest radiograph.

Metastatic gestational trophoblastic disease is problematic both diagnostically and therapeutically.

The disease tends to be diagnosed earlier in patients with antecedent molar pregnancies, usually within 6 months of the previous pregnancy. In contrast, if the preceding pregnancy was normal or ended in abortion, the lesions tend to be diagnosed later—frequently 1–2 years following the pregnancy. Multiple nodules on a chest radiograph in a woman of childbearing age should raise the possibility of metastatic choriocarcinoma. An elevated plasma beta human chorionic gonadotropin (βHCG) level may confirm the diagnosis. Plasma concentrations of βHCG levels are frequently greater than 100,000 IU/L. Choriocarcinoma is managed with chemotherapeutic regimens that usually include methotrexate and actinomycin D. Surgery has a role in patients with solitary pulmonary metastasis resistant to chemotherapy who have no extrapulmonary lesions.

When pulmonary nodules persist despite the return of βHCG levels to normal ($<$ 3 IU/L), the nodules are probably fibrotic. Residual nodules can be assumed to be benign when βHCG levels return to, and remain, normal, the nodules show no increase in size, and other metastatic lesions have resolved. A single report exists of an acquired arteriovenous malformation with resultant hypoxemia within a pulmonary fibrotic residua of a choriocarcinoma metastasis.

Overall survival approaches 70%. Survival is worse in those with pulmonary metastases after a term pregnancy or abortion, because of the longer lead-time between the antecedent pregnancy and diagnosis, allowing for the development of later-stage disease. The main causes of death are cerebral hemorrhage, respiratory failure, and pulmonary embolism.

The present patient underwent lung biopsy, which confirmed the diagnosis of metastatic choriocarcinoma. Her plasma level of βHCG was 108,000 IU/L. She was treated with methotrexate, actinomycin D, and cyclophosphamide, with normalization of her symptoms, chest radiograph, and βHCG plasma levels within 3 months.

Clinical Pearls

1. Choriocarcinoma should be suspected in any woman of childbearing age with multiple pulmonary nodules.

2. The most common type of pregnancy preceding choriocarcinoma is molar pregnancy. Presentation with lung metastasis during a normal pregnancy or following an abortion is rare.

3. The diagnosis is confirmed by the finding of high βHCG levels in a nonpregnant patient.

4. Anticoagulation for pulmonary embolism is contraindicated in the active stage of metastatic choriocarcinoma because of the propensity of spontaneous hemorrhage into metastatic tissue.

5. Persistent pulmonary nodules after therapy that remain stable in size in patients with normal βHCG levels are most likely fibrotic in nature.

REFERENCES

1. Evans KT, Cocksholt WP, Hendrickse P. Pulmonary changes in malignant trophoblastic disease. Br J Radiol 1965, 38:161–171.
2. Libshitz HI, Baber CE, Hammond CV. The pulmonary metastases of choriocarcinoma. Obstet Gynecol 1977;49:412–416.
3. Johnson TR Jr, Comstock CH, Anderson DG. Benign gestational trophoblastic disease metastatic to pleura: unusual case cause of hemothorax. Obstet Gynecol 1979;53:509–511.
4. Kuman J, Ilancheran A, Ratnam SS. Pulmonary metastases in gestational trophoblastic disease: a review of 97 cases. Br J Obstet Gynaecol 1988;95:70–74.
5. Casson AG, McCormack D, Craig I, et al. A persistent pulmonary lesion following chemotherapy for metastatic choriocarcinoma. Chest 1993;103:269–270.

PATIENT 7

A 59-year-old man with a lung mass and recurrent headaches

A 59-year-old man with a heavy smoking history presented with a 3-month cough, right-sided weakness, and progressive headaches. The headache was constant, occasionally associated with nausea, and worsened with straining or coughing. He also noted a 10-pound weight loss.

Physical Examination: Vital signs normal. Head: normal. Fundi: discs flat. Mouth: good dentition. Neck: no lymphadenopathy. Chest: decreased breath sounds over right upper lobe region. Cardiac: normal. Abdomen: no organomegaly. Neurologic: moderate weakness in the right arm and leg.

Laboratory Findings: Hct 41%; WBC 9,700/μl. Electrolytes normal. Chest: below left. Head CT: below right.

Hospital Course: The patient underwent bronchoscopy, which revealed an obstructing mass in the right upper lobe bronchus. Biopsy results determined the mass was an adenocarcinoma.

Question: What are the diagnostic and therapeutic considerations for the patient's intracranial lesion?

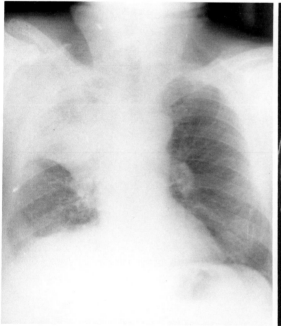 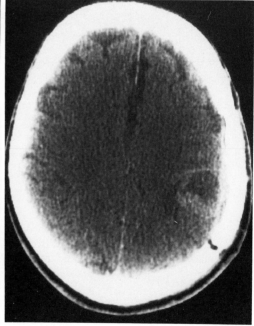

Answer: The patient requires pathologic confirmation that the intracranial lesion is metastatic in nature. Surgical resection in some patients with intracranial metastases may be the most effective form of therapy.

Discussion: Computerized tomographic evidence of an intracranial lesion in a patient with underlying non–small-cell lung cancer presents the clinical possibility of a solitary brain metastasis. Brain metastases have traditionally portended an extremely grave prognosis in patients with intrathoracic malignancies. Recent advances in multimodality approaches to chest malignancies, however, have improved the palliative care of this condition and extended patient survival.

The initial approach requires confirmation of the nature of the intracranial lesion. In the absence of widespread metastases, up to 10% of solitary brain lesions detected by CT in patients with an underlying carcinoma are unrelated to the primary tumor. Most commonly diagnosed disorders that mimic solitary brain metastases include brain abscesses, benign tumors, and primary brain malignancies.

Although the standard traditional approach to patients with solitary brain metastases from any primary tumor has been external beam radiotherapy, recent advances in neurosurgical techniques and neuroimaging have extended therapeutic options to include surgical resection and stereotactic radiosurgery. Selection of the treatment plan for an individual patient is determined by the type and stage of the primary tumor, the location of the intracranial metastases, the extent of debilitating neurosurgical symptoms, and the patient's underlying condition and medical prognosis.

For radiosensitive primary tumors, such as lymphomas and small-cell lung cancers, in patients with intracranial metastases and projected survivals greater than 3 months, external beam radiotherapy remains the treatment of choice. Unfortunately, non–small-cell lung cancers are more radioresistant and require treatment regimens that may expose white matter to radiation injury and produce progressive dementia. Brain metastases from primary melanomas, colon cancers, and renal cell carcinomas are even more radioresistant and should be considered for excisional and stereotactic radiosurgical modalities of care.

Neurosurgical approaches to the removal of solitary brain metastases have advanced largely because of improved imaging techniques that allow pinpoint tumor locations and accurate excisions. Stereotactic techniques create the ability to localize small intracranial tumor deposits and remove them with a minimum of injury to adjacent normal tissue. Computerized tomography with the patient's head secured in a stereotactic frame has been the most commonly employed stereotactic technique, but ultrasound guidance protocols have also been used. Evoked potentials and brain mapping direct the neurosurgeon in preserving functional brain tissue. Patients with solitary brain metastases located in more easily reached intracranial locations can undergo stereotactic excisions under local anesthesia.

Recent controlled studies justify the surgical approach to solitary brain metastases. Patients with non–small-cell lung cancer and solitary brain metastases experience a 19-month survival when treated with surgical excision and cranial external beam radiotherapy compared to 9 months when treated with radiotherapy alone. Other studies evaluating solitary brain metastases in patients with a variety of underlying malignancies demonstrate similar improvements in survival and quality of life when patients are treated with cranial radiotherapy combined with surgery. Patients managed with surgical removal of intracranial metastases ultimately die from progression of the underlying tumor rather than recurrence of the brain lesion.

Surgical excision is especially indicated for patients with single lesions located within the cerebral motor strip because of the risk that external beam radiotherapy will initially worsen motor defects. Surgery is also the preferred therapeutic approach in patients with large intracranial masses, severe symptoms requiring immediate relief, hemorrhagic lesions, easily accessible superficial lesions, and metastases with associated moderate to severe cerebral edema. Solitary brain metastases can be excised during the initial brain biopsy to confirm the nature of an intracranial mass.

Advances in the several techniques of stereotactic radiosurgery allow focused delivery of radiation to specific regions of the brain, which avoids damage to normal tissue as occurs with whole brain irradiation. Increased radiation energy applied to small regions of the brain improves clinical response in patients with brain tumor cell types usually considered resistant to external beam radiotherapy. Precise delivery of radiation additionally creates an opportunity to further treat patients previously managed with maximal doses of external beam radiotherapy. The three major techniques used include proton beam radiotherapy, which applies high energy to tissue sites distant from the particle source, the gamma knife, which employs several different radiation sources to deliver cell-damaging effects to focal regions of the brain, and the linear accelerator, which supplies radiation arcs to the specific areas of the metastasis.

Recent patient series report a 94% rate of tumor control over 9-month observation periods and a

4% initial failure rate in patients with intracranial metastases. Most patients who fail to respond in the region of irradiated brain have underlying non–small-cell lung cancer. Rarely do patients fail therapy because of recurrence in intracranial regions distant from the irradiated site. Radiosurgery is usually well tolerated, with occasional instances of cerebral necrosis requiring surgical resection and cranial nerve injury.

The present patient's chest radiograph showed right upper lobe atelectasis, and the head CT scan revealed a left-sided cerebral mass. He underwent thoracotomy with a lobectomy and mediastinal node dissection. Because of progressively disabling neurologic symptoms, a craniotomy with brain biopsy was performed, which demonstrated metastatic adenocarcinoma. Because the lesion was solitary and well localized, it was surgically removed during the initial neurosurgical procedure. The patient's right-sided weakness persisted but did not progress in the immediate postoperative period.

Clinical Pearls

1. Radiographic evidence of a solitary brain lesion in a patient with an underlying carcinoma requires surgical biopsy in the absence of widespread metastatic disease. Such lesions are unrelated to the primary tumor in 10% of instances.

2. Recent controlled series indicate that quality of life and survival are improved in patients with a solitary brain metastases who are treated with surgical excision combined with radiotherapy compared to radiotherapy alone.

3. External beam radiotherapy remains the procedure of choice for patients with intracranial lymphoma and metastatic small-cell carcinoma.

4. Surgical radiotherapy allows the delivery of high-energy radiation to focal regions of the brain, thereby promoting clinical response and limiting injury to normal white matter in patients with radioresistant tumors.

REFERENCES
1. Sunderson N, Galicich JH. Surgical treatment of brain metastases: clinical and computerized tomography evaluation of the results of treatment. Cancer 1985;55:1382–1388.
2. Loeffler JS, Kooy HM, Wen PW, et al. The treatment of recurrent brain metastases with stereotactic radiosurgery. J Clin Oncol 1990;8:576–582.
3. Patchell RA, Tibbs PA, Walsh JW, et al. A randomized trial of surgery in the treatment of single metastases to the brain. N Engl J Med 1990;322:494–500.
4. Black PM. Solitary brain metastases: radiation, resection, or radiosurgery? Chest 1993;103:367S–369S.

PATIENT 8

A 29-year-old woman with facial and hand swelling

A 29-year-old woman with a long smoking history noted the gradual onset of swelling in her face and hands over the previous 1 month. She otherwise felt well, specifically denying weight loss, fatigue, or fevers. The patient stated that she had a slight nonproductive cough but no hemoptysis. She had no known exposure to tuberculosis but never had a tuberculin skin test.

Physical Examination: Vital signs: normal. General: no acute distress. Head: facial puffiness worse around the eyes. Neck: jugular venous distention; central venous pressure estimated at 12 cm H_2O. Lymph nodes: normal. Chest: vesicular breath sounds with few scattered rhonchi. Cardiac: normal heart sounds; no gallops or murmurs. Abdomen: unremarkable. Extremities: bilateral upper extremity edema; no cyanosis or clubbing.

Laboratory Findings: Hct 35%; WBC 9000/μl with a normal differential. Electrolytes, renal indices, and liver function tests: normal. Chest radiograph: below top. Chest CT: below bottom.

Question: What is the most likely etiology of the patient's presentation?

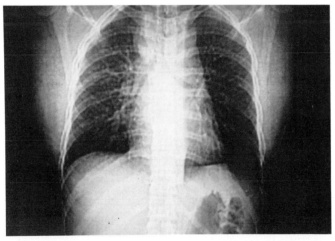

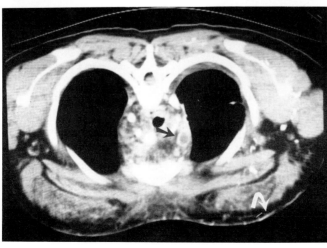

Diagnosis: Fibrosing mediastinitis with superior vena cava syndrome due to histoplasmosis.

Discussion: The onset of the superior vena cava (SVC) syndrome in a previously healthy patient produces striking symptoms that portend serious underlying disease. Bronchogenic carcinoma (usually small cell) is the most common cause of this disorder, accounting for 75% of cases. Lymphoma and metastatic carcinoma contribute an additional 20%. Up to 5% of patients with SVC syndrome have nonmalignant conditions that cause vascular thrombosis or compression of mediastinal vascular structures by inflammatory masses or fibrosis. Mediastinal infection with *Histoplasma capsulatum* is the most common disorder among the inflammatory conditions that produce superior vena caval obstruction.

Mediastinal histoplasmosis can produce SVC syndrome by initiating either granulomatous lymphadenitis or fibrosing mediastinitis. Granulomatous lymphadenitis develops in mediastinal lymph nodes that drain primary areas of lung infection. Enlarged lymph nodes containing caseous material gradually coalesce, forming a single encapsulated mass with a 3–10 cm diameter. Although most patients remain asymptomatic despite radiographic evidence of lymphadenopathy, mediastinal structures in some patients may become compressed, causing SVC syndrome or manifestations of bronchial or esophageal dysfunction.

Fibrosing mediastinitis is virtually always a late manifestation of histoplasma infection characterized by exuberant proliferation of collagen within the mediastinum. The precise pathogenesis of this condition is uncertain but may relate to the leakage of immunogenic material from caseous lymph nodes that elicits an intense fibrotic reaction. Alternatively, an idiosyncratic host response to granulomatous inflammation may initiate ongoing collagen deposition that persists despite adequate sequestration of the fungal organisms. The end result is dense fibrosis with focal areas of calcification and infiltration of fibrocaseous material throughout the mediastinum and into adjacent mediastinal structures.

Patients with fibrosing mediastinitis typically present between the ages of 20 and 40 years, with symptoms determined by the location of the fibrotic inflammatory reaction. If fibrosis does not involve mediastinal structures, the patient may remain asymptomatic. Symptomatic patients commonly present initially with cough, dyspnea, and hemoptysis. Symptoms and signs of SVC syndrome develop in only 16–20% of patients with fibrosing mediastinitis. A paratracheal location of fibrosis has the greatest potential to obstruct the SVC.

The chest radiograph in patients with fibrosing mediastinitis complicated by SVC syndrome usually shows mediastinal masses but occasionally may reveal only minimal abnormalities. A chest CT scan may demonstrate mediastinal fibrosis, lymphadenopathy with partial calcification, evidence of collateral blood flow, and thrombosis of the SVC. The CT scan can also detect compression of other mediastinal structures, such as major bronchi and pulmonary veins, the presence of which worsens the patient's prognosis.

The definitive diagnosis of fibrosing mediastinitis due to histoplasmosis requires demonstration of the organisms in biopsy tissue specimens. Fungal elements within involved lymph nodes, however, are usually nonviable and do not grow in culture, thus requiring special tissue stains for their detection. Most patients, however, can be adequately managed with a presumptive diagnosis in the proper clinical setting when the chest CT shows characteristic features with partially calcified mediastinal masses.

No specific therapy exists for patients with fibrosing mediastinitis complicated by SVC syndrome to prevent progression of the disease. Antifungal agents do not play a role because the fungal organisms are nonviable and no longer actively growing. Palliative surgery is largely unsuccessful, with high operative mortality except in selected patients who may benefit from bronchial reconstruction or venous bypass grafts. The mortality of patients with fibrosing mediastinitis approaches 30%, with most patients dying within 6 years of the onset of symptoms. Occasional patients with SVC syndrome may gradually improve symptomatically as collateral circulation becomes established.

The present patient had classic clinical and radiographic features of fibrosing mediastinitis with SVC obstruction. Her chest CT scan demonstrated fibrosis, adenopathy, and SVC obstruction (note enhancement of the venous wall, arrow in figure). Collateral flow was already established (curved arrow in figure). The patient experienced some improvement with symptomatic care.

Clinical Pearls

1. Fibrosing mediastinitis is virtually always a late consequence of remote infection with *H. capsulatum.*

2. Patients generally present between ages 20 and 40 years with cough, dyspnea, or hemoptysis and an abnormal mediastinum on chest radiograph; however, the radiograph may appear only minimally abnormal in some patients.

3. Histoplasmosis is the most common cause of benign SVC syndrome.

4. The diagnosis of fibrosing mediastinitis can be made presumptively in the proper clinical setting with chest CT showing partially calcified mediastinal masses.

REFERENCES

1. Goodwin RA, Nickell JA, Des Prez RM. Mediastinal fibrosis complicating healed primary histoplasmosis and tuberculosis. Medicine 1972;51:227–246.
2. Goodwin RA, Loyd FE, Des Prez RM. Histoplasmosis in normal hosts. Medicine 1981;60:231–262.
3. Berry DF, Buccigrossi D, Peabody J, et al. Pulmonary vascular occlusion and fibrosing mediastinitis. Chest 1986;89:296–301.
4. Loyd JE, Tillman BF, Atkinson JB, Des Pres RM. Mediastinal fibrosis complicating histoplasmosis. Medicine 1988;67:295–310.
5. Dunn EJ, Ulicny KS Jr, Wright CB, et al. Surgical implications of sclerosing mediastinitis: a report of six cases and review of the literature. Chest 1990;97:338–346.
6. Mathisen DJ, Grillo HC. Clinical manifestations of mediastinal fibrosis and histoplasmosis. Ann Thorac Surg 1992;54:1053–1057.

PATIENT 9

A 62-year-old man with sudden hypotension after pneumonectomy

A 62-year-old man with a long smoking history was admitted for surgical removal of a right lung squamous carcinoma. The tumor was localized to the bronchus intermedius but extended to 2 cm from the carina. At thoracotomy, a large tumor was found wrapped around the right mainstem bronchus and adherent to the right pericardial surface. A pneumonectomy was required along with resection of a portion of the pericardium for complete tumor removal. The patient tolerated the procedure well but suddenly became hypotensive in the recovery room.

Physical Examination: Respirations 25 shallow; pulse 140; blood pressure 60/0. General: cyanotic upper torso and head. Neck: elevated cervical veins. Chest: no breath sounds right chest. Cardiac: absent heart tones.

Laboratory Findings: Chest radiograph: shown below.

Question: What is the cause of the patient's hypotension and the indicated course of action?

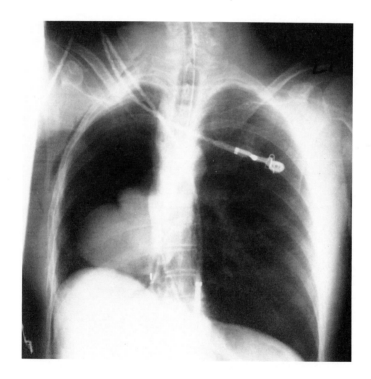

Diagnosis: Cardiac torsion following pneumonectomy.

Discussion: Herniation of the heart through the pericardium with cardiac torsion is a rare but highly lethal condition that occurs in various clinical settings. Also termed incarceration of the heart, volvulus of the heart, and cardiac dislocation, cardiac herniation is invariably fatal when not clinically recognized. It retains a 50% mortality even when diagnosed early and promptly surgically managed.

Cardiac torsion can occur in any condition in which a defect exists in the pericardium through which the heart can herniate. Although described in patients with blunt or penetrating trauma or with congenital pericardial defects, the vast majority of patients with cardiac herniation have undergone an intrapericardial pneumonectomy without closure of the pericardial defect. Typically in the intraoperative or immediate postoperative period during episodes of patient repositioning, coughing, or endotracheal extubation, the heart moves through the pericardial defect into the relatively low pressure region of the pneumonectomy space.

The clinical manifestations of cardiac torsion reflect the altered anatomic position of the heart and its effect on cardiovascular function. The herniated heart can move in one of two configurations: it can undergo acute angulation laterally with the apex abutting the lateral chest wall, or it can rotate posterolaterally with the apex positioned in the region of the posterior costophrenic sulcus. The latter cardiac movement represents an organoaxial volvulus of the heart. With either cardiac configuration, compression of the cardiac outflow tract occurs with or without obstruction of the vena cavae. Also, the right atrium can become twisted and crimped by the edge of the pericardial opening, resulting in further impairment of ventricular filling.

Patients subsequently present with the sudden onset of systemic hypotension. Up to 60% of patients have been reported to demonstrate clinical manifestations of superior vena cava syndrome with cyanotic upper torsos and elevated jugular veins. Although most patients experience cardiac torsion within 24 hours of intrapericardial pneumonectomy, in rare instances patients have developed this complication several weeks after surgery. A delayed presentation is unusual because of the rapid development of cardiac and pericardial adhesions that tether the heart into place.

Cardiac herniation requires rapid diagnosis and immediate initiation of surgical therapy. The goals of surgery are to replace the heart into the pericardial sac and to perform a plastic repair of the pericardial defect. In some patients, tagging of the auricles to the edges of the pericardial defect or enlarging the pericardial wound to prevent cardiac strangulation may be required.

The present patient appeared clinically likely to have a cardiac torsion and underwent a confirmatory chest radiograph, pending return of the thoracic surgeon to the recovery room. The chest radiograph demonstrated herniation of the heart into the right pneumonectomy space. The patient underwent immediate thoracotomy with replacement of the heart into the pericardial sac, which resulted in rapid recovery of his hemodynamic status. The patient was discharged 7 days later without further complications.

Clinical Pearls

1. Cardiac herniation occurs in conditions in which a defect in the pericardium exists. Intrapericardial pneumonectomy is the most commonly associated clinical setting.

2. The occurrence of cardiac herniation is almost entirely limited to the first 24 hours after pneumonectomy.

3. Patients with cardiac torsion present with systemic hypotension with or without associated features of superior vena cava syndrome.

4. Prompt diagnosis and immediate surgical replacement of the heart to within the pericardial sac decrease the mortality to 50%.

REFERENCES
1. Gates GF, Sette RS, Cope JA. Acute cardiac herniation with incarceration following pneumonectomy. Radiology 1970;94:561–562.
2. Patel D, Shrivastav R, Sabety AM. Cardiac torsion following intrapericardial pneumonectomy. J Thorac Cardiovasc Surg 1973;65:626–628.
3. Ohri SK, Siddiqui AA, Townsend ER. Cardiac torsion after lobectomy with partial pericardiotomy. Ann Thorac Surg 1992;53:703–705.

PATIENT 10

A 55-year-old man with productive cough and bilateral upper lobe infiltrates

A 55-year-old white man with chronic obstructive pulmonary disease (COPD) presented with a 3-month history of cough, sputum production, weight loss, and malaise. He denied fever, chills, pleuritic chest pain, or hemoptysis. There was no history of exposure to tuberculosis, and the results of a tuberculin skin test 10 years earlier were negative. The patient had recently retired from a sales position in upstate New York and had moved to coastal South Carolina.

Physical Examination: Temperature 100° F; pulse 88; respirations 20. Skin: no lesions. Lymph nodes: few small anterior cervical nodes. Chest: diminished breath sounds; scattered rhonchi over the anterior chest. Abdomen: no organomegaly. Extremities: no cyanosis, clubbing, or edema.

Laboratory Findings: Hct 39%; WBC 10,800/μl with normal differential; ESR 40 mm/hr. PPD negative; controls: positive. Sputum Gram stain: few PMNs with mixed flora. Sputum AFB smear, partial AFB smear and KOH stain: negative. Chest radiographs: shown below. PFTs: FEV_1/FVC 50%. Fiberoptic bronchoscopy: no endobronchial lesions. BAL stains and cultures: negative. Transbronchial lung biopsy: nonspecific inflammation and fibrosis; cultures pending.

Question: What is the differential diagnosis? What should be the next course of action?

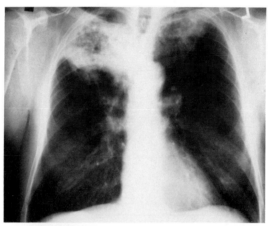

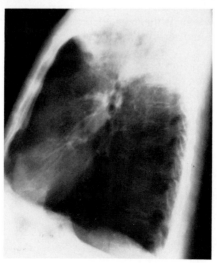

Diagnosis: Primary pulmonary sporotrichosis.

Discussion: Although an unusual cause of pulmonary infection, sporotrichosis is included in the differential diagnosis of upper lobe fibro-nodular and cavitary infiltrates. Caused by the dimorphic fungus, *Sporothrix schenckii*, pulmonary sporotrichosis should be considered when patients from endemic regions (states bordering the Mississippi and Missouri Rivers) present with chronic pulmonary infections and negative evaluations for tuberculosis. The likelihood of sporotrichosis increases if patients have associated skin lesions or an occupational exposure to plants, soil, or wood, which promotes the inhalation of fungal spores. Occupations that appear to place patients at increased risk include forestry and greenhouse work, farming, ranching, and construction work.

Most patients with pulmonary sporotrichosis present between the fourth and fifth decades of life. A predominance of whites and males have been reported. Patients typically have underlying alterations in host defense (alcoholism or diabetes mellitus) or coexisting pulmonary conditions (COPD or tuberculosis) with generalized or localized impairment of airway secretion clearance.

Sporotrichosis is a chronic infection with insidious onset of symptoms. Some patients may have manifestations of the disease several years before the diagnosis is established. The most common symptoms are cough and sputum production. Dyspnea with exertion, pleuritic chest pain, and hemoptysis occur less frequently. Weight loss, fever, and malaise occur in less than half of the patients. Skin lesions characteristic of cutaneous sporotrichosis are not commonly associated with primary pulmonary disease, which is caused by inhalation of the fungus.

The chest radiograph most commonly shows upper lobe infiltrative or fibronodular parenchymal densities, which are usually unilateral in distribution. The infiltrates may progress to cavitation. Hilar and mediastinal adenopathy and pleural effusions occur rarely. The radiographic pattern is not unique and introduces a differential diagnosis of tuberculosis, atypical mycobacteriosis, anaerobic pneumonitis, and infection with other fungal pathogens.

The diagnosis of pulmonary sporotrichosis depends on positive serologic studies or demonstration of the fungus by culture or histologic techniques. *S. schenckii* grows well on simple culture media and has been isolated from expectorated sputum, bronchoscopic specimens, transbronchial biopsy specimens, open lung biopsy specimens, and pleural fluid. The organisms are usually easily identified in tissue as rounded, multiple-budded, yeast-like cells. Gram-positive, cigar-shaped organisms can be identified with a modified Gram stain, using 95% ethanol decolorizer. The direct fluorescent antibody (DFA) technique has been specific in detecting the organism in tissue or in culture. Histopathologically, there may be either caseating or noncaseating granulomas. A positive serologic result using latex agglutination in combination with immunodiffusion appears to be a specific indicator of disease activity.

Because of the small number of cases and lack of comparative clinical trials, ideal therapy for pulmonary sporotrichosis is uncertain. It seems reasonable, based on current information, to give oral iodides or itraconazole for noncavitary disease in immunocompetent patients. Treatment with 1.5–2.0 g of amphotericin B is suggested for cavitary and noncavitary disease in immunocompromised patients. Additional experience with itraconazole may extend its role in the management of this infection. Surgery should be reserved for patients who fail medical therapy; however, drug therapy should be given both before and after surgery in an effort to limit the spread of the infection.

The present patient had a clinical and radiographic presentation compatible with pulmonary sporotrichosis, but none of the clinical features was particularly suggestive of the diagnosis. The tissue samples obtained by transbronchial lung biopsy were positive for *S. schenckii* on DFA staining. Culture of the lung tissue grew *S. schenckii*. After treatment with 1.5 g of amphotericin B, his symptoms resolved and the chest radiograph showed complete clearing.

Clinical Pearls

1. Sporotrichosis should be considered in the differential diagnosis of any patient with upper lobe disease, especially in areas where the disease is endemic, when tests for tuberculosis are negative.

2. Alcoholism and occupational exposure to soil and plants are the most common risk factors.

3. Modified Gram's stain of sputum or bronchial washings, using 95% ethanol decolorizer, frequently reveals the typical gram-positive, cigar-shaped organism.

4. Oral iodides or itraconazole is suggested for noncavitary disease in the immuno-competent patient, whereas amphotericin B should be given for cavitary and noncavitary disease in immunocompromised patients. Surgery should be reserved for patients who fail medical therapy.

REFERENCES

1. Rohatgi TK. Pulmonary sporotrichosis. South Med J 1980;73:1611–1617.
2. Gerding GN. Treatment of pulmonary sporotrichosis. Semin Respir Infect 1986;1:61–65.
3. Pluss JL, Opal SM. Pulmonary sporotrichosis: review of treatment and outcome. Medicine 1986;65:143–153.
4. Breeling JL, Weinstein L. Pulmonary sporotrichosis treated with itraconazole. Chest 1993;103:313–314.
5. Winn RE, Anderson J, Piper J, et al. Systemic sporotrichosis treated with itraconazole. Clin Infect Dis 1993;17:210–217.

PATIENT 11

A 53-year-old man with a pleural effusion after cardiac surgery

A 53-year-old man underwent coronary artery bypass graft surgery because of severe three-vessel coronary artery disease. He had an uncomplicated course until the third day when he began to experience increasing dyspnea and a "heavy" feeling in his right chest. A right-sided thoracentesis was performed after a chest radiograph demonstrated a pleural effusion.

Physical Examination: Temperature 37°, pulse 100, respirations 16, blood pressure 120/56. General: no acute distress. Chest: dullness with decreased breath sounds and fremitus at the right posterior lung base. Cardiac: normal heart sounds, no rub. Abdomen: normal. Extremity: fresh saphenous vein harvest site without evidence of infection.

Laboratory Findings: Hct 32%; WBC 11,500/μl with a normal differential. Electrolytes and renal indices: normal. Pleural fluid: milky fluid; triglycerides 150 mg/dl; cholesterol 20 mg/dl. Chest radiograph: shown below.

Hospital Course: After the initial thoracentesis, the right-sided pleural effusion continued to increase and a chest tube was placed, which drained 800 ml/day. Total parental nutrition was started and the patient's diet was adjusted to limit fat intake.

Question: What therapeutic options exist for the patient?

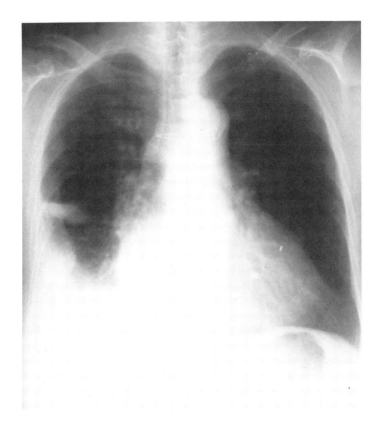

Diagnosis: Postsurgical chylothorax.

Discussion: Chylothorax is a rare but serious complication of several thoracic surgical procedures that occurs with an incidence of 0.2% to 0.56%. Resulting from injury to the thoracic duct in its passage through the mediastinum, chylothorax has been observed more frequently with the advent of more aggressive mediastinal lymph node dissections in patients undergoing lung cancer surgery. Other causes of trauma-related chylothorax include cardiac surgery, esophageal endoscopic sclerotherapy, esophageal surgery, neck hyperextension, and blunt chest trauma. Nontraumatic chylothorax is associated with congenital anomalies of the thoracic duct and various conditions such as lymphoma, carcinoma, acute and chronic mediastinal infections, and radiation fibrosis. Rare instances of chylothorax have been reported in patients with nephrotic syndrome due to movement of chylous ascites across the diaphragm into the pleural space.

Patients with postsurgical chylothorax typically present after the operative procedure with increasing dyspnea, chest heaviness, or cough. Patients with postthoracotomy chest tubes are noted to have varying amounts of excessive pleural drainage that can approach several liters a day. In rare instances, the injury to the thoracic duct may form a fistula with the bronchial tree, in which instance patients present with chyloptysis.

Thoracentesis is key to the diagnosis of chylothorax. The pleural fluid usually has a milky appearance because of its content of triglycerides and chylomicrons. Patients with little or no oral fat intake, however, may present with serosanguinous effusions. A pleural fluid triglyceride concentration greater than 110 mg/dl confirms the diagnosis. The pleural fluid pH is usually between 7.4 and 7.8, fat globules are noted by Sudan III staining, and lymphocyte counts range between 400 and 6800 cells/μl. Pleural fluid drainage in patients with a chest tube changes color after ingestion of butter or cream mixed with a lipophilic dye.

Most patients are treated conservatively after diagnosis of chylothorax. Depending on the size of the pleural effusion and the rate of pleural fluid formation, patients are placed on total parenteral nutrition, low-fat enteral diets, and medium-chain triglyceride supplements, Medium-chained triglycerides offer caloric value but pass directly into the portal circulation, bypassing the intestinal lymphatics, and do not contribute to chyle formation. Rapid pleural fluid formation requires chest tube placement for pleural space drainage. Patients with chest tubes are then observed closely for metabolic imbalance, since the drained chylous fluid contains large amounts of protein, fat, vitamins, and electrolytes. Infectious complications can occur from the loss of lymphocytes in the lymphatic fluid.

With conservative therapy, 50% of chylothoraces resolve spontaneously without additional therapy. In the remaining patients, however, many may require more aggressive intervention if pleural fluid formation does not resolve. The general indications for intervention in patients with posttraumatic chylothorax include: (1) persistent chest tube drainage for more than 14 days; (2) pleural fluid drainage greater than 1,500 ml/day; and (3) unmanageable metabolic complications.

Several interventions are available for patients not responding to conservative management. The first to be used in the 1940s was thoracotomy with thoracic duct ligation at the site of injury, which decreased the mortality of the condition from 45% to less than 2%. Injection of 30% cream through a nasogastric tube during induction of anesthesia or a preoperative lymphangiography CT can assist in localization of the thoracic duct injury. In many patients, however, the site of injury may be difficult to identify or surgically repair, so that the duct is ligated just above the diaphragm where it first enters the chest.

More recently, video-directed thoracoscopy has been applied to the surgical management of chylothorax. Allowing a smaller incision and a shorter postoperative recovery than thoracotomy, thoracoscopy can identify the thoracic duct in its supradiaphragmatic location or at the region of its disruption, and it is ligated with thoracoscopic clips or suture ligatures. Other reports exist of the application of fibrin glue to the region of thoracic duct injury with the assistance of the thoracoscope, sealing the chyle leak and allowing resolution of pleural fluid formation.

Other than direct surgical ligation, other therapeutic interventions include the placement of pleuroperitoneal shunts, pleurodesis with the intrapleural instillation of fibrin glue, talc, or other sclerosing agents, pleurectomy, and mediastinal radiation in patients with underlying mediastinal malignancies. These procedures should be reserved for patients who do not respond to conservative measures and efforts at surgical duct ligation, because they can complicate definitive therapy with thoracotomy or thoracoscopy.

The present patient had pleural fluid findings diagnostic of chylothorax. Despite conservative efforts and later chest tube placement, pleural fluid formation progressed, and the patient underwent a right-sided thoracoscopy with thoracic duct ligation at the site of injury.

Clinical Pearls

1. With conservative therapy, up to 50% of chylothoraces resolve spontaneously.

2. Conservative therapy incorporates low-fat diets, oral supplementation with medium-chain triglycerides, fat-soluble vitamins, and, in patients with rapid pleural fluid formation, chest tube placement and total parenteral nutrition.

3. Surgical intervention should be considered for the following indications: (1) persistent chest tube drainage for more than 14 days; (2) pleural fluid drainage greater than 1,500 ml/day; and (3) unmanageable metabolic complications.

4. Thoracic duct ligation at the site of injury or in its supradiaphragmatic location is definitive therapy. The advent of thoracoscopy provides a less invasive method of duct ligation.

REFERENCES

1. Moss R, Hinds S, Fedullo AJ. Chylothorax: a complication of the nephrotic syndrome. Am Rev Respir Dis 1989;140:1436–1437.
2. Shirai T, Amano J, Takabe K. Thoracoscopic diagnosis and treatment of chylothorax after pneumonectomy. Ann Thorac Surg 1991;52:306–307.
3. Cummings SP, Wyatt DA, Baker JW, et al. Successful treatment of postoperative chylothorax using an external pleuroperitoneal shunt. Ann Thorac Surg 1992;54:276–278.
4. Marts BC, Naunheim KS, Fiore AC, Pennington DG. Conservative versus surgical management of chylothorax. Am J Surg 1992;164:532–535.
5. Kent RB III, Pinson TW. Thoracoscopic ligation of the thoracic duct. Surg Endosc 1993;7:52–53.

PATIENT 12

A 32-year-old woman with vaginal bleeding, respiratory distress, and hypotension following a normal delivery

A 32-year-old woman, gravida 2, para 1, was admitted with spontaneous rupture of membranes during her 41st week of pregnancy. She delivered a healthy child after a normal labor but continued to bleed from her vagina after delivery of the placenta. Manual exploration of the uterus was performed and several small placental fragments were removed. Thirty minutes later, the patient developed severe respiratory distress and hypotension. She was intubated and placed on mechanical ventilation.

Physical Examination: Temperature 96° F; pulse 140; respirations 28, blood pressure 100/60 on dopamine. General: unresponsive. Eyes: pupils equal and reactive to light. Chest: clear. Cardiac: no gallops or murmurs. Abdomen: normal postpartum. Extremities: no cyanosis or edema.

Laboratory Findings: Hct 31%; WBC 30,800/μl; platelets 53,000/μl. Na^+ 137 mEq/L; K^+ 5.8 mEq/L; Cl^- 108 mEq/L; HCO_3^- 7.5 mEq/L; BUN 7 mg/dl; creatinine 1.9 mg/dl. PTT 52 sec; PT 21 sec; fibrinogen 166 mg/dl; D-dimer > 8 μg/ml. ABG (FiO_2 1.0): pH 7.04; PCO_2 20 mmHg; PO_2 220 mmHg. Chest radiograph: endotracheal tube in place; clear lung fields. Swan-Ganz catheter results after fluid resuscitation: RAP 9 mmHg; PAP 37/25 mmHg; PAOP 20 mmHg; CO 5.8 L/min.

Hospital Course: The chest radiograph obtained the following day is shown below.

Question: What is the most likely diagnosis?

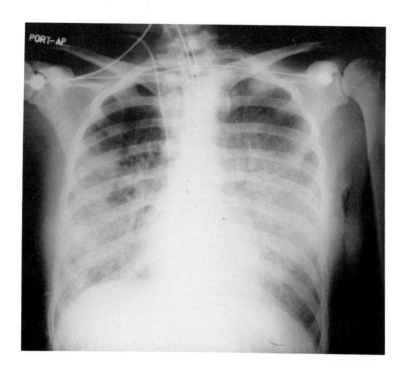

Diagnosis: Amniotic fluid embolism with vaginal hemorrhage due to disseminated intravascular coagulation.

Discussion: Amniotic fluid embolism is an uncommon event that occurs with 1 in 8000 to 1 in 80,000 births. It is largely unpredictable and no measures reliably prevent this condition in mothers undergoing labor and delivery. Fully established amniotic fluid embolism has a mortality of approximately 85% and accounts for 10% of maternal deaths each year in the United States. With improved diagnostic techniques, amniotic fluid embolism may prove to be more common than previously suspected and survival rates may not be as dismal.

The patient traditionally profiled to be at risk for amniotic fluid embolism was an older, multiparous woman who delivered a large baby after a short, tumultuous labor assisted by uterine stimulant drugs. Recent patient series, however, record a tumultuous labor in only 28% of patients with this condition and the use of uterine stimulating agents in 22%. These series also indicate that most babies delivered to mothers with amniotic fluid embolism are only average in size. Although the presence of amniotic fluid in the maternal circulation has no direct effect on the fetus, fetal death can occur if severe hypotension or hypoxemia occur in the mother before the completion of delivery.

Amniotic fluid enters the maternal circulation through disruptions in uterine or decidual vessels. These tears can occur during a cesarean section or in patients with a ruptured uterus or retained placenta. Endocervical vein lacerations or lower uterine tears that occur during normal labor are additional sites of amniotic fluid entry. The volume of amniotic fluid required to enter the circulation in order to cause clinical effects is unknown. Once infused in sufficient quantities, however, amniotic fluid containing fetal elements, such as squamous cells from skin, lanugo hairs, mucin from the gut, and bile-containing meconium, causes multiple end-organ dysfunction.

The onset of amniotic fluid embolism is often sudden and catastrophic without a recognizable prodrome. Although symptoms usually first develop during labor or in the immediate postpartum period, clinical presentations up to 48 hours after delivery have been reported. Most patients present with severe respiratory distress characterized by the sudden onset of dyspnea, tachypnea, and cyanosis with hypoxemia. Chest pain and bronchospasm are less common manifestations of the disease. Up to 25% of patients develop hypotension as the initial clinical event that appears out of proportion to the volume of blood lost during delivery. Ten to 15% of patients have a seizure as the initial event, and an additional 10–15% experience bleeding from an underlying coagulopathy without other associated clinical findings. Regardless of the first expression of the disease, all patients experience cardiorespiratory collapse within minutes of presentation. Patients who survive the initial events often go on to develop pulmonary edema.

Pulmonary artery catheterization performed within 1 hour of symptom onset generally reveals hemodynamic features of pulmonary hypertension and left ventricular failure. The etiology of the left ventricular dysfunction is unclear but may result from a direct depressant effect of amniotic fluid on myocardial contractility, decreased coronary artery blood flow, or the cardiac effects of profound hypoxemia. Intractable hypoxemia and profound pulmonary hypertension may account for 50% of deaths that occur within 1 hour of symptom onset.

Laboratory evidence of a coagulopathy invariably is present among initial survivors. Up to 40–50% of patients have clinically significant bleeding. Possible etiologies of the coagulopathy include thromboplastin-like effects of trophoblastic tissue, induction of platelet aggregation, release of platelet factor III, and activation of the complement cascade by amniotic fluid. In the early postpartum period, intractable vaginal bleeding is the most serious consequence of the coagulopathy.

The diagnosis of amniotic fluid embolism is presumptive in the proper clinical setting, although other disorders causing cardiopulmonary collapse must be considered. These conditions include venous air embolism, pulmonary thromboembolism, myocardial infarction, cardiogenic pulmonary edema, gastric aspiration, bilateral pneumothorax, eclampsia, rupture of the placenta or uterus, hemorrhagic shock, sepsis, and an adverse reaction to local anesthetics. The presence of squamous or trophoblastic cells in the maternal pulmonary circulation during the peripartum period is a nonspecific finding and is not pathognomonic for amniotic fluid embolism.

There is no specific therapy for amniotic fluid embolism. Supportive measures usually require intubation and mechanical ventilation with positive end-expiratory pressure. Hemodynamic monitoring aids fluid management and the adjustment of pressor support. Red cell and fresh frozen plasma transfusion may be required to manage patients with severe coagulopathies and hemorrhage.

The present patient developed the typical features of amniotic fluid embolism. After a short period of ventilator support, her pulmonary edema rapidly resolved and she recovered without sequelae. Her 7-pound, 11-ounce baby experienced no perinatal difficulties.

Clinical Pearls

1. Amniotic fluid embolism is an unpredictable event that usually occurs during labor, delivery, or the early postpartum period, but can develop up to 48 hours postpartum.

2. Sudden respiratory distress is the most common presentation of amniotic fluid embolism. Ten to 15% of patients may present initially with hemorrhage secondary to a coagulopathy.

3. Transient pulmonary hypertension and left ventricular failure followed by cardiogenic pulmonary edema commonly develop in patients who survive more than an hour after onset of symptoms.

4. Squamous or trophoblastic cells normally may be found in the maternal pulmonary circulation during the peripartum period; their presence is not pathognomonic for clinically significant amniotic fluid embolism.

REFERENCES

1. Steiner PE, Lushbaugh CC. Maternal pulmonary embolism by amniotic fluid as a cause of obstetric shock and unexpected deaths in obstetrics. JAMA 1941;117:1245–1254;1340–1345.
2. Morgan M. Amniotic fluid embolism. Anaesthesia 1979;34:20–32.
3. Lee W, Ginsburgh KA, Cotton DB, et al. Squamous and trophoblastic cells in the maternal pulmonary circulation identified by invasive hemodynamic monitoring during the peripartum period. Am J Obstet Gynecol 1986;155:999–1001.
4. Clark SL. New concepts of amniotic fluid embolism: a review. Obstet Gynecol Surv 1990;45:360–368.
5. Clark SL. Successful pregnancy outcomes after amniotic fluid embolism. Am J Obstet Gynecol 1992;167:511–512.

PATIENT 13

A 71-year-old woman with a cavitary pneumonia

A 71-year-old woman was admitted to another hospital for symptoms of pneumonia. Her chest radiograph revealed a right lower lobe infiltrate and sputum cultures grew *Klebsiella pneumoniae*. She was treated with ceftazidime and gentamicin but persisted febrile and toxic appearing for 3 days. She was transferred at her family's request.

Physical Examination: Temperature 103°; respirations 22; pulse 110; blood pressure 124/87. General: anxious-appearing woman frequently coughing purulent, blood-streaked sputum. Chest: dullness with tubular breath sounds at the right posterior lung base. Cardiac: normal heart sounds. Abdomen: no organomegaly.

Laboratory Findings: Hct 34%; WBC 22,800/μl with 95% neutrophils. Sputum Gram stain: multiple neutrophils with 4+ gram-negative rods. Chest radiograph: below top. Chest CT: below bottom.

Question: What complication of pneumonia has occurred?

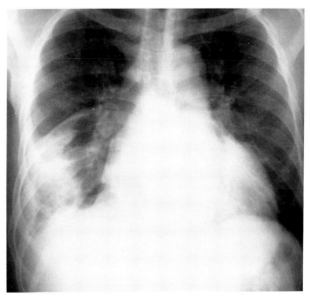

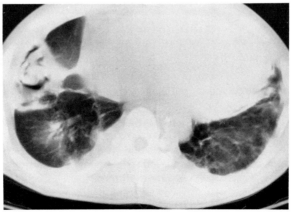

Diagnosis: Progression of bacterial pneumonia to pulmonary gangrene.

Discussion: Pulmonary gangrene is a rare but serious complication of bacterial lobar pneumonia. Also called massive pulmonary necrosis, massive sequestration of the lung, and spontaneous lobar amputation, this condition occurs in patients with severe pulmonry infections with gram-negative pathogens—especially *Klebsiella pneumoniae*— and rarely *Streptococcus pneumoniae*. Recently, pulmonary gangrene has been described in patients with *Pseudomonas aeruginosa* pneumonia and underlying HIV infection.

The clinical progression of pulmonary gangrene begins with an extensive pneumonic infiltration in a patient with signs and symptoms of acute bacterial pneumonia. Despite adequate antibiotic therapy, the pneumonia fails to resolve and arterial thrombosis occurs in the region of the infiltrate. It appears that pulmonary artery thrombosis occurs as a result of bacterial products and the intense parenchymal inflammatory response in the region of the pneumonia. Lung necrosis subsequently occurs followed by the formation of a cavity and sloughing of devitalized lung tissue that creates an intracavitary mass. The term "sphacelus," which comes form the Greek word *sphakelos* meaning "gangrene," has been used to denote the necrotic mass within the lung cavity. Patients at this stage of the disease persist in their toxic appearance and may experience massive, life-threatening hemoptysis.

The radiographic progression of pulmonary gangrene is diagnostic and, when recognized by the clinician, defines the presence of the disease. Initially, patients have lobar pneumonia commonly associated with bulging fissures due to intense inflammatory exudation within the region of infection. Subsequently, multiple small areas of rarefaction develop within the infiltrate followed by formation of a single large cavity containing a movable mass of necrotic tissue. Large masses of tissue nearly filling the cavity produce an "air crescent sign" along the margin of the cavity wall. Occasionally, the characteristic features of pulmonary gangrene are inapparent on a routine chest radiograph and require chest CT for identification.

Conditions other than pyogenic bacterial pneumonias can cause an intracavitary mass with an air crescent sign. Patients with invasive aspergillosis and mucormycosis commonly experience vascular thrombosis from fungal invasion into pulmonary vessels, which causes extensive pulmonary infarction. Chronic necrotizing aspergillosis and pulmonary gangrene in patients with tuberculosis pneumonia can also produce the radiographic appearance of massive pulmonary gangrene.

Recommended management of patients with pulmonary gangrene has varied in reported series but clearly entails aggressive antibiotic therapy for the underlying infection. Once massive necrosis occurs, many clinicians recommend thoracotomy with lobectomy to remove the infarcted tissue, accelerate clinical recovery, and prevent the onset of massive hemoptysis. Reports do exist, however, of successful medical management of pulmonary gangrene with intensive antibiotic therapy without surgery when early liquefaction of the sphacelus and adequate drainage of the abscess cavity are achieved. Patients are left with partial resolution of the pulmonary cavity with varying degrees of lung volume loss on follow-up chest radiographs.

The present patient persisted with a dense area of pulmonary consolidation that contained a cavity on her routine chest radiograph. A chest CT scan demonstrated the typical radiographic features of pulmonary gangrene with an intracavitary mass. She underwent thoracotomy with lobectomy while continuing an intensive antibiotic regimen for the *Klebsiella pneumoniae* pulmonary infection. After a complicated course, she died from respiratory failure, renal insufficiency, and a nosocomial pneumonia.

Clinical Pearls

1. Pulmonary infections with *Klebsiella pneumoniae* or *Streptococcus pneumoniae* account for more than 50% of cases of pulmonary gangrene.

2. The radiographic features of pulmonary gangrene include a large cavity that contains a mass (sphacelus) in the region of a preexisting pneumonic infiltrate.

3. The radiographic appearance of pulmonary gangrene due to pyogenic bacterial infection may also occur in patients with invasive aspergillosis, mucormycosis, chronic necrotizing aspergillosis, and pulmonary tuberculosis.

4. The radiographic appearance of pulmonary gangrene should not be confused with conditions that have a mass within a preexisting cavity, as occurs in patients with aspergillomas or tuberculosis with intracavitary blood clots.

REFERENCES

1. Proctor RJ, Griffin JP, Eastridge CE. Massive pulmonary gangrene. South Med J 1977;70:1144–1146.
2. Gutman E, Rao KVS, Park YS. Pulmonary gangrene with vascular occlusion. South Med J 1978;71:772–775.
3. O'Reilly GV, Dee PM, Otteni GV. Gangrene of the lung: successful medical management of three patients. Radiology 1978;126:575–579.
4. Hammond JMJ, Lyddell C, Potgieter PD, Odell J. Severe pneumococcal pneumonia complicated by massive pulmonary gangrene. Chest 1993;104:1610–1612.
5. Reich JM. Pulmonary gangrene and the air crescent sign. Thorax 1993;48:70–74.

PATIENT 14

A 25-year-old man with chest pain for several weeks

A 25-year-old previously healthy black man presented with a several-week history of bilateral mid-axillary and posterior chest pain. He described the pain as intermittent and occasionally pleuritic. The patient specifically denied cough or dyspnea and had not noted any generalized symptoms.

Physical Examination: Temperature 98° F; pulse 92; respirations 18; blood pressure 110/70. General: appeared well. Chest: dull to percussion with decreased fremitus and breath sounds at both lung bases more on the left than right. Cardiac: normal. Abdomen: no hepatosplenomegaly. Extremities: no cyanosis, clubbing, or edema.

Laboratory Findings: Hct 35%; WBC 5500/μl with normal differential. Electrolytes, hepatic function tests, and renal indices: normal. Spirometry: FVC 70% of predicted; FEV_1 80% of predicted; FEV_1/FVC ratio 82%. PPD: negative with negative controls. Chest radiograph: below left. Pleural fluid analysis: below right. Pleural biopsy: noncaseating granulomas. AFB and KOH stains: negative.

Question: What is the cause of the patient's chest pain?

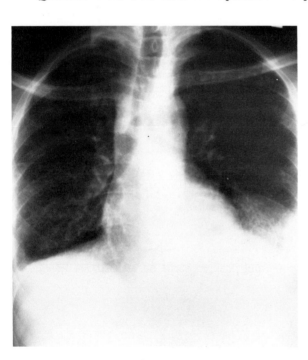

Pleural Fluid Analysis

Appearance: Serous

Nucleated cells: 4050/μl

Differential:
    90% lymphocytes
    10% mononuclear cells

RBC: 200/μl

Protein: 3.3 g/dl (serum 6.9 g/dl)

LDH: 150 IU/L (serum 240 IU/L)

Glucose: 95 mg/dl (serum 110 mg/dl)

pH: 7.40

Cytology: negative

Stains: Gram, KOH, AFB negative

Cultures: negative

Diagnosis: Sarcoidosis of the pleura.

Discussion: Considering how frequently the lungs are involved in patients with sarcoidosis, pleural disorders are a much less common manifestation of the disease. Clinical series report an incidence of pleural involvement from < 1% to 35% in patients with sarcoidosis. If the few studies with the higher incidences are excluded from analysis, however, most investigations indicate that 2–3% of patients with sarcoidosis experience pleural complications. These complications include pleural effusions, radiographic evidence of pleural thickening, and pneumothorax.

Pleural disease occurs most commonly during stages II and III sarcoidosis. Pleural complications, however, can also develop with stage 0 or I disease and may rarely represent the initial presentation of the disease. Of the pleural complications, pleural effusions usually occur in patients with earlier stages of sarcoidosis and represent a relatively good prognosis. Patients with pleural thickening or pneumothoraces tend to have more extensive disease and a progressive course.

The average age of patients with pleural sarcoidosis is 38 years. Males and females are affected equally. Interestingly, pleural abnormalities occur more commonly on the right, although up to one-fourth of patients have both hemithoraces involved. The typical sarcoid pleural effusion appears radiographically small and may resolve spontaneously. However, massive and bilateral effusions may also occur. Pleural fluid analysis reveals that the pleural fluid can be either a transudate or an exudate. Most effusions contain a predominance of lymphocytes, although some exudates may be essentially devoid of cells. The lymphocytosis may reflect the long duration of the effusion before clinical detection and the performance of thoracentesis. The helper/suppressor T lymphocyte ratio of pleural fluid has been reported to be five times higher than the ratio found in peripheral blood, which is similar to the relationship between bronchoalveolar lavage fluid and peripheral blood in patients with sarcoidosis. This observation suggests similarities in the pathogenesis of pleuritis and alveolitis in sarcoidosis.

Pleural sarcoidosis is a diagnosis of exclusion that requires a careful consideration of clinical and laboratory findings. Histologic confirmation of noncaseating granulomas on pleural biopsy specimens with negative pleural fluid and pleural tissue stains and cultures in a patient with a clinically compatible history is usually sufficient to make the diagnosis. A presumptive diagnosis may be made in patients with pleural thickening without effusions if the underlying diagnosis of sarcoidosis is well established and the chest radiograph is typical of pleural sarcoid disease.

Pleural effusions either resolve spontaneously or respond to corticosteroids within a few weeks to months of the initiation of therapy. Effusions may recur during a steroid taper or following discontinuation of the drug. The optimal dose and duration of therapy for sarcoid pleural effusions are unknown.

The present patient had a transbronchial lung biopsy that demonstrated noncaseating granulomas compatible with sarcoidosis; stains and cultures were negative. He was treated with 40 mg of prednisone daily for 3 weeks and tapered to discontinuance over the following 3 months. The chest pain resolved after several days and the effusions after 3 weeks of therapy. He had no recurrences of pleural disease over the next year.

Clinical Pearls

1. Pleural effusions, pleural thickening, and pneumothorax occur in about 3% of patients with sarcoidosis.

2. Pleural effusions most commonly affect patients with stage II or III sarcoidosis but may also occur in stages 0 or I, and rarely appear as the initial manifestation of the disease.

3. A typical sarcoid pleural effusion is a small unilateral exudate with lymphocytosis; however, effusions may be massive, bilateral, transudative, and contain no cells.

4. Pleural sarcoidosis is a diagnosis of exclusion when noncaseating granuloma with negative stains and cultures are found on pleural biopsy.

REFERENCES

1. Chusid EL, Siltzbach LE. Sarcoidosis of the pleura. Ann Intern Med 1974;81:190–194.
2. Wilen SB, Rabinowitz JG, Ulreich S, Lyons HA. Pleural involvement in sarcoidosis. Am J Med 1974;57:200–209.
3. Beckman JF, Zimmet SM, Chun BK, et al: Spectrum of pleural involvement in sarcoidosis. Arch Intern Med 1976;136:323–330.
4. Groman GS, Castele RJ, Altose MD, et al: Lymphocyte subpopulations in sarcoid pleural effusion. Ann Intern Med 1984;100:75–76.
5. Soskel NT, Sharma OP. Pleural involvement in sarcoidosis: case presentation and detailed review of the literature. Semin Respir Med 1992;13:492–514.

PATIENT 15

A 24-year-old woman with pulmonary edema after labor and delivery

A 24-year-old woman was admitted with uterine contractions during the 28th week of her pregnancy. Her prenatal examinations had gone well, and she denied previous cardiopulmonary disease or illicit drug abuse. The patient was started on intravenous terbutaline to inhibit labor. Initially the drug was successful, but the contractions returned 12 hours later and she delivered her child after discontinuation of tocolytic therapy. Twenty-four hours later, she experienced cough, severe shortness of breath, and pink frothy sputum that required intubation and mechanical ventilation.

Physical Examination: Temperature 100°; respirations 28; pulse 120; blood pressure 150/89. Neck: no jugular venous distention. Chest: diffuse crackles. Cardiac: grade II/VI systolic ejection murmur left lower sternal border; no S3.

Laboratory Findings: Hct 34%; WBC 7000/μl with normal differential; platelets normal. Electrolytes and renal indices normal. PT 12 sec; PTT 24 sec. ABG (40% FiO$_2$): PO$_2$ 59 mmHg; PCO$_2$ 31 mmHg; pH 7.49. Chest radiograph: shown below.

Question: What is the likely cause of this patient's respiratory deterioration?

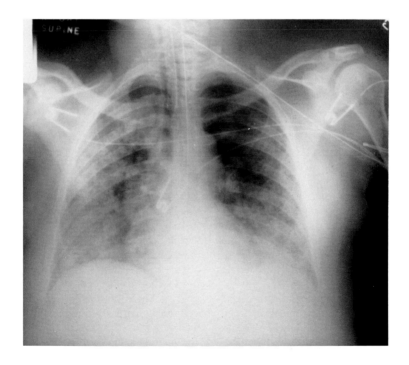

Diagnosis: Pulmonary edema due to tocolytic therapy.

Discussion: Normal intrauterine pregnancy initiates a series of physiologic events that result in major alterations in intravascular volume. By the third trimester of pregnancy, blood volume increases by 45% compared to prepregnancy values. Additionally, intracapillary pressure rises, intravascular oncotic pressure falls secondary to hemodilution, and cardiac output increases by 1–1.5 L/min. Many of these hemodynamic alterations are a consequence of decreased excretion of water and sodium that occurs in the supine position from the effects of the gravid uterus.

In the clinical setting of these pregnancy-related hemodynamic changes, the initiation of tocolytic therapy with intravenous beta-agonist drugs has been associated with the acute onset of pulmonary edema. These agents are used to suppress premature uterine contractions through their effects on increasing intracellular cyclic adenosine monophosphate (cAMP) and relaxing smooth muscle. Although the most commonly used drugs for this purpose—terbutaline, ritodrine, salbutamol, albuterol, and isoxsuprine—are relatively beta 2-specific, they still have the potential to initiate cardiovascular changes and cause varying degrees of pulmonary edema.

Pulmonary edema from tocolytic therapy typically occurs during oral or intravenous use or within 24 hours after the discontinuation of beta-agonist drugs. Respiratory difficulties may first appear within 12 hours of delivery when tocolytic therapy has failed to prevent labor. Patients at increased risk for this complication are multiparous or have coexisting factors, such as localized or systemic infections, silent cardiac disease, or treatment with magnesium sulfate or corticosteroids.

The clinical manifestations include dyspnea with or without chest pain, cough, and pink or frothy sputum. The chest examination demonstrates bilateral crackles and the cardiac examination is usually unrevealing. The chest radiograph shows bilateral alveolar infiltrates characteristic of pulmonary edema.

The pathogenesis of pulmonary edema caused by tocolytic therapy remains incompletely defined. Reported instances in which patients were evaluated by placement of a Swan-Ganz catheter provide conflicting data, with some patients having normal and others elevated pulmonary artery occlusion pressures. It is thus unclear whether tocolytic-induced pulmonary edema is noncardiogenic or cardiogenic in origin.

There are several putative mechanisms, however, whereby beta-agonist therapy may induce pulmonary edema. Because beta-agonists increase the release of antidiuretic hormone (ADH) and decrease water and sodium excretion, they may aggravate the already-expanded intravascular volume of pregnancy. Instances of tocolytic-related pulmonary edema with normal pulmonary occlusion pressures, however, argue against this mechanism. Direct myocardial toxicity from beta-agonists akin to the myocardial injury observed in patients with pheochromocytomas has been suggested as a mechanism, but echocardiograms obtained during episodes of pulmonary edema have not demonstrated left ventricular dysfunction. It is also possible that fluid infusions used to manage the systemic vasodilatation of drug therapy with beta-agonists present a volume overload when vasoconstriction occurs after discontinuation of tocolytic therapy. A pulmonary capillary leak phenomenon may also participate in pathogenic mechanisms. Although exact mechanisms remain elusive, pulmonary edema may occur from varying degrees of heart failure, pulmonary vasoconstriction, capillary leak syndrome, intravascular volume overload, and reduced serum oncotic pressure.

The onset of pulmonary edema in the peripartum period requires consideration of a differential diagnosis that includes amniotic fluid or venous air embolism, aspiration of gastric contents, sepsis, preeclampsia with pulmonary edema, and peripartum cardiomyopathy. A recently described entity of pulmonary edema in the postpartum period that occurs in cocaine addicts who are treated with bromocriptine to suppress lactation should also be considered. Tocolytic-related pulmonary edema is suggested by the absence of abnormalities of clotting and the rapid improvement of pulmonary edema (usually not requiring intubation and mechanical ventilation). Once diagnosed, patients should be managed with supplemental oxygen and close observation, with intubation and ventilatory support for severe degrees of respiratory failure. Diuretic therapy may improve the clinical course in patients with volume overload but may cause hypotension in the presence of intravascular volume depletion.

The present patient had tocolytic-related pulmonary edema that was managed with ventilatory support, mild diuresis, and careful observation. She rapidly improved within several hours and was successfully extubated the following day. The patient's infant did well after management for respiratory distress in the neonatal ICU.

Clinical Pearls

1. Pulmonary edema related to tocolytic therapy occurs most often after intravenous infusions of beta-agonist drugs but also has been reported during oral therapy.

2. Pulmonary edema can occur after discontinuation of beta-agonist therapy or in the postpartum period when tocolytic therapy is unsuccessful in preventing labor.

3. It is unclear whether tocolytic-related pulmonary edema is cardiogenic or noncardiogenic in origin. Data from Swan-Ganz catheterization studies are conflicting in nature.

4. Bromocriptine therapy to suppress lactation can also cause postpartum pulmonary edema in cocaine-addicted mothers through effects on central dopamine receptors.

REFERENCES

1. Milos M, Aberle DR, Parkinson BT, et al. Maternal pulmonary edema complicating beta-adrenergic therapy of preterm labor. AJR 1988;151:917–918.
2. Pisani R, Rosenow EC III. Pulmonary edema associated with tocolytic therapy. Ann Intern Med 1989;110:714–718.
3. Mabie WC, Hackman BB, Sibai BM. Pulmonary edema associated with pregnancy: echocardiographic insights and implications for treatment. Obstet Gynecol 1993;81:227–234.

PATIENT 16

A 56-year-old man with a slowly enlarging peripheral lung nodule

A 56-year-old man presented with a 10-month history of a nonproductive cough. He denied dyspnea, hemoptysis, chest pain, weight loss, or fatigue. The patient believed he had some minimal exposure to asbestos during his career as a structural engineer but denied other occupational exposures or known contacts with tuberculosis. The patient had a 7 pack/year smoking history but had discontinued smoking 20 years earlier.

Physical Examination: Temperature 98.6°; pulse 68; respirations 16; blood pressure 150/95. Skin: normal. Chest: normal. Extremities: no clubbing or edema.

Laboratory Findings: CBC and electrolytes: normal. ESR 9 mm/hr. Chest radiograph (below left): a right lower zone peripheral lesion that had increased in size since the last exam 5 years earlier. Chest CT: shown below right (prone view).

Question: What is the most likely cause of the patient's enlarging mass?

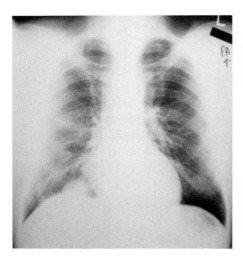 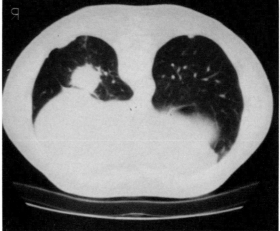

Diagnosis: Rounded atelectasis.

Discussion: Rounded atelectasis is a rare, non-malignant lesion that represents a form of peripheral lobar collapse occurring almost exclusively in patients with asbestos exposure. It is a serendipitous finding in most instances, with patients presenting without chest symptoms or with other pulmonary manifestations of asbestos exposure.

Two theories exist for the pathogenesis of rounded atelectasis. The most commonly cited hypothesis is that peripheral lobar collapse occurs as a result of benign asbestos pleural effusion. The pleural effusion, if sufficiently large, causes a portion of lung to float and separate from the parietal pleura. The pleural fluid compresses a focal area of the lung, creating a cleft or groove between atelectatic and aerated regions. Organization of fibrinous exudate within the cleft promotes the deposition of mature fibrous tissue that fixes the cleft and maintains the underlying parenchymal atelectasis.

A second hypothesis contends that a region of asbestos-induced inflammation on the visceral pleura leads to a localized focus of fibrosis. As the fibrous tissue matures, it contracts and pulls the underlying pleura with it, producing a "bunching" effect on the visceral pleura. The pleura eventually buckles into the lung, producing a cleft. The buckling action produces localized atelectasis because the elastic tissue framework of the alveolar septae is intimately connected with the pleural internal elastic lamina.

Areas of rounded atelectasis appear at thoracotomy as subpleural, palpable masses covered with a grayish-white coating. The surgeon can peel off fibrous tissue in several layers. As each layer is removed, the lung expands until full reinflation occurs, resulting in a normal appearance of lung tissue. Occasionally, the fibrous tissue penetrates into the pulmonary parenchyma. In most cases the lesions are found opposite a parietal pleural plaque.

Radiographically, rounded atelectasis usually presents as a round, sharply marginated 2.5- to 5-cm pleural-based mass lesion. The mass forms an acute angle with the pleura, indicating its intrapulmonary location. Volume loss is usually present. The comet tail sign, the *sine qua non* of rounded atelectasis, is a curvilinear shadow extending from the lower border of the mass to the hilum that represents blood vessels and bronchi.

The differential diagnosis of a slowly enlarging parenchymal or pleural mass includes carcinomas (usually adenocarcinoma or bronchoalveolar cell carcinoma), mesotheliomas, hamartomas, granulomas, and bronchogenic cysts. If serial radiographs are available, rounded atelectasis often can be distinguished from malignancy by the growth rate. Rounded atelectasis often develops within weeks and the vast majority of lesions do not increase in size over time. Many resolve spontaneously or with resolution of the pleural effusion. There has been a single report of a patient with enlarging rounded atelectasis over 12 months. It is unclear whether the enlargement was due solely to rounded atelectasis, as a large surrounding hematoma was found at thoracotomy and may have accounted for the radiographic enlargement.

A CT scan confirms the intrapulmonary location of the mass and more clearly delineates the presence of lung interposed between the chest wall and the mass. The major CT signs of rounded atelectasis include (1) a rounded peripheral lung mass; (2) a mass most dense at its periphery; (3) central air bronchograms; (4) a mass that forms an acute angle with the pleura; (5) pleural scarring adjacent to the mass; (6) vessels and bronchi curving toward the mass as a "comet tail"; and (7) the presence of at least two sharp margins caused by the curving lung structures. In the present case, the CT (previous page) demonstrated a 3 cm irregular spiculated mass abutting the right hemidiaphragm in the right lower lobe. There was evidence of pleural thickening in this region, and several small pleural plaques were also identified.

In the majority of patients with rounded atelectasis, the radiographic and clinical features described above are sufficient to diagnose the condition and limit further diagnostic testing to serial radiographic follow-up. A negative needle aspiration may add confidence to the diagnosis. In unusual instances, thoracotomy may be necessary to exclude malignancy.

Treatment is seldom necessary because most patients are asymptomatic. Decortication should be reserved for the rare patient with an atelectatic lesion large enough to compromise respiratory function.

The unusual enlargement of the lesion in the present patient raised concern about potential malignancy; therefore, a right lower lobe basilar segmentectomy was performed. The pathology was compatible with rounded atelectasis without evidence of malignancy. He has done well after 3 years of follow-up.

Clinical Pearls

1. Rounded atelectasis is an unusual form of peripheral lobar collapse that occurs almost exclusively from asbestos exposure.

2. The comet tail sign, a curvilinear shadow of the bronchovascular bundle, is pathognomonic for rounded atelectasis.

3. It is extremely unusual for rounded atelectasis to enlarge radiographically, as most lesions remain stable; some lesions regress or resolve.

4. An appropriate clinical history and compatible radiographic findings usually obviate the need for invasive diagnostic procedures.

REFERENCES

1. Hanke R, Kretzschmar R. Round atelectasis. Semin Roentgenol 1980;15:174–182.
2. Dernevik L, Gatzinsky P, Hultman E, et al. Shrinking pleuritis with atelectasis. Thorax 1982;37:252–258.
3. Doyle TC, Lawler GA. CT features of rounded atelectasis of the lung. AJR 1984;143:225–228.
4. Dernevik L, Gatzinsky P. Pathogenesis of shrinking pleuritis with atelectasis—"rounded atelectasis." Eur J Respir Dis 1987;71:244–249.
5. Silverman SP, Marino PL. Unusual case of enlarging pulmonary mass. Chest 1987;91:457–458.

PATIENT 17

A 62-year-old man with a cavitary infiltrate and acid-fast bacilli

A 62-year-old man with a 3-month history of weight loss presented with a 7-day history of cough and low-grade fever. He had a long smoking history and carried a diagnosis of emphysema. Ten years earlier he had undergone repair of an abdominal aortic aneurysm.

A chest film revealed a left upper lobe infiltrate (below left), and the patient was hospitalized for parenteral cefuroxime therapy. Sputum culture showed oral flora and diphtheroids. After 10 days of therapy, his symptoms persisted and he was transferred for further evaluation.

Physical Examination: Temperature 102°; pulse 120; respirations 23. Lymph nodes: palpable 1- to 2-cm nodes along the cervical chains. Chest: decreased breath sounds with amphoric breathing over the left upper lung zone. Cardiac: grade 2/6 systolic ejection murmur.

Laboratory Findings: Hct 32%; WBC count: 13,000/μl with 87% PMNs, 9% bands, and 4% lymphocytes. Electrolytes, renal indices, and liver function tests: normal. Sputum Gram stain: multiple organisms; acid-fast stain: rare, weakly staining bacilli. Chest radiograph: below right.

Question: What diagnosis is most probable? How would you proceed?

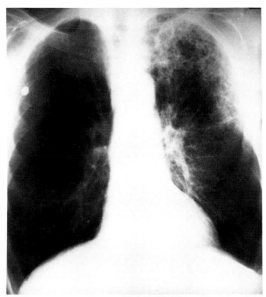 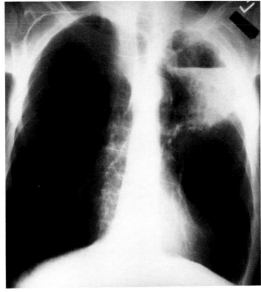

Diagnosis: Cavitary pneumonia caused by *Rhodococcus equi* in a patient with the acquired immunodeficiency syndrome (AIDS).

Discussion: *R. equi*, an aerobic bacterium, is a well-known pathogen in veterinary medicine. First described in 1923 as a cause of pneumonia in foals, *R. equi* is a common cause of suppurating pulmonary infections in horses, cattle, swine, and sheep; occasionally it contributes to visceral abscesses, such as those that occur in lymphadenitis, mediastinitis, and endometriosis. The predilection for infection in grazing animals appears to be explained by the organism's reservoir in soil.

Rarely cultured from healthy persons, *R. equi* is an opportunistic pathogen that causes necrotizing pneumonia with cavitary infiltrates, pleural effusions, and thoracic empyema in immunocompromised patients. Infection in humans was first associated with hematologic malignancies, organ transplantation, and immunosuppressive therapy.

Recently, *R. equi* cavitary lung suppuration has emerged as an important disorder in patients with AIDS, who may also have bacteremia and infection in the intestines and retroperitoneal, axillary, and pelvic lymph nodes. Subcutaneous and intracranial abscesses may result from hematogenous spread in a pattern reminiscent of nocardial disease. The opportunistic nature of *R. equi* disease in patients with human immunodeficiency virus type 1 (HIV-1) infection may alert the clinician to underlying immunocompromise in patients with undiagnosed AIDS. Indeed, it has been suggested that *R. equi* infection be included as a diagnostic criterion for AIDS.

Patients present with generalized weakness, fever, cough productive of scant sputum, dyspnea, and pleuritic chest pain. About 50% of patients report some contact with farm animals or contaminated soil. The chest film reveals a dense infiltrate, typically in the upper lung zone, that may be accompanied by pleural thickening or effusion. The infiltrates tend to cavitate over 2–4 weeks, leaving large, shaggy-walled lung abscesses with air-fluid levels. Persistence of a dense, mass-like infiltrate has been described in a patient with AIDS in whom the differential diagnosis included Kaposi's sarcoma and pulmonary lymphoma.

The pathogenesis of *R. equi* infection is unclear, but humans appear to contract the disease most commonly through the respiratory tract. An alimentary port has also been implicated in patients with AIDS in whom intestinal and abdominal lymphatic disease developed in the absence of pulmonary infection. The organism is an intracellular pathogen; in biopsy specimens, it is found "packed" with macrophages that are surrounded by mononuclear cell invasion and tissue necrosis.

At present, it is uncertain how *R. equi* causes such extensive lung necrosis, since it does not release tissue-destructive enzymes.

The diagnosis of pneumonia requires careful consideration of *R. equi* infection in any immunocompromised patient with cavitary lung disease. The organism may be recovered in expectorated sputum, but bronchoscopy, thoracentesis, or biopsy of infected lymph nodes is usually required. *R. equi* appears on Gram stain as a gram-positive organism with variable shapes ranging from coccoid to bacillary clubbed forms.

Previously classified as a *Corynebacterium*, the organism may be mistaken for a diphtheroid or bacillus species and considered a contaminant or commensal. It differs from *Corynebacterium*, however, in its formation of mucoid, salmon-pink colonies and its nonfermentative and comparatively inactive metabolism.

R. equi also stains weakly acid-fast, which may cause diagnostic confusion with tuberculosis in patients with cavitary lung disease and positive acid-fast sputum smears. However, recognition that *Mycobacterium tuberculosis* rarely causes cavitary infiltrates in patients with AIDS facilitates diagnosis. Acid-fast stains of feces are commonly performed in patients with AIDS. The presence of weakly staining coccobacillary forms on these stains should prompt consideration of *R. equi* infection.

Cure of *R. equi* lung infection requires prolonged use of antibiotics, drainage of empyemas, and consideration of resection of infected lung tissue. Despite aggressive therapy, the mortality associated with pneumonia from *R. equi* is 25%. Nearly all human isolates are resistant to penicillin. Erythromycin, chloramphenicol, aminoglycosides, vancomycin and, occasionally, tetracycline have been the most commonly used drugs that demonstrate in vitro and clinical efficacy. Recent data from the Centers for Disease Control indicate that all reported isolates from patients with HIV infection are sensitive to amoxicillin-clavulanate, ampicillin-sulbactam, gentamicin, or imipenem. Less than 5% of isolates were resistant to erythromycin, rifampin, tetracycline, or trimethoprim-sulfamethoxazole. General recommendations exist for combination therapy with two agents to be continued several months beyond clinical and roentgenographic resolution and conversion of sputum specimens to negative on culture. Patients should be observed closely for signs of relapse, which often occurs.

The present patient's sputum Gram stain was positive for diphtheroid organisms that subsequently grew *R. equi* in culture. He was treated with erythromycin and vancomycin, with partial resolution of the lung cavity during the ensuing 4 months. Apparently because of blood transfusions received 10 years earlier for his aortic surgery, his blood tested positive for HIV-1.

Clinical Pearls

1. A cavitary infiltrate in an immunocompromised patient suggests *R. equi* infection.

2. The initial clue to the diagnosis of pulmonary *R. equi* disease may be a sputum laboratory report of "diphtheroid commensals."

3. The presence of weakly staining coccobacillary organisms on acid-fast smears of fecal specimens obtained from patients with AIDS requires the exclusion of intestinal infection with *R. equi*.

REFERENCES

1. Van Etta LL, Filice GA, Ferguson RM, et al. *Corynebacterium equi:* a review of 12 cases of human infection. Rev Infect Dis 1983;5:1012–1018.
2. Bishopric GA, d'Agay MF, Schlemmer B, et al. Pulmonary pseudotumour due to *Corynebacterium equi* in a patient with the acquired immunodeficiency syndrome. Thorax 1988;43:486–487.
3. Weingarten JS, Huang DY, Jackman JD Jr. *Rhodococcus equi* pneumonia: an unusual early manifestation of the acquired immunodeficiency syndrome (AIDS). Chest 1988;94:195–196.
4. Lasky JA, Pulkingham N, Powers MA, Durack DT. *Rhodococcus equi* causing human pulmonary infection: review of 29 cases. South Med J 1991;84:1217–1220.
5. Magnani G, Elia GF, McNeil MM, et al. *Rhodococcus equi* cavitary pneumonia in HIV-infected patients: an unsuspected opportunistic pathogen. J Acquired Immune Deficiency Syndrome 1992;5:1059–1064.
6. McNeil MM, Brown JM. Distribution and antimicrobial susceptibility of *Rhodococcus equi* from clinical specimens. Eur J Epidemiol 1992;8:437–443.

PATIENT 18

A 52-year-old woman with a pleural effusion for 10 years

A 52-year-old woman was referred for evaluation of dyspnea on exertion, cough, and a long-standing pleural effusion. Ten years earlier, she experienced an illness characterized by pneumonitis, pericarditis, and myocarditis followed shortly after by facial, arm, and leg edema with a right pleural effusion. Cardiac catheterization at that time was normal. She had been managed with diuretics but continued to experience leg swelling and required six thoracenteses over the years for relief of dyspnea. The patient also reported difficulties with sinus infections since childhood.

Physical Examination: Temperature 98.2°, pulse 88, respirations 20, blood pressure 118/66. Appearance: healthy appearing. Skin: telangiectasia of the right neck and upper chest. Chest: dullness with decreased fremitus on the right. Cardiac: normal. Extremities: no cyanosis or clubbing, 1+ pretibial edema, nails short with cross-ridging and onycholysis.

Laboratory Findings: Hct 37%; WBC 4500/μl with normal differential, ESR 12 mm/hr. FVC 1.68 liters (55% of predicted); FEV_1 1.37 liters (59% of predicted); FEV_1/FVC ratio 81%. Chest radiograph: below left. Pleural fluid analysis: below right.

Question: What is the most likely diagnosis? What would you recommend to the patient at this time?

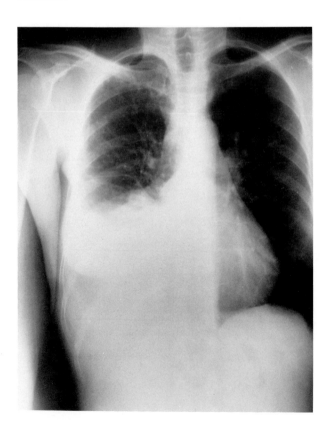

Pleural Fluid Analysis

Appearance: serosanguinous

Nucleated cells: 1376/μl

Differential:
  96% lymphocytes
  4% mononuclear cells

RBC: 8000/μl

Protein: 3.4 g/dl (serum 6.7 g/dl)

LDH: 40 IU/L (serum 70 IU/L)

Glucose: 99 mg/dl

pH: 7.41

Amylase: 54 IU/L (serum 70 IU/L)

Rheumatoid factor: negative

Triglycerides: 45 mg/dl

Cytology: negative

Culture: negative

Diagnosis: Yellow nail syndrome.

Discussion: The duration of a pleural effusion may give some insight into its etiology. Pleural effusions that persist for a year or more may be due to yellow nail syndrome (YNS), trapped lung (usually from rheumatoid pleurisy or tuberculosis), or a cholesterol effusion (seen with a trapped lung, commonly due to rheumatoid disease or tuberculosis). Effusions that last several months, but less than a year, include benign asbestos pleural effusions, uremic pleurisy, post cardiac injury syndrome, fungal pleural effusions, actinomycosis, malignant effusions, and effusions from radiation pleuritis. Pleural effusions due to trapped lung, rheumatoid pleurisy, asbestos pleural effusion, cholesterol effusion, and YNS may escape detection because many patients with these conditions have few or no symptoms.

YNS, first described 30 years ago, consists of a triad of yellow nails, lymphedema, and respiratory tract illness that occurs slightly more commonly in women than men. Respiratory manifestations include pleural effusions, bronchiectasis, recurrent pneumonias, bronchitis, or sinusitis. The condition results from an abnormality of the lymphatic vessels with impaired drainage leading to subungual edema, lymphedema of the extremities, and pleural effusions. Lymphangiograms show a paucity of hypoplastic or dilated lymphatics.

The age of onset of symptoms ranges from as early as birth to as late as age 65, with the median age being 40 years. Yellow nails are the initial finding in one-third of patients. Nails grow at approximately half the rate of the lower limits of normal nail growth. Other nail abnormalities include overcurvature (transversely or longitudinally), thickening, onycholysis, cross-ridging, and loss of lunulae and cuticles. Women frequently cover their unsightly nails with opaque nail polish, which may obscure the finding from the unwary clinician. Lymphedema develops in approximately 80% of patients during the course of the illness and represents the initial symptom in about one-third of patients. Edema can be pitting or nonpitting and may be confined to the fingertips.

Approximately 60% of patients with YNS develop pleuropulmonary symptoms during the course of their disease, whereas a third of patients present with a respiratory manifestation. Pleural effusions have been noted in 36% of reported cases. Patients often give a history of recurrent attacks over many years of bronchitis, bronchiectasis, sinusitis, pneumonia, or pleuritis. Symptoms seldom appear simultaneously and the full triad is not always present.

Pleural effusions may be unilateral or bilateral, and the volume of pleural fluid varies from small to massive. In most patients, the fluid is straw-colored but may be sanguinous. The protein concentration ranges between 3.5 and 4.5 g/dl and the LDH concentration is often greater than 200 IU/L. Nucleated cell counts are usually greater than $2000/\mu l$ with a predominance ($> 80\%$) of lymphocytes. The glucose is equivalent to serum, and the pH approximates 7.40.

Therapy for YNS is generally symptomatic. Local steroid injections and oral vitamin E have been reported to be successful in treating the yellow nails. Following thoracentesis, fluid typically recurs over a few days to several months. Chemical pleurodesis and pleurectomy may prevent fluid reaccumulation in patients with symptomatic pleural effusions. In at least one patient, the yellow nails reverted to normal following pleurectomy. Spontaneous partial or complete recovery of nail abnormalities occurs in 30% of patients who may experience occasional relapses. Lymphedema and pleural effusions are persistent and spontaneous recovery has not been reported.

The present patient fulfilled the clinical diagnosis of YNS. She was managed expectantly for episodes of sinusitis. It was suggested that pleurodesis could be considered if the pleural effusions and severity of the dyspnea progressed to limit her activities.

Clinical Pearls

1. Yellow nail syndrome should be considered in the differential diagnosis of a pleural effusion that has been present for months or years.

2. A history of bronchiectasis, bronchitis, or sinusitis in association with chronic pleural effusion should suggest the diagnosis.

3. Slow nail growth is the most consistent nail finding. Women often cover the unsightly nails with opaque nail polish, which may obscure the diagnosis from the unwary observer.

4. The triad of yellow nails, lymphedema, and respiratory tract disease is rarely present at initial presentation. Pleural effusion usually is a late manifestation and does not regress spontaneously.

REFERENCES

1. Hiller E, Rosenow EC III, Olsen AM. Pulmonary manifestations of the yellow nail syndrome. Chest 1972;61:452–458.
2. Beer DJ, Pereira W Jr, Snider GL. Pleural effusion associated with primary lymphedema: a perspective on the yellow nail syndrome. Am Rev Respir Dis 1978;117:595–599.
3. Nordkild P, Kromann-Andersen H, Struve-Christiensen E. Yellow nail syndrome: the triad of yellow nails, lymphedema, and pleural effusions. Acta Med Scand 1986;219:221–227.

PATIENT 19

A 66-year-old woman with respiratory failure after cardiac surgery

A 66-year-old woman with a history of congestive heart failure presented with the rapid onset of shortness of breath. Her family stated that the patient first noted a burning sensation around her lips while eating dinner that progressed to swelling of her tongue. Several minutes later, the patient lost the ability to speak and experienced marked difficulty inhaling. Her only medications were digoxin and enalapril.

Physical Examination: Temperature 99°; pulse 132; blood pressure 189/92; respirations 32. General: labored breathing with inspiratory stridor. Head: markedly swollen tongue protruding from the patient's mouth. Chest: decreased breath sounds. Cardiac: normal. Extremities: no swelling.

Laboratory Findings: Hct 36%; WBC 8000/μl with a normal differential. Na^+ 134 mEq/L; K^+ 4.3 mEq/L; Cl^- 101 mEq/L; HCO_3^- 25 mEq/L; BUN 23 mg/dl; Cr 1.9 mg/dl. ABG (5 L/min nasal cannula): pH 7.32, PCO_2 43 mmHg, PO_2 125 mmHg. Chest radiograph: normal. EKG: normal.

Question: What is the underlying condition? How should the patient be managed?

Diagnosis: Upper airway obstruction from angioedema induced by angiotensin-converting enzyme (ACE) inhibitor therapy.

Discussion: The advent of drugs in the family of ACE inhibitors has markedly improved the management of hypertension and congestive heart failure. Although generally considered more effective and better tolerated than beta-blockers and diuretics, ACE inhibitors cause various complications such as dry persistent cough, headaches, dizziness, and varying degrees of systemic hypotension. They also may worsen renal function in patients with underlying renal artery stenosis and in patients managed concomitantly with loop diuretics.

ACE inhibitors also have been reported to cause a less common complication of facial and cervical angioedema that can progress to severe upper airway obstruction when structures of the oropharynx are involved. Both enalapril and captopril have been associated with this adverse reaction, which occurs in 0.1–2% of treated patients. ACE inhibitor–induced angioedema may develop within days or several months after the first initiation of therapy. Patients typically note swelling of facial features that progresses to difficulty with speech, dysphagia, and dyspnea due to upper airway obstruction. Inspiratory stridor and obvious soft tissue swelling of facial and oropharyngeal structures are common clinical findings. Patients may progress to respiratory failure that requires emergency intubation. Risk factors are not clearly defined, but patients with preexistingly narrowed airways due to obesity, previous airway intubation, or neck surgery may be at increased risk. A relationship of angioedema to drug dose has not been established.

The pathogenesis of angioedema initiated by ACE inhibitors is inferred from their known effects on bradykinin metabolism. These agents inhibit kinin II, which is the primary degradative enzyme for bradykinin. Initiation of ACE inhibitor therapy may consequently interfere with bradykinin metabolism and increase tissue concentrations of this inflammatory mediator. In certain individuals, angioedema may ensue from the effects of bradykinin on promoting endothelial permeability, increasing venular pressure, and stimulating the release of other inflammatory mediators. Since bradykinin has been considered a potential etiologic agonist in inducing ACE inhibitor–induced cough, it is interesting to speculate that persistent coughing and angioedema in ACE inhibitor–treated patients may be part of a continuum of the same disorder. Serum concentrations of C1 esterase inhibitor and C4 have been found to be normal in patients with this form of angioedema.

ACE inhibitor–induced angioedema should be treated with discontinuation of ACE inhibitor therapy and urgent initiation of corticosteroids and antihistamines. Although patients generally rapidly recover, intubation may be required to maintain a patent airway until swelling resolves.

The present patient appeared severely fatigued from the high work of breathing through a narrowed upper airway and required orotracheal intubation. She was treated with corticosteroids and antihistamines. The swelling resolved during the next 12 hours and the patient underwent an uncomplicated extubation.

Clinical Pearls

1. Angioedema of facial and neck structures can develop after several days or months of the first initiation of therapy with ACE inhibitor drugs.

2. Swelling of oropharyngeal structures can cause severe upper airway obstruction, requiring intubation until angioedema resolves.

3. Although the etiology of ACE inhibitor–induced angioedema is not clearly defined, drug interference with the metabolic degradation of bradykinin may play a role.

4. Patients with ACE inhibitor–induced angioedema are treated with corticosteroids and antihistamines; intubation may be required until airway swelling resolves.

REFERENCES

1. Jain M, Armstrong L, Hall J. Predisposition to and late onset of upper airway obstruction following angiotensin-converting enzyme inhibitor therapy. Chest 1992;102:871–874.
2. Roy TM, Byrd RP Jr, Fields CL. Upper airway obstruction following angiotensin-converting enzyme inhibitor therapy [letter]. Chest 1993;104:1310.

PATIENT 20

A 67-year-old man with lung nodules while receiving methotrexate for a skin disorder

A 67-year-old man presented with a several-week history of sinus congestion and nonproductive cough. He had undergone removal of a malignant colon polyp 7 years earlier, but serial colonoscopies had remained negative since then. The patient had a positive tuberculin test 18 years earlier and received 1 year of isoniazid prophylaxis. Because of difficulties with pityriasis rubra pilaris, he had been taking methotrexate 15–25 mg/week for the past 3 months. The patient had not traveled outside of South Carolina in the previous year, but had lived in Tennessee and Indiana in the past.

Physical Examination: Vital signs: normal. Skin: diffuse erythema consistent with pityriasis rubra pilaris. Head: no sinus tenderness. Neck: no adenopathy. Chest: clear to auscultation.

Laboratory Findings: Hct 37%; WBC 5300/μl with 57% neutrophils, 17% lymphocytes, 14% monocytes, 12% reactive lymphocytes. ESR: 2 mm/hr. Chest radiographs: multiple 1.5 to 2.0 cm nodules (arrows) in the right middle and right lower lobes that were not present on a radiograph 2 years earlier.

Question: What disorder should be included in this patient's differential diagnosis?

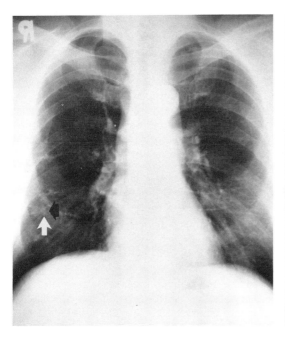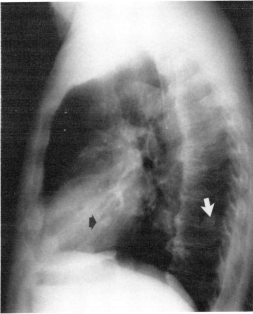

Diagnosis: *Mycobacterium avium intracellulare* infection.

Discussion: In addition to its use in patients with rheumatoid arthritis and various severe skin disorders, methotrexate is being used for a growing list of indications. With a wider application of this agent, clinicians are becoming more familiar with its spectrum of adverse reactions. Although methotrexate is usually well tolerated, patients may experience transient elevations in liver function tests, nausea, and stomatitis. Pulmonary complications of either acute pneumonitis or progressive fibrosis are well described but occur in an idiosyncratic fashion with an unknown pathogenesis. Pulmonary toxicity was previously thought to occur only in patients receiving more than 20 mg/week. More recent reports, however, indicate that nearly 6% of patients taking lower doses of the drug will experience pulmonary toxicity.

Opportunistic infection is another complication of low-dose methotrexate therapy that has been reported increasingly more frequently in patients with normal leukocyte counts. To date, a total of 25 cases of opportunistic infection in patients taking low-dose methotrexate have been reported in the English literature. Nineteen of the 25 reported patients had opportunistic infections originating in the lungs. The most prevalent opportunistic infection reported is *Pneumocystis carinii* pneumonia, accounting for 10 of the 25 (40%) cases. Other pathogens include *Histoplasma capsulatum, Cryptococcus neoformans, Nocardia brasiliensis, Herpes zoster, Varicella zoster,* and *Mycobacterium avium intracellulare.*

A minimal duration of methotrexate therapy is apparently necessary before opportunistic infection occurs. A review of 124 patients taking low-dose methotrexate for rheumatoid arthritis reported no infectious complications before completion of 12 weeks of therapy; all of the existing reports of opportunistic infection occurred in patients completing at least 11 weeks of treatment with the drug. The present patient had received 12 weeks of methotrexate therapy when his symptoms began.

Despite a low incidence of bone marrow suppression in patients receiving low-dose methotrexate, changes in immune function have been described. Patients receiving as little as 7.5 mg/week of methotrexate may experience B-cell suppression and inhibition of B-cell differentiation due to increased numbers of T8 lymphocytes and natural killer cells. No significant decrease in the number of circulating B-lymphocytes is seen. In addition, use of nonsteroidal anti-inflammatory drugs may increase serum levels of methotrexate by decreasing renal excretion of methotrexate and cause greater immunosuppression than otherwise expected.

The differential diagnosis for the present patient with new pulmonary nodules and a nonproductive cough would include metastatic cancer, infection due to mycobacteria, fungus, or other opportunistic pathogens, and methotrexate lung toxicity. He underwent open lung biopsy, which revealed caseating granulomas with acid-fast organisms. Tissue cultures grew *Mycobacterium avium intracellulare.* The patient's methotrexate was discontinued, and he received 18 months of therapy with isoniazid, rifampin, and ethambutol. There was complete radiographic resolution of the lung nodules without recurrence over 2 years of observation.

Clinical Pearls

1. Opportunistic infection can complicate low-dose methotrexate therapy anytime after 11 weeks of therapy, even with normal leukocyte counts.

2. The most common opportunistic infection reported with low-dose methotrexate is *Pneumocystis carinii* pneumonia.

3. Pulmonary toxicity with low-dose methotrexate (less than 20 mg/week) occurs in 5.5% of patients and can present as either acute pneumonitis or fibrosis.

4. Nonsteroidal anti-inflammatory drugs decrease renal excretion of methotrexate, potentially increasing serum levels of methotrexate and increasing the risk for toxicity.

REFERENCES

1. Carson CW, Cannon GW, Egger MJ, et al. Pulmonary disease during the treatment of rheumatoid arthritis with low-dose pulse methotrexte. Semin Arthritis Rheum 1987;16:186–195.
2. Olsen NJ, Callahan LF, Pincus T. Immunologic studies of rheumatoid arthritis patients treated with methotrexate. Arthritis Rheum 1987;30:481–488.
3. Fehlauer CS, Carson CW, Cannon GW, et al. Methotrexate therapy in rheumatoid arthritis: two-year retrospective followup study. J Rheumatol 1989;16:307–312.
4. Shiroky JB, Frost A, Skelton JD, et al. Complications of immunosuppression associated with weekly low-dose methotrexate. J Rheumatol 1991;18:1172–1175.
5. LeMense GP, Sahn SA. Opportunistic infection during treatment with low-dose methotrexate. Am J Respir Crit Care Med 1994:150:259–260.

PATIENT 21

A 55-year-old woman with hemoptysis and a cavitary lung mass

A 55-year-old woman with an extensive smoking history presented with right-sided chest pain. Nine months earlier, she noted a nonproductive cough and fatigue that had progressed in severity. She denied alcohol consumption, recent dental work, loss of consciousness, fever, or chills.

Physical Examination: Temperature 99°; pulse 110; respirations 25; blood pressure 120/76. General: mild dyspnea with intermittent coughing productive of blood-streaked sputum. Mouth: good dentition. Chest: dullness at right posterior lung base; egophony. Cardiac: normal heart sounds.

Laboratory Findings: Hct 31%; WBC 8900/μl, platelets 230,000/μl. Electrolytes, renal indices, liver function tests: normal. Chest radiographs: shown below.

Hospital Course: After initiation of clindamycin, the patient underwent bronchoscopy with transbronchial biopsy and percutaneous needle aspiration of the cavitary mass in the right lower lobe, both of which demonstrated necrotic debris. Because of the sudden onset of massive hemoptysis, the patient underwent thoracotomy and removal of the right lower lobe. The surgical pathology demonstrated intense inflammation and tissue with histologic features of squamous cell carcinoma and spindle-cell sarcoma.

Question: What is the underlying cause of the patient's cavitary lung lesion?

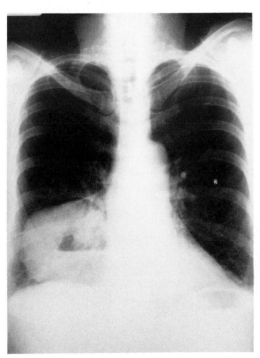 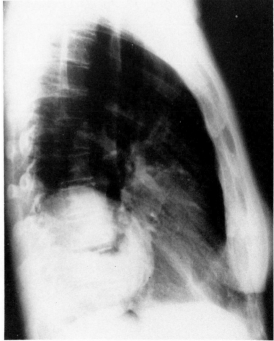

Diagnosis: Peripheral primary lung carcinosarcoma with necrosis and cavitation.

Discussion: Carcinosarcomas are extremely aggressive biphasic tumors composed of an admixture of malignant epithelial and sarcomatous components. Representing less than 0.3% of all primary lung cancers, carcinosarcomas have been described in the upper respiratory tract, esophagus, breast, skin, uterus, gallbladder, and skin. The lung is the fourth most common site to be affected.

In the combined reports to date, the carcinomatous component of the tumor is a squamous cell carcinoma in 70% of patients, with an adenomatoid cell type or undifferentiated pattern in 20% and 10% of patients, respectively. The sarcomatous component is a spindle-cell type and may contain foci of leiomyosarcoma, chondrosarcoma, osteosarcoma, fibrosarcoma, or immature cellular forms.

The pathogenesis of carcinosarcomas remains unclear despite more than a century of conjecture. The possibility that a primary carcinoma initiates a pseudosarcomatous tissue reaction is unlikely because of the reported instances of distant metastases of the sarcomatous component of the disease. Presently, controversy exists as to whether carcinosarcomas represent the collision of two distinct primary tumors or a single tumor derived from a pluripotential cell that undergoes sarcomatous and carcinomatous differentiation. Results of tumor tissue immunostaining studies appear to favor the latter hypothesized mechanism.

Carcinosarcomas more commonly present in men in their fifth to seventh decades of life. A strong association with smoking has been observed. Presenting symptoms depend on whether the tumor occurs as a central or peripheral lesion. Central, endobronchial polypoid tumors initiate symptoms of airway obstruction with cough, postobstructive pneumonitis, hemoptysis, and dyspnea. Peripheral tumors undergo progressive enlargement until patients experience chest pain from pleural invasion or symptoms related to distant metastases. Rare reports exist of hypertrophic osteodystrophy and extensive pleural involvement that simulates a malignant mesothelioma.

No distinctive radiographic features suggest the diagnosis of carcinosarcoma. As with other primary lung cancers, carcinosarcomas occur more commonly in the upper lung zones, and endobronchial sites of involvement cause radiographic features similar to other airway tumors. Peripheral carcinosarcomas typically present as circumscribed masses 2–8.5 cm in diameter with occasional involvement of the pleura or radiographic evidence of cavitation. Hilar or mediastinal lymphadenopathy is commonly present.

An accurate preoperative diagnosis is rarely made because of the difficulty in sampling both histologic components of the tumor. Furthermore, the tumor necrosis that carcinosarcomas commonly undergo makes attempts at percutaneous needle or transbronchial biopsy techniques unrewarding. Classification of the tumor as a carcinosarcoma requires careful immunostaining often supplemented by electron microscopy of surgical specimens.

Patients with carcinosarcomas have a poor prognosis. The median duration of survival after diagnosis is 6 months, with 6% of patients surviving 5 years. Patients with central compared to peripheral tumors have a more favorable prognosis most likely because they present earlier in the course of the disease. The carcinomatous component of the tumor tends to metastasize to regional lymph nodes. The sarcomatous component eventually undergoes distant metastasis in up to 40% of patients.

Because of the aggressive nature of the tumor, patients should be considered for curative resection whenever possible, although extension to regional lymph nodes portends a poor surgical result. The small patient series reported to date do not allow conclusions about the value of adjuvant radiation therapy or systemic chemotherapy for patients with unresectable disease.

The present patient's resected tumor had pathologic features of a pleomorphic neoplasm with the immunostaining characteristics of a carcinosarcoma. She recovered from thoracotomy but was found to have extensive pelvic metastases. Chemotherapy was initiated, but the patient followed a progressive downhill course and expired 3 months later.

Clinical Pearls

1. Carcinosarcomas represent less than 0.3% of all primary lung cancers and contain distinct components of carcinomatous and sarcomatous cellular differentiation.

2. It is still unclear whether carcinosarcomas arise from the collision of two distinct tumors or from sarcomatous and carcinomatous differentiation of a single pluripotential malignant cell.

3. Carcinosarcomas are aggressive tumors that metastasize in two patterns; the carcinomatous component spreads to regional lymph nodes, and the sarcomatous component undergoes widespread metastasis.

REFERENCES

1. Humphrey PA, Scroggs MW, Roggli VL, Shelburne JD. Pulmonary carcinomas with a sarcomatoid element: an immunocytochemical and ultrastructural analysis. Hum Pathol 1988;19:155–165.
2. Cupples J, Wright J. An immunohistological comparison of primary lung carcinosarcoma and sarcoma. Pathol Res Pract 1990;186:326–329.
3. Sümmermann E, Huwer H, Seitz G. Carcinosarcoma of the lung, a tumour which has a poor prognosis and is extremely rarely diagnosed. Thorac Cardiovasc Surg 1990;38:247–250.
4. Engel AF, Groot G, Bellot S. Carcinosarcoma of the lung. A case-history of disseminated disease and review of the literature. Eur J Surg Oncol 1991;17:94–96.
5. Miller DL, Allen MS. Rare pulmomary neoplasms. Mayo Clin Proc 1993;68:492–498.

PATIENT 22

An asymptomatic 70-year-old man with a calcified pleural mass

A 70-year-old man with a long smoking history was referred for evaluation of a left pleural mass noted on a routine chest radiograph. He was otherwise well, denying any pulmonary or systemic symptoms. The patient did report a 2- to 3-month exposure to asbestos approximately 40 years earlier.

Physical Examination: Temperature 98.4°; pulse 74; respirations 20; blood pressure 132/76. General: healthy appearing. Chest: decreased breath sounds, dullness to percussion, and decreased fremitus over the left lateral chest.

Laboratory Findings: CBC: normal. Electrolytes and renal indices: normal, total protein: 7.1 g/dl, LDH 144 IU/L. Chest radiograph (below top): large, left calcified pleural density with overlying rib thickening. Chest CT (below bottom): fluid collection within a thick, fibrocalcific rind and overlying rib enlargement.

Question: What is the most likely cause of the pleural effusion?

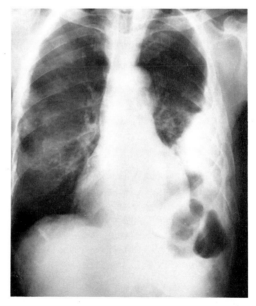

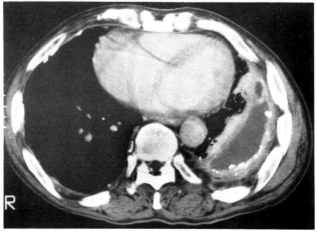

Diagnosis: Chronic tuberculous empyema.

Discussion: Tuberculous pleurisy is a relatively common manifestation of tuberculosis, occurring in 5% of patients with active disease. Most patients with pleural involvement present with pleural effusions that follow a self-limited course, resolving with or without treatment over 6–16 weeks. After recovery, the chest radiograph usually reveals a normal pleural space or minimal pleural thickening.

Rarely, primary tuberculous effusions fail to resolve and progress to a chronic suppurative form of infection termed tuberculous empyema. During the prechemotherapy era, tuberculous empyemas occurred with much greater frequency often in association with trapped lungs secondary to therapeutic pneumothoraces. In some patients, tuberculous empyemas may initiate marked pleural thickening that virtually isolates the tubercle bacilli and the inflammatory response within the pleural space. Consequently, patients with chronic tuberculous empyema may remain relatively asymptomatic for years. Patients may come to clinical attention because of a routine chest radiograph or the development of complications, such as a bronchopleural fistula or empyema necessitans. The onset of a bronchopleural fistula is a particularly important complication in that it allows tubercle bacilli from the empyema to mix with respiratory secretions and converts the patient to an infectious state.

Today, tuberculous empyema occurs most commonly in the setting of inadequate medical therapy. The markedly thickened and calcified pleura surrounding the cavity of tuberculous empyema presents a barrier to the intrapleural penetration of antituberculous drugs. Inadequate drug concentrations in regions of actively dividing tuberculous bacilli promote the emergence of resistant organisms. Although drug concentrations have not been measured in tuberculous empyema fluid, reports exist of treatment failures and conversion to resistant strains in patients treated with adequate chemotherapeutic regimens. These observations stress the importance of initiating therapy with a four-drug regimen using maximum tolerated doses and close monitoring of the clinical response, including serial cultures of infected fluids and drug susceptibility testing.

Examination of pleural fluid establishes the diagnosis of tuberculous empyema by revealing grossly purulent fluid that is smear positive for acid-fast bacilli and subsequently cultures *Mycobacterium tuberculosis.* Tuberculous empyemas usually have nucleated cell counts greater than $100,000/\mu l$ with a neutrophil predominance (usually $> 95\%$). The pleural fluid is usually acidotic (< 7.20) with a low glucose concentration (< 20 mg/dl). The pleural fluid protein concentration is greater than 5 g/dl and the LDH is greater than 1000 IU/L. The CT scan reveals a thick, calcified pleural rind often associated with overlying rib thickening, both of which suggest the presence of a "chronic active" tuberculous empyema.

In addition to chemotherapy, patients require pleural space drainage. Virtually all patients have a trapped lung that complicates lung reexpansion. Repeated thoracenteses until the empyema fluid converts to a sterile pleural exudate during a course of antituberculous chemotherapy is a therapeutic option in some patients. Empyemectomy and decortication should be considered in patients who are acceptable surgical candidates, who fail medical therapy, or have a symptomatic trapped lung.

The present patient underwent a large-volume thoracentesis that returned purulent material positive on stain and culture for *M. tuberculosis.* He was treated with isoniazid, rifampin, pyrazinamide, and ethambutol.

Clinical Pearls

1. Chronic tuberculous empyema may develop as a manifestation of untreated or inadequately treated tuberculosis and be present for years without causing symptoms.

2. Findings on a routine chest radiograph or the development of a bronchopleural fistula or empyema necessitans usually brings the patient to clinical attention.

3. The diagnosis of chronic tuberculous empyema should be suggested by a thick, calcific pleural rind and rib thickening on chest CT. The diagnosis is established by aspirating pus from the pleural space that is smear and culture positive for acid-fast bacilli.

4. A four-drug regimen using maximum doses combined with pleural space drainage (repeat thoracenteses or empyemectomy and decortication) is necessary for adequate resolution.

REFERENCES

1. Hulnick DH, Naidich DP, McCauley DI. Pleural tuberculosis evaluation by computed tomography. Radiology 1983;149:759–765.
2. Niehart RE, Hof DG. Successful nonsurgical treatment of tuberculous empyema in an irreducible pleural space. Chest 1985;88:792–794.
3. Iseman MD, Madsen LA. Chronic tuberculous empyema with bronchopleural fistula resulting in treatment failure and progressive drug resistance. Chest 1991;100:124–127.
4. Gotfried MH. An asymptomatic pleural mass in a 72-year-old man. Chest 1994;106:572–574.

PATIENT 23

A 72-year-old woman with a left lower lung zone mass

A 72-year-old woman with a known history of carcinoma of the breast was admitted for evaluation of substernal chest pain that had begun 2 hours earlier. The pain radiated to her left shoulder and was associated with mild shortness of breath and nausea. In the emergency department, intravenous morphine improved her symptoms.

Physical Examination: Temperature 98°; pulse 110; respirations 18; blood pressure 150/92. General: no acute distress. Skin: normal. Lymph nodes: few shotty left anterior cervical nodes. Chest: few basilar crackles. Cardiac: grade II/VI systolic ejection murmur. Abdomen: normal bowel sounds.

Laboratory Findings: Hct 36%; WBC 5,600/μl. ECG: ischemic ST changes in lateral precordial leads. Chest radiographs: left lower lung zone mass (arrows).

Questions: What test would most rapidly give a specific diagnosis for the intrathoracic mass?

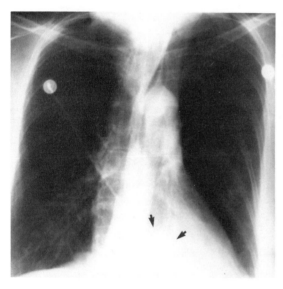 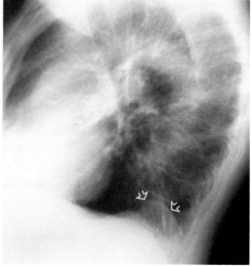

Answer: A CT scan demonstrated the pathognomonic features of a small asymptomatic Bochdalek hernia.

Discussion: Bochdalek hernias occur in the posterior-medial thorax in up to 1 in 2500 live births and result from embryologic abnormalities of diaphragmatic development. Initially, the embryo has a single pleuroperitoneal cavity that is divided within the seventh to eighth weeks of intrauterine life by formation of the membranous and muscular portions of the diaphragm. These diaphragmatic leafs undergo fusion that is occasionally incomplete in the region of the pleuroperitoneal canal. A Bochdalek hernia forms through this transdiaphragmatic defect when complete closure of the canal fails to occur.

Neonates with Bochdalek hernias commonly present with signs and symptoms of respiratory distress when large intrathoracic herniations of abdominal viscera and omentum cause ipsilateral lung compression near the time of birth. In some instances, persons with small herniations remain asymptomatic and present later in life. The impression regarding the prevalence of adult Bochdalek hernias has undergone recent revision with the availability of thoracic CT scanning. Analysis of CT scans obtained for various indications determine that up to 6% of patients have asymptomatic Bochdalek hernias, which is a prevalence 100-fold greater than previously thought.

Bochdalek hernias in adults are most commonly detected as incidental findings on posteroanterior or lateral chest radiographs. The hernia appears as a focal, smooth bulge 4–5 cm anterior to the posterior diaphragmatic insertion. It was previously considered that Bochdalek hernias occur nine times more commonly in the left diaphragm.

Recent patient series using CT scanning, however, indicate that Bochdalek hernias have only a twofold left-sided predominance. Symptomatic patients most often present with gastrointestinal complaints when incarcerated loops of herniated bowel undergo partial obstruction or intrathoracic strangulation. Rare reports exist of patients with strangulated colons that perforate and present as pyopneumothoraces.

The differential diagnosis of a radiographically apparent Bochdalek hernia includes a diaphragmatic eventration, a pleural-based pulmonary mass, supradiaphragmatic fat, and an intrathoracic lipoma. A chest CT scan can confirm the diagnosis and avoid additional diagnostic studies by demonstrating the diaphragmatic defect and the low density of the hernia, which usually contains fat. The pathognomonic CT features of a Bochdalek hernia include a rounded mass on the posteromedial aspect of the hemidiaphragm that has a low attenuation coefficient. The diaphragmatic musculature is discontinuous adjacent to the hernia and assumes a V-shaped configuration around the diaphragmatic defect. The hernia is observed to extend continuously from the peritoneal cavity to the intrathoracic space. Occasionally, the relationship between the diaphragm and Bochdalek hernia is difficult to discern, wherein thoracic MR imaging can confirm the diagnosis.

The present patient improved with medical management of her myocardial ischemia. A CT scan demonstrated the characteristic features of a Bochdalek hernia that required no further care.

Clinical Pearls

1. Neonates with Bochdalek hernias present with respiratory symptoms caused by compression of the ipsilateral lung from herniated abdominal viscera and omentum.

2. Up to 6% of patients evaluated for various complaints with chest CT scans have radiographic evidence of Bochdalek hernias.

3. Bochdalek hernias occur most commonly in the left hemithorax 4–5 cm anterior to the posterior diaphragmatic insertion.

4. Bochdalek hernias contain fat and appear as low-density masses. The CT scan confirms the diagnosis by demonstrating a discontinuous diaphragm in the region of the hernia defect and continuous extension of intraabdominal structures from the peritoneal cavity to the intrathoracic space.

REFERENCES

1. Gale ME. Bochdalek hernia: prevalence and CT characteristics. Radiology 1985;156:449–452.
2. Shin MS, Mulligan SA, Baxley WA, HO K-J. Bochdalek hernia of diaphragm in the adult: diagnosis by computed tomography. Chest 1987;92:1098–1101.
3. Sinha M, Gibbons P, Kennedy SC, Matthews HR. Colopleural fistula due to strangulated Bochdalek hernia in an adult. Thorax 1989;44:762–763.
4. Brooks AP, McLean A, Reznek RH. Diaphragmatic (Bochdalek) hernias simulating pulmonary metastases on computed tomography. Clin Radiol 1990;42:102–104.
5. Uchino A, Yoshida N, Ohnari N, Ohno M. Asymptomatic Bochdalek hernia diagnosed by magnetic resonance imaging. Radiat Med 1990;8:58–60.

PATIENT 24

A 67-year-old man with a left-sided chest mass

A 67-year-old man undergoing a routine health evaluation felt well except for a several-year history of intermittent epigastric pain occasionally associated with nausea and vomiting. He had a history of coronary artery disease, atrial fibrillation, and a gunshot wound in World War II.

Physical Examination: Vital signs: normal. Chest: well-healed scar in left lower thoracic cage. Cardiac: normal. Abdomen: normal.

Laboratory Findings: Chest radiograph: below left. CT scan: below right.

Question: What diagnosis would explain the abnormality on the chest radiograph and the patient's intermittent symptoms?

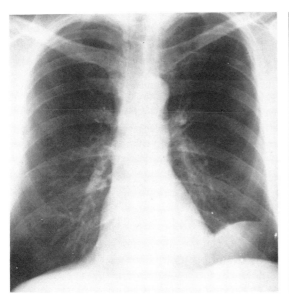 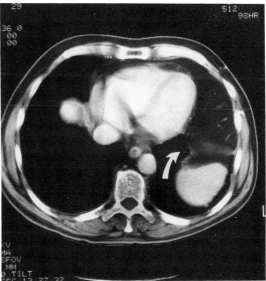

Diagnosis: Traumatic diaphragmatic hernia.

Discussion: Diaphragmatic hernias, defined as the transdiaphragmatic evisceration of abdominal contents into the thorax, can occur from either a congenital or acquired diaphragmatic defect. The vast majority of acquired defects result from blunt abdominal trauma or penetrating injuries to the diaphragm caused by gunshot or stab wounds. Motor vehicle accidents are the most common cause of blunt trauma resulting in diaphragmatic hernias, although other causes, such as falls or sporting injuries, have also been reported. In these conditions, a sudden increase in the pleuroperitoneal pressure gradient ruptures the diaphragm at points of potential weakness where embryologic fusion of the diaphragmatic membranes occur. This "explosive" mechanism of injury results in a larger diaphragmatic defect in patients with diaphragmatic hernias caused by blunt trauma in contrast to penetrating injuries. The association with trauma also explains why acquired diaphragmatic hernias are more common in men than women and have a peak incidence of 35 years, when men are at greatest risk for traumatic injuries.

Diaphragm rupture should be considered in any patient who sustains a penetrating injury to the thoracoabdominal region below the fourth thoracic rib anteriorly and above the umbilicus. It also should be suspected in patients with severe blunt trauma who require surgical exploration for visceral injury. From 3–8% of such patients will be found to have diaphragmatic hernias. Because the liver may buttress the right diaphragm, left diaphragm rupture occurs more frequently in patients with blunt trauma.

Once rupture has developed, the omentum may bulge through the muscular rent and prevent primary diaphragmatic closure. Negative intrapleural pressure promotes further ascent of intraabdominal organs into the thorax. This progressive transdiaphragmatic herniation can occur immediately after the initial injury (described as "early" herniation) or weeks, months, or even years after the traumatic event ("late" herniation). Transdiaphragmatic hernias may not become apparent in trauma patients requiring positive pressure ventilation until extubation, when inspiratory intrapleural pressure again becomes negative.

The associated injuries typically define the clinical presentation of the patient with trauma sufficiently severe to cause early diaphragmatic injury. These patients commonly sustain injuries to the spleen, liver, long bones, pelvis, and head. Patients with late diaphragmatic herniation usually present with signs and symptoms of intestinal obstruction or strangulation. The liver is the most common organ to herniate through the right diaphragm; the stomach, colon, small bowel, and spleen herniate most frequently on the left. Symptoms and signs of late diaphragmatic herniation include respiratory distress and dullness to percussion with decreased breath sounds and audible bowel sounds over the chest.

The chest radiograph may suggest the diagnosis. Helpful radiologic findings include: (1) a curvilinear visceral shadow mimicking an abnormally high diaphragm; (2) contralateral shift of the heart and mediastinum; (3) atelectasis in the lung superior to the "elevated" hemidiaphragm; (4) fracture of lower ribs; and (5) gastric or colon gas markings extending above the normal level of the diaphragm. A nasogastric tube projecting above the level of the diaphragm is also suggestive. Contrast studies of the upper or lower gastrointestinal tract are confirmatory. Other imaging techniques that assist in the diagnosis include computed tomography, magnetic resonance imaging, and liver scans showing a thoracic position of liver. Discovery in the thorax of peritoneal lavage fluid or air from a diagnostic pneumoperitoneum is confirmatory. Laparoscopy and thoracoscopy have also been used with success.

Recognition and surgical correction of traumatic diaphragmatic rupture are imperative. The surgical approach (abdominal or thoracic) for repair in early rupture is partly dictated by other visceral injuries. In the late setting, the thoracic approach is preferred, as adhesions between the eviscerated structures and the thoracic contents are usually present.

The present patient's chest radiograph demonstrated an opacity in the left base that silhouetted the apex of the heart; bullet fragments overlying the region of the left hemidiaphragm were also apparent. CT showed eventration of omental fat (curved arrow, previous page). Thoracotomy revealed an 8-cm omental mass herniating through a 2-cm left diaphragm defect, incurred by the gunshot wound the patient received in World War II. The hernia was reduced and the patient has done well without further abdominal complaints.

Clinical Pearls

1. In early traumatic diaphragmatic herniation, a high index of suspicion is necessary because the clinical presentation is manifested predominantly by the associated organ injuries.

2. The positive intrapleural pressure associated with mechanical ventilation may delay herniation of abdominal organs in patients with diaphragmatic rupture.

3. A patient who presents with symptoms and signs of intestinal obstruction or strangulation should be questioned about remote trauma because diaphragmatic herniation may occur years after injury.

4. Because the liver may buttress the right diaphragm, massive herniation on the right is less common.

5. Recognition and surgical correction of traumatic diaphragmatic rupture are imperative.

REFERENCES

1. Johnson CD. Blunt injuries of the diaphragm. Br J Surg 1988;75:226–230.
2. Gelman R, Mirvis SE, Gens D. Diaphragmatic rupture due to blunt trauma: sensitivity of plain chest radiographs. AJR 1991;156:51–57.
3. Maddox PR, Mansel RE, Butchart EG. Traumatic rupture of the diaphragm: a difficult diagnosis. Injury 1991;22:299–302.

PATIENT 25

A 62-year-old man with respiratory failure and a bronchopleural fistula

A 62-year-old man presented with fever, weight loss, and cough productive of yellow sputum. Six months earlier he had undergone right upper lobectomy because of squamous cell carcinoma. His postoperative course was complicated by a persistent bronchopleural fistula that eventually resolved after 2 weeks of chest tube drainage.

Physical Examination: Temperature 38°C; pulse 95/min; respirations 20/min; blood pressure 120/75 mmHg. Chest: dullness and decreased breath sounds over posterior right upper chest. Cardiac: normal. Abdomen: normal bowel sounds.

Laboratory Findings: WBC 15,000/μl; Hct 31%; electrolytes, creatinine, and liver function tests: normal. ABG (RA): pH 7.36; PCO_2 37 mmHg; PO_2 76 mmHg. Pulmonary function studies: FEV_1 = 3.2 L; FVC = 4.0 L; $FEV_1\%$ = 80%. Chest radiograph (below left): loculated pleural effusion with air-fluid levels in the right apical lung zone.

Course: The clinical presentation suggested a persistent postoperative bronchopleural fistula with a loculated empyema. After thoracentesis confirmed the presence of pus, the patient underwent a limited thoracotomy with open drainage, chest tube placement, and thoracoplasty for obliteration of the empyema space. One day after surgery, while still intubated, the patient developed a left-sided infiltrate (below right), marked subcutaneous emphysema, and a chest tube air leak. Severe hypoxemia (PO_2 = 49 mmHg on F_iO_2 100%) was managed by the addition of increasing levels of PEEP to 15 cm H_2O, which was associated with worsening hypoxemia and an increasing chest tube air leak.

Question: What approach to mechanical ventilation might improve gas exchange in this patient?

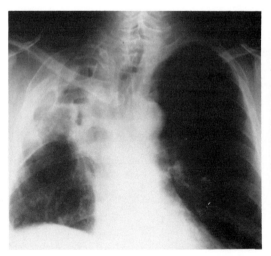
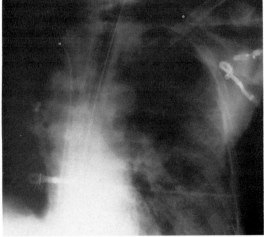

Answer: Intubation with a double-lumen endotracheal tube and independent lung ventilation.

Discussion: Positive pressure ventilation with the addition of positive end-expiratory pressure (PEEP) improves oxygenation in the majority of patients with bilateral diffuse lung disease through the recruitment of collapsed or partially inflated alveolar structures. Patients with predominantly unilateral lung disease, however, usually do not benefit from positive airway pressure and may actually experience worsening of gas exchange with PEEP. Regional inequalities in pulmonary time constants underlie this paradoxical response.

Regional time constants are a function of lung compliance and airway resistance. Simply stated, mechanically applied positive pressure tidal volumes follow intrapulmonary paths of least resistance, seeking airways with low resistance and alveoli with high compliance. In unilateral lung disease, the preferential route of a ventilator-supplied breath is to the normal, unrestricted lung. Similarly, application of PEEP primarily affects regions with high compliance, causing alveolar overdistention and pulmonary microvascular compression in the normal lung, thereby diverting blood flow to the diseased lung, which has the higher intrapulmonary shunt. The resultant imbalance of ventilation and perfusion aggravates hypoxemia and risks barotrauma to the normal lung if progressively higher levels of PEEP are applied.

Ventilatory support of patients with unilateral lung disease is further complicated by the presence of a large bronchopleural fistula contralateral to the diseased lung. As exemplified by the present patient, application of increasing levels of PEEP intensifies the chest tube air leak, thereby preventing recruitment of collapsed alveolar units in the lung with the increased shunt.

Independent lung ventilation with dual ventilators provides a therapeutic approach for improving oxygenation in patients with profound respiratory failure from asymmetric lung disease. Airway cannulation with a double-lumen endotracheal tube isolates the right and left airways and allows application of tailored tidal volumes and levels of PEEP uniquely appropriate for the differing functional characteristics of each lung. Although anecdotal reports establish that this form of ventilation can correct severe hypoxemia in this clinical setting, improved patient outcome requires a complete understanding of both double-lumen endotracheal tubes and dual ventilator management.

Constructed of polyvinyl chloride, double-lumen endotracheal tubes have a distal "bronchial" port and a proximal "tracheal" port with a soft cuff above each opening. Insertion of a left-sided tube into the left mainstem bronchus allows ventilation of the left lung through the bronchial lumen and the right lung through the tracheal lumen, with lung isolation provided by inflation of the double cuffs. Although right-sided, double-lumen endotracheal tubes are available for patients unable to undergo cannulation of the left mainstem bronchus, their use is complicated by the proximity of the right upper lobe orifice to the bronchial cuff, which frequently causes right upper lobe atelectasis.

Proper placement of double-lumen endotracheal tubes requires careful attention to technique. An appropriately sized tube—usually a 39 French for women and 41 French for men—is advanced through the glottis with the curved tip positioned anteriorly. The tube is rotated 90° toward the bronchus to be intubated as the tip approaches the carina. Once mild resistance is met, the bronchial and tracheal cuffs are inflated and position checked by auscultation. When properly placed, alternating ventilation through the bronchial or tracheal ports produces isolated left-sided or right-sided breath sounds, respectively. Difficult instances of airway placement can be aided with the fiberoptic bronchoscope.

Complications of double-lumen endotracheal tubes include airway trauma during difficult intubations and inadequate ventilation or barotrauma resulting from initial tube misplacement or subsequent malposition through tube migration. Rupture of the bronchus or distal trachea can occur from overinflation of either cuff. Long-term patient management is complicated by the small caliber of the tube lumens, which impedes adequate airway suctioning. This small caliber furthermore promotes intrinsic PEEP in patients with high minute ventilations because of the increased resistance presented for expiratory flow.

No established guidelines exist for initiating ventilatory parameters in patients undergoing independent lung ventilation. Ventilators are often linked electronically to provide synchronized rates, although asynchronous ventilation works equally as well. Synchronization, however, simplifies interpretation of pulmonary artery catheter waveforms and cardiac output data.

Overlying objectives to independent lung ventilation include equalization of the mechanical differences in compliance and functional residual capacity between the two lungs to prevent disadvantageous shifts of pulmonary blood flow. These goals require application of varying tidal volumes and levels of PEEP to each lung guided by overall gas exchange in addition to individual peak airway pressures and compliance curves. In unilateral lung disease with hypoxia complicated by contralateral bronchopleural fistulas, application of PEEP to the high-shunt lung may sufficiently improve overall oxygenation and elimination of carbon dioxide to allow lower tidal volumes and airway pressures in the lung with the air leak. Novel approaches employing double-lumen endotracheal tubes include high-frequency ventilation to the lung with a bronchopleural fistula combined with contralateral conventional ventilation.

The present patient was intubated with a left-sided, double-lumen endotracheal tube to allow synchronous independent lung ventilation. Application of 15 cm H_2O PEEP with a tidal volume of 500 ml to the left lung and a tidal volume of 300 ml without PEEP to the right lung improved gas exchange and decreased the degree of chest tube air leak. The patient's condition worsened, with a severe left-sided pneumonia that eventually involved the right lung, and he died 7 days later.

Clinical Pearls

1. Left-sided, double-lumen endotracheal tubes are preferred over right-sided tubes for independent lung ventilation because of a lower risk of right upper lobe obstruction.

2. Patients ventilated with double-lumen endotracheal tubes require monitoring for intrinsic PEEP because of the increased resistance to expiratory air flow imparted by the tube's narrow internal dimensions.

3. Independent lung ventilation can be provided with or without synchronization of dual ventilators; synchronous ventilation, however, simplifies interpretation of pulmonary artery catheter data.

REFERENCES

1. Powner SD, Eross B, Grenvik A. Differential lung ventilation with PEEP in the treatment of unilateral pneumonia. Crit Care Med 1977;5:170–172.
2. Benjaminsson E, Klain M. Intraoperative dual-mode independent lung ventilation of a patient with bronchopleural fistula. Anesth Analg 1981;60:118–119.
3. Baumann MH, Sahn SA. Medical management and therapy of bronchopleural fistulas in the mechanically ventilated patient. Chest 1990;97:721–728.

PATIENT 26

A 68-year-old man with a 3-month history of right chest pain

A 68-year-old man presented with right-sided, dull chest pain that had become progressively more severe during the previous 3 months. The patient noted dyspnea with exertion and increasing fatigue. He had been well except for mild hypertension controlled for the past 10 years with a beta blocker. He retired from the insurance business at age 62. He had smoked cigarettes for 20 years but quit 18 years earlier.

Physical Examination: Temperature 99° F; pulse 96, respirations 28; blood pressure 140/80. General: thin, appeared chronically ill. Chest: decreased expansion, dull percussion, decreased fremitus, and decreased breath sounds on right.

Laboratory Findings: Hct 35%; WBC 9200/μl. Electrolytes and renal indices: normal, liver function tests: normal. Chest radiograph: below left. Pleural fluid analysis: below right.

Question: What is the most likely cause of the patient's chest pain?

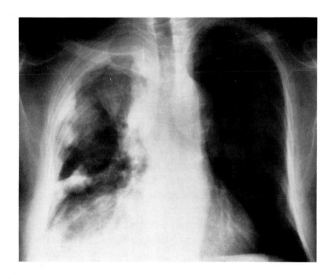

Pleural Fluid Analysis

Appearance: serosanguinous

Nucleated cells: 4500/μl

Differential:
  20% PMNs
  40% mononuclear cells
  40% lymphocytes

RBC: 8000/μl

Protein: 4.2 gm/dl (serum 6.8 gm/dl)

LDH: 600 IU/L (serum 200 IU/L)

Glucose: 45 mg/dl (serum 110 mg/dl)

pH: 7.20 (7.43)

Amylase: 70 IU/L (serum 130 IU/L)

Cytology: negative

Smears: Gram, KOH, and AFB: negative

Cultures: negative

Diagnosis: Diffuse malignant mesothelioma.

Discussion: The presence of a mononuclear predominant, low glucose, low pH pleural effusion presents a limited differential diagnosis that includes pleural malignancy, tuberculous pleurisy, or rheumatoid pleurisy. The absence of arthritis makes rheumatoid pleurisy unlikely, considering that only 6% of patients develop pleural effusions before the onset of articular manifestations of the disease. Chronic unremitting chest pain, dyspnea, and cough further limit the differential diagnosis in that these symptoms are not prominent features of tuberculous pleurisy. Additionally, most patients with tuberculous pleural effusions have pleural fluid lymphocytosis in the range of 90 to 95%, and pleural fluid acidosis is observed in only 20% of patients. The combination of a low pleural fluid pH, glucose, and mononuclear cell predominance in an elderly patient with unremitting dull chest pain suggests the diagnosis of pleural malignancy and, more specifically, diffuse malignant mesothelioma.

Patients with malignant mesothelioma virtually always present with symptoms, the most common being chest pain and dyspnea. In contrast, up to 25% of patients with carcinomatous and lymphomatous pleural metastases may be asymptomatic at the time of diagnosis. Chest pain is the presenting complaint in only 25% of patients with carcinoma of the pleura. Furthermore, pleural effusions with a low pH and low glucose occur in only 30% of patients with pleural carcinomatosis compared to 60% of patients with mesotheliomas. A low pH and glucose predict a worse prognosis in mesothelioma as well as in carcinoma of the pleura.

The radiographic findings of a large pleural effusion and nodular pleural densities without contralateral mediastinal shift suggest the diagnosis of mesothelioma. The absence of contralateral shift results from the spreading nature of the tumor that encases the lung, creating a restrictive abnormality, and invades the hilum, producing bronchial obstruction and atelectasis.

Pleural effusions tend to occur early in the course of mesothelioma, are unilateral, more common on the right, and moderate to large in volume; however, effusions can be massive and bilateral. As the disease progresses, the fluid becomes reabsorbed or organized and the mediastinum shifts ipsilaterally. Multiple pleural adhesions have been noted in some patients. The effusion may be serous or bloody and is always exudative, in contrast to carcinoma and lymphoma, in which the effusion may be transudative early in the course of the disease in 3–19% of patients. The high incidence of pleural effusions with a low pH and low glucose in mesothelioma is explained by the extensive tumor bulk of the pleura that impairs glucose transfer into and hydrogen ion efflux from the pleural space.

The association of asbestos exposure and diffuse malignant mesothelioma was originally proposed by Wagner in South Africa in 1960 and later substantiated by others. The relationship of the level of asbestos exposure to the risk of mesothelioma has not been established, but such risk is not as closely related to dose as it is for pulmonary fibrosis (asbestosis) and asbestos-related lung cancer. No relationship exists to cigarette smoking. Asbestos exposure is the most important risk factor for malignant mesothelioma, but chronic inflammation and other minerals, such as erionite, have rarely been implicated. In as many as 20–30% of patients, no definite asbestos exposure can be confirmed.

A substantial quantity of tissue is necessary for diagnosis, usually obtained at thoracoscopy or open biopsy. Histochemistry, immunochemistry, and ultrastructural studies often are needed to differentiate malignant mesothelioma from metastatic adenocarcinoma.

No treatment has proven efficacy for prolonging survival in patients with diffuse malignant mesothelioma. Palliation may be achieved with chemical pleurodesis or tumor debulking and pleurectomy in those with symptomatic pleural effusions.

In the present patient, a history of asbestos exposure could not be elicited. The diagnosis was confirmed at thoracoscopy. He died 9 months following diagnosis after receiving supportive care only.

Clinical Pearls

1. Patients with mesothelioma are virtually always symptomatic at the time of diagnosis, with chest pain being the most common symptom.

2. Absence of contralateral mediastinal shift with a large effusion and pleural nodules on chest radiograph suggest the diagnosis.

3. Sixty percent of patients at the time of diagnosis of a diffuse malignant mesothelioma have a pleural effusion with a low pH and low glucose, a finding associated with a worse prognosis.

REFERENCES

1. Wagner JC, Sleggs CA, Marchand P. Diffuse pleural mesothelioma and asbestos exposure in northwestern Cape Province. Br J Ind Med 1960;260–271.
2. Taryle DA, Lakshminarayan S, Sahn SA. Pleural mesotheliomas: an analysis of 18 cases and review of the literature. Medicine 1976;55:153–162.
3. Alexander E, Clark RA, Colley DP, et al. CT of malignant pleural mesothelioma. Am J Roentgenol 1981;137:287–291.
4. Dewar A, Valente M, Ring NP, et al: Pleural mesothelioma of epithelial type and pulmonary adenocarcinoma: an ultrastructural and cytochemical comparison. J Pathol 1987;152:309–316.
5. Gottehrer A, Taryle DA, Reed CE, et al. Pleural fluid analysis in malignant mesothelioma: prognostic implications. Chest 1991;100:1003–1006.

PATIENT 27

A 58-year-old woman with bilateral nodular infiltrates

A 58-year-old woman presented with a 1-month history of progressive dyspnea and cough productive of yellowish sputum. Several months earlier, she was diagnosed by open lung biopsy as having bronchiolitis obliterans and organizing pneumonia, for which she was taking 60 mg of prednisone per day. At the onset of dyspnea 1 month earlier, the patient had undergone a negative evaluation of a localized left upper lobe infiltrate and was treated empirically with oral antibiotics.

Physical Examination: Temperature 100°; pulse 110; respirations 25; blood pressure 120/60. General: moderate respiratory distress; cushingoid appearance. Skin: no lesions. Fundi: normal. Chest: bilateral rales without pleural rubs. Cardiac: I/VI systolic murmur. Abdomen: obese without organomegaly.

Laboratory Findings: Hct 31%; WBC 13,500/μl with 90% granulocytes. Electrolytes and renal indices: normal. Sputum: 4+ polymorphonuclear cells; mixed bacteria that included gram-negative rods and branching gram-positive filamentous organisms. Chest radiograph: shown below.

Question: What condition is a likely cause of the patient's pulmonary infiltrates?

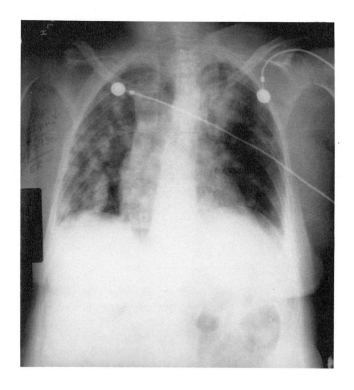

Diagnosis: Pulmonary nocardiosis.

Discussion: Nocardiosis is a suppurative infection that occurs most commonly in the lung but is associated with a high incidence of disseminated disease. Caused by an aerobic actinomycete found in soil, the vast majority of infections ocur with the species *Nocardia asteroides*, with less than 10% of disease resulting from *N. brasiliensis* or *N. caviae*.

Previously considered a rare disease, it is presently estimated that up to 500–1000 cases occur in the United States each year, with 85% of patients having serious pulmonary or systemic infections. Although 15% of patients have no clinically evident underlying disease, the most common predisposition for nocardiosis is an alteration of mechanical, cellular, or humoral immune defense mechanisms. Associated conditions include steroid and cytotoxic therapy, organ transplantation, solid and hematologic malignancies, alcoholism, chronic obstructive pulmonary disease, alveolar proteinosis, infection with human immunodeficiency virus, dysgammaglobulinemias, pancytopenias, and chronic granulomatous disease of childhood.

Most patients contract nocardial infections through inhalation, although inoculation of the skin can result in local cutaneous abscesses, and a gastrointestinal route has been suspected as a cause of disseminated disease. Once within the distal airways, *Nocardia* species undergo phagocytosis by alveolar macrophages, which cannot reliably kill the ingested intracellular pathogens. Eradication requires an inflammatory response with concerted activities of leukocytes, lymphocytes, and tissue macrophages. Failure of this response results in tissue necrosis, formation of poorly encapsulated abscesses that promote tissue spread of infection, and occasional granuloma formation. Despite its inhalational route of infection, person-to-person or animal-to-animal transmission has not been demonstrated, although some evidence suggests a nosocomial mode of spread.

As occurs with actinomycosis, there is an interesting predominance of males in most reported series. Most patients present with fever, cough with or without sputum production, pleuritic chest pain, and dyspnea with variable degrees of anorexia and weight loss. A slowly progressive, subacute clinical course may suggest the diagnoses of tuberculosis, a fungal infection, or neoplastic disease. Occasional patients with vascular erosion present with massive hemoptysis. The presence of an immunocompromising condition in a patient with progressive pulmonary infiltrates and abscess formation despite use of broad-spectrum antibiotics should suggest nocardiosis as a likely clinical diagnosis.

Pulmonary nocardiosis has an inclination to undergo hematogenous spread early in the course of the disease. Although any tissue may be involved, central nervous system, cutaneous, or other soft tissue sites of infection are common. Central nervous system nocardiosis involving the brain, meninges, and spinal cord accounts for 20–38% of disseminated disease. Patients may present with headache, lethargy, seizures, peripheral paresthesias, nuchal rigidity, confusion, or aphasia. Contiguous spread from the lung to the pleura, mediastinum, chest wall, or pericardium occurs less commonly than in patients with actinomycosis but can cause a thoracic empyema, superior vena cava syndrome, and purulent pericarditis.

Nocardiosis has a varying, nonspecific radiographic appearance. Classic manifestations include interstitial or alveolar infiltrates with or without associated pleural effusions. The infiltrates may not be confined to a segment or lobe and often assume the appearance of a well-defined, solid mass. Cavitary infiltrates or upper lobe disease mimicking classic pulmonary tuberculosis in an immunosuppressed host is suggestive of the disease. As in the present patient, multiple nodular infiltrates with or without cavitation also may occur. Patients with HIV infection commonly present with cavitary disease of the upper lobe.

The diagnosis of pulmonary nocardiosis often is confirmed by culture and examination of sputum specimens. *Nocardia* species appear in Gram stain preparations as branching gram-positive beaded filaments 0.5–1.0 microns in diameter. On modified Ziehl-Neelsen or Kinyoun stains, *Nocardia* appears weakly acid fast, which separates it from the bacteria that cause actinomycosis. Because *Nocardia* species may grown in 48 hours but often require 1–3 weeks, the microbiology laboratory must be alerted to the possible diagnosis so that culture plates will not be prematurely discarded. Negative sputum examinations indicate a need for bronchoscopy with bronchoalveolar lavage, transbronchial lung biopsy, percutaneous needle aspiration, or other invasive procedure. Cerebrospinal fluid and blood have a low yield for recovery of the organism. Tissue specimens require preparation with a Brown-Brenn modification of the Gram stain because hematoxylin and eosin or periodic acid–Schiff stains usually cannot demonstrate *Nocardia* infection.

Occasionally, *Nocardia* species are isolated from sputum samples in the absence of clinically evident disease. Because these pathogens are rarely commensals, immunocompromised patients with positive sputum cultures should receive therapy as if they had active disease. Patients without clinically evident predisposing conditions should undergo a careful evaluation to exclude clinically occult pulmonary or extrapulmonary sites of infection.

Sulfonamides are the agents of first choice for patients with pulmonary nocardiosis. Surgical adjunctive therapy may be required for drainage of empyemas and resection of extensive suppurative lung disease. Although no clinical data demonstrate any differences in outcome between the various sulfonamide drugs, combination therapy with trimethoprim-sulfamethoxazole (TMP-SMX) is now most commonly employed. Serum sulfa levels are maintained between 12 and 15 mg/dl, with some reduction in drug dose after 6 weeks or when clinical evidence of improvement occurs. Second-line drug regimens are reserved for patients—such as many of those with HIV disease—who cannot tolerate sulfonamide therapy. Limited experience exists with these secondary regimens, but in vitro sensitivity testing and sporadic reports indicate the potential value of cefuroxime, ceftriaxone, cefotaxime, amikacin, netilimicin, minocycline, imipenem, cycloserine, and some of the carboxyquinolones. Combination regimens using doxycycline and amikacin, imipenem and TMP/SMX, or imipenem and cefotaxime have been effective in scattered reports, but extensive experience with combination therapy is lacking.

Absolute recommendations for ideal therapeutic combinations in sulfonamide-intolerant patients cannot be made, and drug regimens should be guided by sensitivity testing. Although standardized susceptibility testing for *Nocardia* species is not available, the disk diffusion method correlates well with results from broth microdilution minimum inhibitory concentration (MIC) techniques. Results of susceptibility testing, however, are no guarantees of clinical response. Patients with major infections should be continued on antimicrobial therapy for 6–12 months. Lifelong maintenance therapy may be required in patients with ongoing immunocompromise. All patients should be evaluated by CT or MRI brain imaging to exclude clinically occult intracranial disease.

The present patient's sputum and blood were positive on culture for *Nocardia asteroides*. She was intubated and started on therapy with TMP-SMX. Ten days later, she was converted to erythromycin, amikacin, and imipenem after failing to respond to treatment. She subsequently developed multiorgan failure with sepsis and succumbed to the disease.

Clinical Pearls

1. Although pulmonary nocardiosis occurs primarily in patients with compromised mechanical, cellular, or humoral host defense mechanisms, up to 15% of patients have no clinically evident underlying disease.

2. Human-to-human transmission of nocardiosis has not been clearly demonstrated. Because epidemiologic data suggest the possibility of a nosocomial mode of spread, however, reasonable caution warrants separation of infected patients from others with immunocompromising conditions.

3. The presence of a classic upper lobe, cavitary infiltrate in a patient with HIV infection should suggest the possibility of nocardiosis.

4. *Nocardia* species isolated from sputum specimens should never be dismissed as commensals. Immunosuppressed patients should receive appropriate therapy, and nonimmunosuppressed, asymptomatic patients should undergo exclusion of clinically occult disease.

REFERENCES

1. Heffner JE. Pleuropulmonary manifestations of actinomycosis and nocardiosis. Semin Respir Dis 1988;3:352–361.
2. Wilson JP, Turner HR, Kirchner KA, Chapman SW. Nocardial infections in renal transplant recipients. Medicine 1989;68:38–57.
3. Berkey P, Bodey GP. Nocardial infection in patients with neoplastic disease. Rev Infect Dis 1989;2:407–412.
4. Conant EF, Wechsler RJ. Actinomycosis and nocardiosis of the lung. J Thorac Imaging 1992;7:75–84.

PATIENT 28

A 41-year-old Vietnamese woman with a solitary pulmonary nodule and a positive PPD

A 41-year-old woman presented for evaluation of a solitary pulmonary nodule. The nodule was noted on a chest radiograph obtained in the evaluation of a positive PPD (15-mm induration) during her recent immigration from Vietnam. The patient had no respiratory or constitutional complaints and denied ever having smoked cigarettes.

Physical Examination: Temperature 98.5° F; heart rate 68; respiratory rate 14; blood pressure 112/68. Lymph nodes: negative. Chest: clear. Cardiac: normal.

Laboratory Findings: Hemogram, electrolytes, and renal indices: normal. Liver function tests: normal. Urinalysis: normal. HIV test: negative. Chest radiograph (below top): 2-cm, well-circumscribed nodule in the left lower lobe behind the cardiac silhouette. Chest CT (below bottom): noncalcified nodule.

Question: What is the differential diagnosis? How should the patient be evaluated?

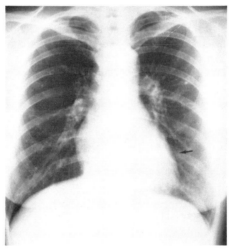

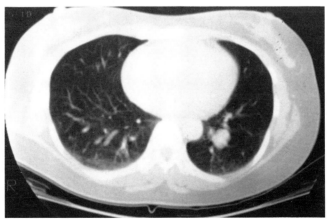

Diagnosis: Sclerosing hemangioma of the lung.

Discussion: Considering all of the solitary pulmonary nodules that undergo clinical evaluation, approximately 60% prove to be benign. Of the benign lesions, more than 80% are granulomas and 13% are hamartomas. The remaining etiologies of benign solitary pulmonary nodules include bronchogenic cysts, benign fibrous mesotheliomas, resolved pulmonary infarctions, rounded atelectasis, sclerosing hemangiomas, hyalinizing granulomas, pulmonary sequestrations, infestations by *Dirofilaria immitis,* echinococcal cysts, and arteriovenous malformations.

Sclerosing hemangioma of the lung is a benign neoplasm of undetermined origin that was first described by Leibow and Hubbell in 1956. Since that time, over 150 cases have been reported in the English literature. Described in patients ranging in age from 4 to 83 years, sclerosing hemangiomas occur predominantly in women (80%) in their fourth to seventh decades of life. Nodules are most often identified by screening chest radiographs because more than 75% of patients are asymptomatic. When symptoms do occur, hemoptysis is the most common presenting complaint and develops in 12% of patients. Massive hemoptysis, however, has not been reported in this condition. Cough (9% of patients), chest pain ($< 2\%$), fever ($< 1\%$), and fatigue ($< 1\%$) have also been reported in patients with sclerosing hemangiomas.

Sclerosing hemangiomas are usually solitary and peripheral but multiple lesions can occur in a unilateral or bilateral distribution. These tumors have been reported in all lobes with equal frequency. The lesion is slow growing and can be as large as 8 cm in diameter; however, over two-thirds of tumors are < 3 cm at the time of excision. Although doubling times of 660–1250 days have been noted, sclerosing hemangiomas have been reported to remain unchanged for as long as 5 years. After resection of single or multiple nodules, recurrence of the disease has not been reported.

Only a single report documents ipsilateral hilar node metastases.

Sclerosing hemangiomas appear as well-circumscribed, noncalcified nodules on routine chest radiographs and CT scans. Rarely, the nodule may demonstrate an air crescent sign. A single report describes enhancement of the nodule after intravenous infusion of contrast material. An accompanying pleural effusion has been reported in only one patient with a sclerosing hemangioma.

The diagnosis of sclerosing hemangioma most often requires resection and histologic examination of the nodule. Only a single report indicates that the diagnosis may be made by percutaneous thin needle aspiration. The pathologic specimen is remarkable for a sharply demarcated but nonencapsulated tumor that contains foci of hemorrhage. The gross specimen is firm to the touch. The four histologic patterns observed include solid, hemorrhagic, papillary and sclerotic. Although most tumors contain a mixed pattern of several histologic types, one pattern usually predominates. The presence of distinct round tumor cells within the stroma is a constant finding in all patterns. These cells are uniform and bland appearing, and contain round to oval nuclei with fine chromatin and inconspicuous nucleoli. Mitotic figures are rare. The tumor has been mistaken for carcinoid, hamartoma, bronchoalveolar cell carcinoma, and small cell carcinoma.

On the basis of the present patient's positive PPD, country of origin, and nonsmoking history, a tuberculous granuloma appeared to be the most likely diagnosis on clinical presentation. A percutaneous fine needle aspirate was obtained but was nondiagnostic; culture of the aspirate for tuberculosis and fungi was negative. The patient then underwent thoracoscopic wedge resection of the nodule that confirmed the diagnosis of a sclerosing hemangioma. She had an uncomplicated postoperative course and has demonstrated no evidence of tumor recurrence during 6 months of follow-up.

Clinical Pearls

1. Most solitary pulmonary nodules undergoing clinical evaluation are benign, and > 80% of benign lesions are due to granulomatous disease.

2. The most common nongranulomatous cause of benign lung nodules is hamartoma, which represents approximately 13% of benign lesions.

3. Sclerosing hemangioma most commonly presents as a small, solitary, peripheral, well-circumscribed lesion on a screening chest radiograph in an asymptomatic middle-aged woman.

4. The most common presenting symptom is hemoptysis, which occurs in only 12% of patients.

5. Sclerosing hemangioma of the lung is a benign, slow-growing tumor that requires surgical resection for diagnosis.

REFERENCES

1. Leibow AA, Hubbell DS. Sclerosing hemangioma (histiocytoma, xanthoma) of the lung. Cancer 1956;9:53–75.
2. Katzenstein ALA, Gmelich JT, Carrington CB. Sclerosing hemangioma of the lung: a clinicopathologic study of 51 cases. Am J Surg Pathol 1980;4:343–356.
3. Midthun DE, Swensen SJ, Jett JR. Approach to the solitary pulmonary nodule. Mayo Clin Proc 1993;68:378–385.

PATIENT 29

A 59-year-old man with respiratory failure after cardiac surgery

A 59-year-old man with mild chronic obstructive pulmonary disease and refractory ventricular arrhythmias developed left lower quadrant discomfort that progressed 2 days later to severe pain, rebound, and fever. A diverticular abscess was diagnosed and the patient underwent an uncomplicated laparotomy and partial colectomy. Eighteen hours after surgery, dyspnea was noted that rapidly progressed to severe hypoxemia, and the patient required intubation with mechanical ventilation. The patient's preoperative medications included occasional inhaled albuterol, digoxin, amiodarone, furosemide, and lorazepam.

Physical Examination: Temperature 102°; pulse 120; blood pressure 120/65; respirations 22. Chest: diffuse crackles. Cardiac: soft S4. Abdomen: surgical incision; minimal incisional tenderness; no bowel sounds.

Laboratory Findings: Hct 36%; WBC 12,000/μl with normal differential. Electrolytes and renal indices: normal. ABG (100% oxygen): pH 7.45; PCO$_2$ 32 mmHg; PO$_2$ 62 mmHg. Chest radiograph: shown below.

Question: What is a probable cause of the patient's respiratory failure?

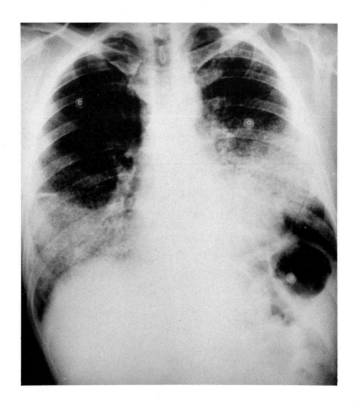

Diagnosis: Postoperative amiodarone pulmonary toxicity.

Discussion: Amiodarone is a triiodinated class III antiarrhythmic drug that is highly effective against otherwise refractory atrial and ventricular arrhythmias. First introduced as an antianginal agent, initial experience in Europe profiled amiodarone as a nearly ideal drug because of its high antiarrhythmic efficacy, once-daily dosing, and absence of negative inotropic effects. However, greater use of amiodarone in the United States with a higher dosing schedule of 400 mg/day subsequently brought to light serious adverse reactions, such as skin discoloration, corneal microdeposits, thyroid dysfunction, peripheral neuropathy, hepatic dysfunction, and pulmonary toxicity. Adverse pulmonary reactions are a particularly serious manifestation of amiodarone toxicity, occurring in 5–15% of treated patients. Once established, amiodarone pulmonary toxicity has a 5–10% rate of mortality.

Amiodarone pulmonary toxicity may be chronic or acute. Chronic toxicity is more common, presenting as a slow and insidious progression of dyspnea, cough, weight loss, and pulmonary infiltrates. The infiltrates are typically diffuse, bilateral interstitial or alveolar in nature, but one-third of patients may present with well-localized lobar, nodular, mass-like, or cavitary lesions. Pleural thickening may accompany the infiltrates but frank pleural effusions are rare. Lung biopsy specimens demonstrate interstitial fibrosis, focal areas of hemorrhage, and organizing pneumonia. Bronchoalveolar lavage (BAL) samples reveal foamy histiocytes that may represent alveolar macrophages or transformed type II pneumocytes laden with lamellated phospholipid inclusion bodies.

The acute form presents with the rapid onset of dyspnea, cough, hypoxemia, and occasional high fevers that may suggest an infectious condition such as bacterial pneumonia. In some instances, fulminant respiratory failure occurs with the clinical features of adult respiratory distress syndrome. The radiographic infiltrates have a more alveolar appearance compared with the chronic form of the disease.

Several reports exist of acute respiratory failure ascribed to amiodarone toxicity in patients who have undergone surgical procedures, such as insertion of an automatic internal cardiac defibrillator or myocardial resection for malignant arrhythmias. These patients initially do well in the early postoperative period but then experience the rapid onset of dyspnea, hypoxemia, and pulmonary infiltrates within 12–36 hours of surgery. Most patients with postoperative reactions to the drug have not experienced any evidence of amiodarone toxicity before surgery. No correlation appears to exist between the preoperative dose of the drug or duration of therapy and the risk of postoperative respiratory failure.

Although several theories exist regarding the pathogenesis of amiodarone pulmonary toxicity, exact mechanisms remain incompletely defined. Potential mechanisms include hypersensitivity reactions, direct toxicity from high lung tissue drug concentrations, impairment of phospholipase activity with excessive pulmonary phospholipid deposition, and generation of toxic oxygen metabolites. The last mechanism may be important in postoperative amiodarone toxicity in that high intraoperative inspired oxygen concentrations may be the triggering event for accelerating oxidant production and promoting injury to alveolar membranes. This theory is supported by recent reports of unilateral pulmonary edema in the lung exposed to high oxygen concentrations in amiodarone-treated patients who undergo surgery with single-lung ventilatory techniques. Several of the potential mechanisms for amiodarone toxicity may exist in that patients recovering from postoperative acute reactions have been later rechallenged with the drug without incurring the chronic form of the disease.

The diagnosis is one of exclusion in that no diagnostic clinical, radiographic, or pathologic features of the disease exist. Cellular constituents of BAL fluid are highly variable and insufficiently specific to make the diagnosis. Pathologic findings of lamellar bodies characteristic of amiodarone toxicity are not diagnostic because they occur in drug-treated patients even in the absence of pulmonary toxicity. The diagnosis can be supported by CT in patients with localized infiltrates by the demonstration of markedly increased radiographic densities within the infiltrate, which occur from high lung tissue concentrations of the iodinated compound.

Amiodarone should be discontinued or reduced in dosage in patients with clinical manifestations of pulmonary toxicity. Corticosteroids and plasmapheresis have been used with anecdotal success, but their role in amiodarone toxicity remains unclear. The risk of pulmonary reactions to amiodarone can be decreased by limiting the dose to less than 400 mg/day. Patients with advanced age, lower pretreatment measurements of lung diffusion (DLCO), and higher plasma concentrations of desethylamiodarone, an amiodarone metabolite, are at increased risk for pulmonary toxicity. Considering the potential for postoperative reactions, patients should be drug-free as long as possible preoperatively and informed about the risks of pulmonary toxicity. Patients with malignant ventricular arrhythmias who cannot be maintained preoperatively off of amiodarone should be managed with low inspired oxygen concentrations during surgery.

The present patient experienced progressive respiratory failure despite initiation of corticosteroid therapy and expired 5 days after surgery. Autopsy demonstrated characteristic pathologic features of amiodarone toxicity and no evidence of pulmonary infection or thromboembolic disease.

Clinical Pearls

1. Chronic amiodarone pulmonary toxicity has a varied radiographic appearance that includes diffuse interstitial or alveolar infiltrates and localized lobar, nodular, mass-like, or cavitary lesions.

2. Even in the absence of preoperative manifestations of pulmonary toxicity, patients treated with amiodarone are at increased risk for acute respiratory failure after surgical procedures.

3. The diagnosis of amiodarone pulmonary toxicity must be made by exclusion. Lung biopsy findings and the nature of BAL cellular constituents are not sufficiently specific to assist diagnosis.

4. Patients treated with amiodarone should be supported during surgery with the lowest concentration of inspired oxygen necessary to maintain adequate systemic oxygenation.

REFERENCES

1. Kuhlman JE, Teigen C, Ren H, et al. Amiodarone pulmonary toxicity: CT findings in symptomatic patients. Radiology 1990;177:121–125.
2. Pollak PT, Sharma AD, Carruthers SG. Relation of amiodarone hepatic and pulmonary toxicity to serum drug concentrations and superoxide dismutase activity. Am J Cardiol 1990;65:1185–1191.
3. Greenspon AJ, Kidwell GA, Hurley W, Mannion J. Amiodarone-related postoperative adult respiratory distress syndrome. Circulation 1991;84(Suppl III):III-407–III-415.
4. Herndon JC, Cook AO, Ramsay AE, et al. Postoperative unilateral pulmonary edema: possible amiodarone pulmonary toxicity. Anesthesiology 1992;76:308–312.
5. Ohar JA, Jackson F, Dettenmeier PA, et al. Bronchoalveolar lavage cell count and differential are not reliable indicators of amiodarone-induced pneumonitis. Chest 1992;102:999–1004.

PATIENT 30

A 49-year-old man with pulmonary embolism and an enlarging pleural effusion

A 49-year-old man presented with a painful and swollen left leg, dyspnea, right pleuritic chest pain, and hemoptysis. Two weeks earlier, a concrete block had fallen on his left leg, causing an extensive hematoma over his thigh.

Physical Examination: Temperature 100°F; pulse 100; respirations 32; blood pressure 130/80. Chest: dullness to percussion; decreased fremitus; and diminished breath sounds with scattered crackles over the right lung base. Cardiac: normal. Extremities: edema and erythema of the left leg distal to the groin.

Laboratory Findings: Hct 38%; WBC 11,000/μl. PT 12 sec; PTT 30 sec. Platelets: 285,000/μl. Chest radiograph: shown below left. ECG: sinus tachycardia. ABG (RA): pH 7.47; PCO_2 32 mmHg; PO_2 78 mmHg. Lung scan: three segmental mismatches and a matched defect in the right lower lung zone, indicating a high probability of pulmonary embolism. Pleural fluid analysis: shown below.

Hospital Course: Ninety-six hours after intravenous heparin was initiated, the patient experienced sudden worsening of dyspnea. A repeat chest radiograph showed an increase in the right pleural effusion. Thoracentesis revealed frankly bloody fluid with a hematocrit of 23%. A PTT was 1.5 times control.

Question: What is the most likely diagnosis, the best method of substantiating the diagnosis, and the appropriate management?

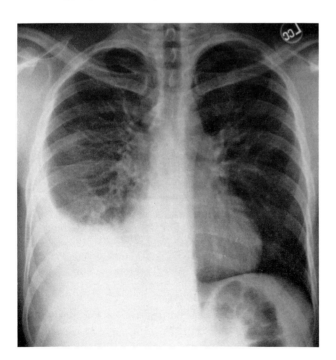

Initial Pleural Fluid Analysis

Appearance: serosanguinous

Total protein: 3.8 g/dl

LDH: 290 IU/L

Nucleated cells:
  7500/μl
  80% neutrophils
  20% mononuclear cells

Glucose: 100 mg/dl

pH: 7.32

Gram stain: negative

Cytology: pending

Diagnosis: Spontaneous hemothorax associated with heparin therapy for pulmonary embolism with infarction.

Discussion: Hemorrhage is the most common of the clinically important complications of heparin therapy. Other complications that occur early in the course of anticoagulation include heparin-associated thrombocytopenia and anaphylaxis. The severity of hemorrhagic complications varies from soft tissue ecchymoses with little more than cosmetic importance to major bleeding that can result in a fatal outcome. The incidence of heparin-associated hemorrhage reported in different clinical series ranges from virtually nonexistent to almost one in three patients.

The most common sites of heparin-associated bleeding include the gastrointestinal and genitourinary tracts, wounds, retroperitoneum, and muscle. Pulmonary and pleural space hemorrhages are surprisingly rare, considering that up to 70% of pleural effusions associated with pulmonary embolism are hemorrhagic and half of such effusions are associated with pulmonary infarction.

Hemothorax complicating anticoagulation therapy was first reported approximately 50 years ago. Since that time, additional reports have described this complication in patients ranging in age from 22–79 years. There has been a slight predominance of women, which is in concert with the increased frequency of hemorrhagic complications of anticoagulation in elderly women. Some reports have documented therapeutic prolongation of the PT and PTT, whereas some patients have had coagulation parameters well above the therapeutic range. In almost all instances, hemothorax developed without other associated bleeding sites.

Hemothorax usually occurs within the first week of heparin therapy, with the earliest report being 4 days after the start of anticoagulation. Early intrapleural bleeding has generally occurred ipsilateral to the patient's presenting chest pain caused by the pulmonary embolism. Thoracotomy or autopsy examinations most commonly demonstrate a localized hemorrhagic pulmonary infarction without a specific bleeding site in patients with heparin-induced hemothorax. There have been two reports of hemothorax occurring in patients on long-term oral anticoagulation; the hemothoraces occurred on the contralateral side of the initial chest pain.

Up to 40–50% of patients with pulmonary embolism have pleural effusions. These effusions occupy less than a third of the hemithorax and may be either transudates or exudates. Transudates, presumably caused by atelectasis, represent approximately 25% of these effusions. Exudates, caused by pulmonary ischemia or infarction, typically appear hemorrhagic. Pleural effusions related to pulmonary embolism almost always present on the admission chest radiograph or develop within the first 24 hours of hospitalization. In the absence of radiographic evidence of pulmonary infarction, the effusions usually reach a maximum volume within 2 or 3 days and completely resolve in 5–10 days. In patients with radiographic evidence of pulmonary infarction, the effusions may take 2 weeks or longer to resolve, possibly due to continued slow bleeding from the infarction.

With or without radiographically evident pulmonary infarction, however, the effusion should not increase in size after the first few days of the acute event and initiation of effective anticoagulation. Therefore, an anticoagulated patient with pulmonary embolism in whom increasing pleural effusion develops a few days after admission requires an immediate thoracentesis. The differential diagnosis of the enlarging effusion includes recurrent pulmonary embolism, an incorrect diagnosis (such as pneumonia), or hemothorax.

If the thoracentesis fluid is frankly bloody with a pleural fluid/peripheral blood hematocrit ratio ≥ 0.5, the diagnosis of hemothorax is established. In this setting, heparin should be discontinued immediately and the pleural space drained by tube thoracostomy. Chest tube drainage relieves dyspnea, monitors bleeding, possibly tamponades the bleeding site by reexpanding the lung, and prevents the development of an organized clot and pleural fibrosis.

If anticoagulation has been initiated only recently, a vena cava filter is required to prevent recurrent pulmonary embolism. Since most patients with heparin-associated hemothorax have had therapeutic coagulation studies, coagulation parameters rapidly return to normal when the heparin infusion is discontinued. Therefore, the use of protamine sulfate is usually unnecessary. In a patient with a markedly prolonged PTT, however, judicious use of protamine sulfate may be indicated if the chest tube demonstrates ongoing bleeding.

In the present patient, the second thoracentesis demonstrated a hemothorax due to heparin therapy. After discontinuation of heparin, placement of a chest tube, and insertion of an inferior vena cava filter, the patient recovered without reinitiation of anticoagulation therapy or further complications. He remains well after 1 year of follow-up.

Clinical Pearls

1. Spontaneous hemothorax is a rare but potentially lethal complication of heparin anticoagulation in patients with pulmonary infarction.

2. In the patient with pulmonary embolism and a pleural effusion that increases in size 3 or 4 days following initiation of heparin therapy, immediate thoracentesis is warranted to exclude hemothorax, an alternative diagnosis, or recurrent embolism.

3. If heparin-induced hemothorax is diagnosed, heparin should be discontinued immediately, chest tube drainage instituted, and a vena cava filter placed.

REFERENCES

1. Simon HB, Daggett WM, Desanctis RW. Hemothorax as a complication of anti-coagulant therapy in the presence of pulmonary infarction. JAMA 1969;208:1830–1834.
2. Bynum LJ, Wilson JE. Characteristics of pleural effusions associated with pulmonary embolism. Arch Intern Med 1976;136:159–162.
3. Rostand RA, Feldman RL, Block ER. Massive hemothorax complicating heparin anti-coagulation for pulmonary embolus. South Med J 1977;70:1128–1130.
4. Bynum LJ, Wilson JE III. Radiographic features of pleural effusions in pulmonary embolism. Am Rev Respir Dis 1978;117:829–834.
5. Heffner JE. Pleural effusions secondary to pulmonary thromboembolism. Semin Respir Med 1987;9:59–64.

PATIENT 31

A 59-year-old woman with sudden onset of shortness of breath and stridor

A 59-year-old woman was brought to the emergency department from a restaurant where she had developed the sudden onset of shortness of breath. She denied previous episodes of shortness of breath or cardiopulmonary disorders, but the degree of dyspnea prevented further history taking.

Physical Examination: Temperature 99° F; pulse 125; respirations 32; blood pressure 150/92. General: moderate to severe dyspnea with stridor. Skin: diffuse diaphoresis. Neck: trachea midposition; bulky fullness in supraclavicular notch and medial right supraclavicular fossa. Chest: decreased breath sounds at both bases. Cardiac: grade I/IV systolic ejection murmur. Abdomen: normal bowel sounds; mild tenderness in epigastrium; palpable liver edge at costal margin. Extremities: no clubbing or edema.

Laboratory Findings: Hct 41.6%, WBC 17,400/μl. Electrolytes and renal indices: normal. ABG (2 L/min nasal cannula O_2): PO_2 84; PCO_2 56; pH 7.27. Chest radiographs: shown below.

Question: What is the etiology of this patient's respiratory failure? How would you improve her condition?

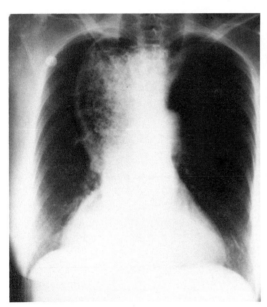 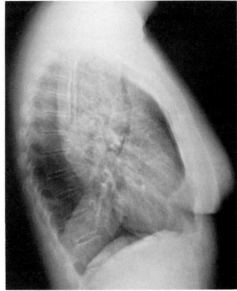

Diagnosis: Achalasia with upper airway obstruction from a food-filled megaesophagus.

Discussion: Achalasia is a functional disorder of swallowing characterized by increased tone of the lower esophageal sphincter (LES) and absence of coordinated esophageal peristalsis. Literally meaning "failure to relax," the primary lesion of achalasia appears to be deinnervation of the inhibitory nerves that dilate the LES and allow food boluses to enter the stomach. Eventually, functional obstruction of the gastroesophageal junction and ensuing esophageal aperistalsis induce massive enlargement of the esophagus (megaesophagus), which then serves as a warehouse for liquids and stagnant food during their slow transit to the stomach. Patients present at variable stages of achalasia from childhood to advanced age, with painless dysphagia commonly compounded by heartburn, weight loss, and regurgitation of esophageal contents.

Recurrent and often silent aspiration of liquids and undigested food predisposes patients with achalasia to several well-established pulmonary complications, which include pneumonia, lung abscess, atelectasis, bronchiectasis, and nocturnal bronchospasm. The potential for achalasia to cause upper airway obstruction with acute respiratory failure in patients with megaesophagus is less widely recognized.

The pathogenesis of airway obstruction relates to the physiologic characteristics of the upper esophageal sphincter (UES). During swallowing, this sphincter opens in response to low intraluminal pressures applied from the pharyngeal side. Once food enters the esophagus and the sphincter closes, however, the UES resists pressures as high as 100 cm H_2O from the esophageal side. This partial "one-way" valve may then prevent belching and regurgitation, leading to further overdistension of the esophagus. As the process relentlessly progresses, the expanding megaesophagus may then compress the trachea against the bony thoracic inlet.

Airway obstruction is typically rapid in onset after a meal when the engorged esophagus expands into the tightly confined cervical anatomy. Intense dyspnea with air swallowing or positive pressure face mask (Ambu bag) ventilation may further insufflate the esophagus and aggravate the degree of respiratory failure. Accompanying compression of venous structures may cause superior vena cava syndrome with evidence of venous hypertension in neck structures. Esophageal dilatation limited to the thorax may present more insidiously, with progressive stridor and dyspnea that simulate a mediastinal tumor. Rarely, the megaesophagus stretches the recurrent laryngeal nerves and causes bilateral vocal cord paralysis, which is an additional cause of upper airway obstruction.

Patients with achalasia and upper airway obstruction present in respiratory distress with distended neck veins and arterial blood gases that demonstrate hypoxic and hypercapnic respiratory failure in severe instances. A soft, bulky neck mass that compresses with palpation represents the distended megaesophagus and suggests the diagnosis. Patients who collapse while struggling for breath may regurgitate and aspirate esophageal contents in the supine position, thereby obscuring the initial underlying event.

Chest radiographs usually show a widened mediastinum composed of the esophagus with its smooth borders bulging into the right hemithorax and following a sigmoid curve toward the diaphragm. Alimentary contents lend a characteristically "mottled" appearance to the esophagus, which commonly contains an air-fluid level. The trachea bows anteriorly on the lateral view and demonstrates a long, regular narrowing. The aryepiglottic folds and retropharynx may appear edematous when visualized acutely during attempts at laryngoscopic intubation.

The emergent approach to patients with achalasia and acute upper airway obstruction depends on the severity of respiratory symptoms. Patients with adequate respiratory reserve improve rapidly after a nasogastric tube or fiberoptic endoscope decompresses the esophagus. Patients with severe respiratory insufficiency, however, may deteriorate if blind attempts at nasogastric tube placement further compromise the upper airway or induce regurgitation and aspiration. In this situation, tracheal intubation should precede esophageal decompression efforts; extrinsic compression of the airway below the glottis may require a smaller than usual endotracheal tube size.

After recovery from respiratory failure, patients require treatment directed at lowering LES tone to decompress the esophagus and prevent a recurrence of airway obstruction. Medical therapy with calcium channel blockers and nitrates rarely provides significant relief in severe achalasia. Bougienage results in only temporary relief of dysphagia, lasting less than a week. Most patients with a previous episode of upper airway obstruction require pneumatic dilatation of the LES or esophagomyotomy. Although esophagomyotomy improves dysphagia symptoms in 85% of patients, it is often reserved for patients who have failed several pneumatic dilatations since this procedure may be successful long term in 65% of attempts.

The present patient underwent placement of a large-bore nasogastric tube that removed 300 ml of stagnant food and syrupy liquid. She improved immediately with resolution of respiratory distress and stated that her dyspnea had developed immediately after finishing a large pancake breakfast. She reported a long history since childhood of achalasia that was largely controlled with calcium channel blockers, but denied previous episodes of airway obstruction. At esophagoscopy, the recesses of the megaesophagus were explored but patulent folds prevented identification of the LES, thereby obviating pneumatic dilatation. She subsequently underwent esophagomyotomy through a lateral thoracotomy incision.

Clinical Pearls

1. Patients with severe achalasia and megaesophagus may present with postprandial upper airway obstruction from compression of the trachea at the thoracic inlet.

2. Cervical venous congestion and a compressible bulge in the neck in a patient with respiratory distress are signs of achalasia with airway obstruction. Radiographic features of a sigmoid megaesophagus with anterior dislocation of the trachea confirm the diagnosis.

3. Patients with adequate respiratory reserve respond rapidly to esophageal decompression with a nasogastric tube.

4. Patients with severe respiratory failure should initially undergo tracheal intubation with a small endotracheal tube (size 7 or less) to facilitate passage through the subglottic region of tracheal compression.

REFERENCES

1. Travis KW, Saini VK, O'Sullivan PT. Upper-airway obstruction and achalasia of the esophagus. Anesthesiology 1981;54:87–88.
2. Carlsson-Norlander B. Acute upper airway obstruction in a patient with achalasia. Arch Otolaryngol Head Neck Surg 1987;113:885–887.
3. Dominguez F, Hernandez-Ranz F, Boixeda D, Valdazo P. Acute upper-airway obstruction in achalasia of the esophagus. Am J Gastroenterol 1987;82:362–364.
4. Reynolds JC, Parkman HP. Achalasia. Gastroenterol Clin North Am 1989;18:223–255.
5. Westbrook JL. Oesophageal achalasia causing respiratory obstruction. Anaesthesia 1992;47:38–40.

PATIENT 32

A 19-year-old man with acute chest pain after smoking "crack" cocaine

A 19-year-old man presented with intense substernal chest pain immediately after smoking "crack" cocaine. He also noted a new "cracking or popping" noise in his chest. The patient denied dyspnea, hemoptysis, or arm pain.

Physical Examination: Temperature 99.3° F; pulse 86; respirations 18; blood pressure 114/64. General: uncomfortable with chest pain. Neck: normal. Chest: normal. Cardiac: a "crunching" sound localized over the left anterior chest wall synchronous with the heart beat. Abdomen: normal. Extremities: no cyanosis or edema.

Laboratory Findings: CBC: normal. Chest radiographs (shown below): lucent stripes in the superior mediastinum indicating a pneumomediastinum.

Question: What is the most likely etiology of the patient's problem?

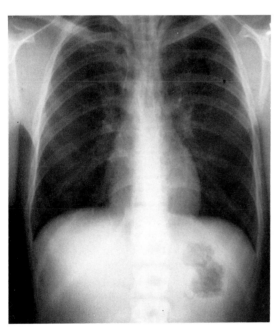 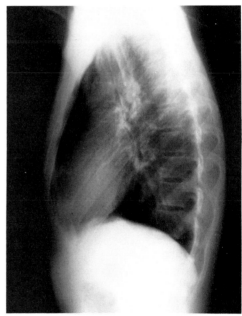

Diagnosis: "Crack" cocaine-induced pneumomediastinum.

Discussion: The illicit use of cocaine has increased dramatically in the United States over the last decade. With this more widespread usage has come a greater awareness of the diverse medical complications associated with this drug. The cardiovascular and neurologic adverse reactions represent some of the more profound manifestations of cocaine abuse, with clinical presentations that include myocardial ischemia and infarction, cardiac arrhythmias (both brady and tachy), sudden death, aortic dissection, peripheral vasoconstriction with hypertension, stroke, seizures, hyperpyrexia, and psychosis. Pulmonary complications have emerged as equally important and potentially life-threatening manifestations of cocaine self-administration.

The list of pulmonary disorders associated with cocaine are diverse and often vary with the method of drug administration. For instance, all routes of cocaine administration can result in noncardiogenic pulmonary edema or respiratory arrest. Inhalation of free-base cocaine ("crack"), however, is more likely to cause diffuse alveolar hemorrhage with massive hemoptysis. And most intriguing, a deep inhalation of free-base cocaine often assisted by a mouth-to-mouth positive pressure boost from a "buddy" to enhance the drug high has been associated with pneumomediastinum and pneumothorax.

It appears that pneumothorax results from the positive intrathoracic pressure and violent coughing that occur when abusers of cocaine use a deep inhalation technique. It has been conjectured that the cocaine alkaloid may have a direct toxic effect on pulmonary membranes and contribute to alveolar rupture. Additionally, interstitial pressure may be decreased during vigorous inhalation, leading to a further increase in the raised alveolar-interstitial pressure gradient initiated by cocaine's vasoconstrictive effects on blood vessels adjacent to the alveoli. When the pressure difference between alveoli and interstitium reaches a critical level, alveolar rupture occurs.

Once alveolar rupture occurs, air enters the perivascular interstitium and dissects within the bronchovascular sheath to the mediastinum. Dissection from the mediastinum to the pericardial sac may occur through the pericardial reflections of the pulmonary vessels. Air in the mediastinum may also move upward through fascial planes into the cervical and supraclavicular subcutaneous soft tissue, presenting as subcutaneous empysema. A pneumothorax may occur when mediastinal collections of air rupture through the mediastinal parietal pleura into the pleural cavity.

Typically, pneumomediastinum related to cocaine abuse occurs in a young male with acute, sharp, substernal chest pain, Hamman's sign, and dyspnea. Other features include neck pain and swelling, sore throat, hoarseness, cardiovascular compromise, and subcutaneous emphysema. These symptoms can occur immediately or several hours after cocaine use.

Hamman's sign is a crunching sound accentuated with systolic contraction of the heart. Half of the patients with cocaine-induced pneumomediastinum have been reported to have Hamman's sign. Although originally thought to be pathognomonic of pneumomediastinum, a "crunching" sound also may be heard in patients with pneumothorax or with a dilated esophagus, stomach, or colon.

The chest radiograph in patients with pneumomediastinum demonstrate gas collections within mediastinal structures. On frontal views, mediastinal air deflects the pleura laterally along the left heart border, creating a lucent stripe of air medially bounded by a lateral, vertical pleural line. A "continuous diaphragm" sign, wherein the central portions of the diaphragm are visualized behind the heart, may also be apparent. Air lucencies may surround the aorta, vena cava, or trachea. The lateral radiograph may show air within mediastinal tissue planes and surrounding the cardiac shadow. Radiographic resolution usually lags behind clinical improvement.

Most spontaneously breathing patients with an isolated pneumomediastinum follow an uncomplicated course with spontaneous resolution within several days of presentation. Simple observation is indicated, although careful consideration should be given to occult, underlying etiologies, such as a ruptured esophagus, that require urgent diagnosis and care. Some physicians hospitalize patients with isolated pneumomediastinum; others observe reliable patients without serious underlying cardiopulmonary disease as outpatients. Follow-up chest radiographs are advised in order to exclude progression of the pneumomediastinum or the occurrence of a pneumothorax. During convalescence, patients should be advised to avoid strenuous activities, particularly Valsalva maneuvers.

The present patient's chest radiograph demonstrated a pneumomediastinum. He was hospitalized for observation and supplemental oxygen. The chest pain and Hamman's sign resolved within 24 hours, and the chest radiograph showed gradual resolution over 3 days.

Clinical Pearls

1. Cocaine inhalation with a Valsalva maneuver may cause an increased alveolar-interstitial pressure gradient with alveolar rupture that results in a pneumomediastinum, pneumothorax, or pneumopericardium.

2. The route of air entry from a ruptured alveolus into the pleural space follows a course along bronchovascular sheaths into the mediastinum and through ruptures in the paramediastinal visceral pleura.

3. Most cases of cocaine-induced pneumomediastinum resolve spontaneously and do not require intervention. Follow-up chest radiographs are recommended to exclude progression of the pneumomediastinum and a complicating pneumothorax.

REFERENCES

1. Salzman GA, Khan F, Emory C. Pneumomediastinum after cocaine smoking. South Med J 1987;80:1427–1429.
2. Ettinger NA, Albin RJ. A review of the respiratory effects of smoking cocaine. Am J Med 1989;87:664–668.
3. Heffner JE, Harley RA, Schabel SI. Pulmonary reactions from illicit substance abuse. Clin Chest Med 1990;11:151–162.
4. Seaman ME. Barotrauma related to inhalational drug use. J Emerg Med 1990;8:141–149.
5. Baumann MH, Sahn SA. Hamman's sign revisited: pneumothorax or pneumomediastinum? Chest 1992;102:1281–1282.

PATIENT 33

A 58-year-old man with dyspnea, hypotension, and an expanding chest wall mass

A 58-year-old man with a 50-pack-year smoking history presented with dyspnea and a rapidly expanding right, parasternal chest wall mass. He first noted retrosternal chest "aching" 3 months earlier that was soon accompanied by low-grade fevers, coughing, night sweats, lethargy, and weight loss. Two weeks before admission he had developed a "bump" near this sternum that grew to the size of a "lemon." Onset of shortness of breath prompted medical evaluation.

Physical Examination: Temperature 98.6°; pulse 110/min; respirations 25/min; blood pressure 90/60 (10 mmHg pulsus paradoxicus). Mouth: gingivitis. Neck: dilated neck veins. Thorax: 4 × 5 cm firm, right parasternal mass; normal overlying skin. Chest: scattered rales; left pleural rub. Cardiac: depressed heart tones; no pericardial rubs or murmurs.

Laboratory Findings: Hct 31%; WBC 33,000/μl; Na$^+$ 122 mEq/L; K$^+$ 5.4 mEq/L; Cl$^-$ 85 mEq/L; HCO$_3^-$ 20 mEq/L; BUN 99 mg/dl; creatinine 2.8 mEq/L. Sputum: mixed flora. EKG: nonspecific changes. Chest radiograph (below): enlarged cardiac silhouette; left upper lobe infiltrate.

Hospital Course: A sample from the mass obtained by needle aspiration was sent to the laboratory for cytologic and microbiologic analysis. The patient rapidly developed increasing dyspnea, hypotension, and pulsus paradoxicus. A cardiac echo demonstrated a thickened pericardium, a pericardial effusion, and evidence of pericardial tamponade.

Question: What is the most likely clinical diagnosis?

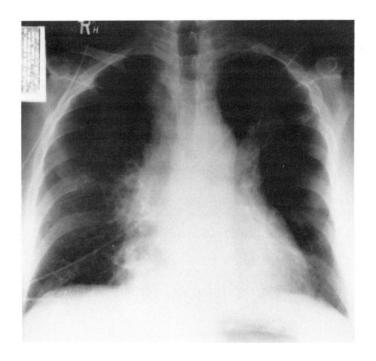

Diagnosis: Pericardial actinomycosis with pericardial tamponade.

Discussion: Thoracic actinomycosis is an acute and chronic suppurative infection that involves the lungs, pleura, chest wall, and mediastinal structures. The resulting inflammatory response is characterized by fibrotic scarring, tissue destruction, abscess formation, and sinus tracts that extend across anatomic barriers. Although caused by any of the five species of the genus *Actinomyces (A. israelii, A. naeslundii, A. viscosus, A. meyeri, A. odontolyticus)* or the related species *Propionibacterium propionicus, Actinomyces israelii* is the most common human pathogen related to the disease.

The bacteria associated with actinomycosis are filamentous, gram-positive, rod-shaped organisms that are strictly anaerobic, commensal habitants of the oropharynx and gastrointestinal tract. They gain access to the lower airway through aspiration of bacteria-laden oropharyngeal contents. Of low pathogenicity themselves, actinomycosis-related bacteria establish infection in anaerobic regions of the lung devitalized by the combined influences of atelectasis, airway foreign bodies or particulate matter, and preexisting aspiration pneumonitis caused by other bacterial species. Common bacteria associated with actinomycosis lung infection include *Actinobacillus actinomycetemcomitans, Haemophilus* spp., fusobacterium, anaerobic and other streptococci, micrococci, staphylococci, *Eikenella corrodens,* and *Bacteroides* spp.

Risk factors for thoracic actinomycosis include alcoholism and other conditions that promote altered mental status and an increased incidence of aspiration. The presence of periodontal and dental disease appears to promote pulmonary infection by increasing the prevalence and quantity of actinomycosis-related species in oral secretions. Also, chest trauma, surgical manipulation of thoracic structures, and compromised mucociliary clearance, as occur in patients with chronic bronchitis or bronchiectasis, are risk factors for the disease. Thoracic actinomycosis does not occur as a result of defects in humoral or cell-mediated immunity because of the low virulence of the pathogens that depend on a breakdown of local barriers of defense in regions of devitalized tissue.

Once established in the lower airway, a focus of actinomycosis progresses slowly, with patients presenting after weeks or months with an indolent illness. The characteristic features of weight loss, cough, chest pain, anemia, and intermittent fever may simulate a neoplastic conditon such as lung cancer and present the differential diagnosis of an unresolved pneumonia. An endobronchial focus of actinomycotic infection with its associated desmoplastic tissue reaction is particularly likely to lead to a misdiagnosis of bronchogenic carcinoma until culture and tissue biopsy analyses are completed.

Thoracic actinomycosis is classically known for its inclination to extend across anatomic boundaries and destroy chest wall structures, resulting in sinus tracts or chest wall masses. The chest wall masses may appear inflamed or have normal overlying skin, as occurred in the present patient. Chest wall involvement has diminished during the last several decades with earlier and more effective antibiotic therapy for aspiration pneumonia. Regions of pleural thickening or pleural effusions are additional associated findings of pulmonary infection.

Only 2% of patients with thoracic actinomycosis progress to involvement of cardiac structures. The route of spread occurs most commonly by local extension from an adjacent pulmonary or mediastinal infection, although rare patients may develop endocardial infection after bloodstream dissemination. The most common sites of infection are the pericardium in 80% of patients, the myocardium in 50%, and endocardial structures such as cardiac valves in 35%.

Patients with cardiac actinomycosis range in age from 24–57 years and 84% are men, which is similar to the unexplained four-to-one male predominance of thoracic actinomycosis in general. The disease is insidious with a mean duration from onset of symptoms to presentation of 25 weeks. Fever may be absent during the initial presentation but occurs sometime during the course of the disease in the majority of patients. Up to 30% of patients will have a pericardial friction rub and 80% will have clinically apparent primary disease in the thorax with contiguous spread to the heart. Chest wall masses in this patient population, however, occur only rarely.

Impressions about the cardiovascular manifestations of cardiac actinomycosis have changed during the last several decades. Early descriptions emphasized that cardiac tamponade was a rare finding and that most patients presented with congestive heart failure. In the antibiotic era, however, congestive heart failure is an unsual manifestation, with tamponade occurring in 53% of patients and constrictive or adhesive pericarditis in 37%. Cardiac arrhythmias are uncommon except for atrial fibrillation, which results as a consequence of pericarditis.

Cardiac involvement should be suspected in patients with cardiovascular dysfunction and clinical manifestations of thoracic actinomycosis. Common radiographic manifestations of thoracic disease include extension of the pulmonary lesion into the chest wall, wavy periostitis or frank destruction of ribs, extension through an interlobar fissure, and vertebral destruction with erosion of both the transverse processes and vertebral bodies. The pulmonary infiltrate may or may not be cavitated and frequently appears as a mass like density. Pleural thickening and pleural effusions are other typical findings. The chest CT scan may more clearly define mediastinal or chest wall invasion from an adjacent pulmonary infiltrate and demonstrate a thickened pericardium or pericardial effusion in patients with cardiac infection. Echocardiography may also define the presence of pericardial abnormalities. When abnormal, the electrocardiogram shows features typical of pericarditis.

Pericardiocentesis in patients with cardiac actinomycosis may demonstrate purulent pericardial fluid in 53% of instances or serosanguinous fluid with a preponderance of neutrophils. Only 20% of patients have positive fluid culture results. Gram stain of pericardial fluid may detect the branching, filamentous rods, although a tendency to fragment and stain unevenly may give the bacteria the appearance of gram-positive cocci. Sulfur granules—1- to 2-mm granules that are yellow-white irregular masses of the organism embedded in a matrix—occur in 25% of actinomycosis pericardial fluid and strongly support the diagnosis. Actinomycosis-related bacteria do not stain with acid-fast preparations, in contrast to *Nocardia* species, which are weakly acid fast.

If noncardiac sites are unavailable for culture or biopsy in patients with unrevealing pericardial fluid results, pericardial biopsy and tissue culture may provide the diagnosis in 26% of patients with cardiac actinomycosis. Sulfur granules within tissue specimens have peripheral clubbing, which is an inflammatory host reaction to the infection, and confirm the diagnosis. Sulfur granules are difficult to find in tissue biopsy specimens and may require close examination of multiple serial

sections. Isolation of actinomycosis-related pathogens from sputum may not be helpful because of the commensal nature of these bacteria.

The therapy of cardiac actinomycosis depends on a combination of surgical resection and drainage with prompt initiation of antimicrobial therapy. Treatment is started with intravenous penicillin G (12 to 20 million units/day) for 4–6 weeks followed by 6–12 months of oral phenoxymethylpenicillin or amoxicillin. The prolonged course of therapy is required because the infection occurs in poorly vascularized, indurated tissue that prevents adequate antibiotic penetrance. Alternative therapy in penicillin allergic patients includes tetracycline, erythromycin, clindamycin, chloramphenicol, and third-generation cephalosporins. Over 80% of patients with pericardial actinomycosis require surgical or catheter drainage of pericardial fluid, with one-half of patients requiring a pericardiectomy. A lack of clinical response suggests the presence of undrained abscesses, necrotic tissue, or a polymicrobial infection with resistant pathogens. With aggressive therapy, up to 90% of patients survive cardiac actinomycosis.

The aspirate from the present patient's parasternal mass demonstrated branching, gram-positive bacteria that subsequently grew *A. israelii*. A chest CT at the level of the heart (see figure below left) demonstrated a thickened pericardium (arrows) and bilateral pleural effusions. A CT section at the level of the ascending aorta (see figure below right) showed extension of the intrathoracic actinomycosis infection through the chest wall (arrow). The patient's hypotension resolved with insertion of a pericardial catheter. After initiation of intravenous penicillin, performance of a pericardiectomy, insertion of chest tubes, and mediastinal debridement, the patient recovered completely during a prolonged hospitalization.

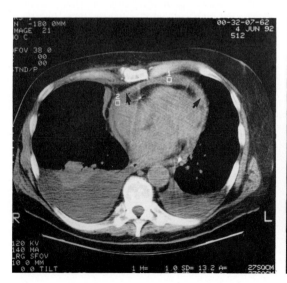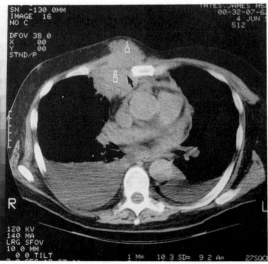

Clinical Pearls

1. Actinomycosis is not a disease associated with systemic alterations of humoral or cell-mediated host defense mechanisms. Alterations of local intrapulmonary defense mechanisms, as occur in aspiration pneumonia, however, are important mechanisms for promoting thoracic infection with these low-virulence pathogens.

2. Only 2% of patients with thoracic actinomycosis have cardiac involvement. Eighty-percent of patients with cardiac disease have pericardial infection, 50% have myocardial infection, and 35% have involvement of the cardiac valves.

3. More than 50% of patients with cardiac actinomycosis present with pericardial tamponade, with 37% having constrictive or adhesive pericarditis.

4. Cardiac actinomycosis requires combined therapy with prompt initiation of antibiotics and evaluation for pericardial drainage or resection. Up to 90% of patients survive when treated aggressively with a drainage procedure.

5. The chest CT characteristically demonstrates a pericardial effusion and a thickened pericardium in patients with pericardial actinomycosis.

REFERENCES

1. Heffner JE. Pleuropulmonary manifestations of actinomycosis and nocardiosis. Semin Respir Med 1988;3:352–361.
2. Orloff JJ, Fine MJ, Rihs JD. Acute cardiac tamponade due to cardiac actinomycosis. Chest 1988;93:661–663.
3. Slutzker AD, Claypool WD. Pericardial actinomycosis with cardiac tamponade from a contiguous thoracic lesion. Thorax 1989;44:442–443.
4. Fife TD, Finegold SM, Grennan T. Pericardial actinomycosis: case report and review. Rev Infect Dis 1991;13:120–126.
5. Heffner JE, Harley RA. Thoracic actinomycosis. Semin Respir Med 1992;13:247–255.

PATIENT 34

A 37-year-old man with lacrimal gland enlargement and hemoptysis

A 37-year-old man was referred by an ophthamologist for evaluation of hemoptysis. He had been undergoing care for lacrimal gland enlargement during the previous 4 months. The patient denied respiratory complaints until he noted blood-streaked sputum within the past 24 hours.

Physical Examination: Temperature 98.1°; respirations 24. Eyes: bilateral lacrimal gland enlargement (below top); no conjunctivitis or proptosis. Head: no sinus tenderness. Chest: minimal rhonchi over the right lung field. Cardiac: normal. Neurologic: unremarkable.

Laboratory Findings: Hct 27%; WBC 6,200/μl; platelets 298,000/μl. Electrolytes: normal. BUN 28 mg/dl. PT and PTT: normal. Urinalysis: 21–50 RBC/hpf. Chest radiograph: below bottom.

Question: What diagnosis can explain the patient's clinical presentation?

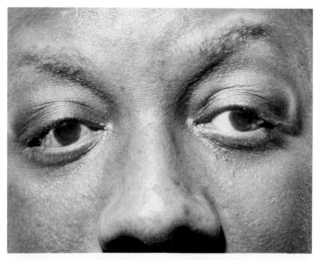

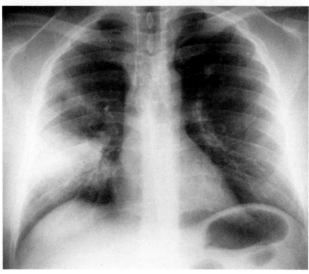

Diagnosis: Wegener granulomatosis (WG).

Discussion: The major differential diagnosis of a clinical presentation of hematuria and hemoptysis includes the pulmonary renal syndromes of WG, Goodpasture syndrome, Churg-Strauss syndrome, rapidly progressive glomerulonephritis, and polyangiitis overlap syndrome. The presence of ophthalmologic findings narrows the diagnostic possibilities and strongly suggests WG.

WG was first described as a distinct clinical entity in the 1930s by Friedrich Wegener. Characterized by necrotizing granulomas of the upper or lower respiratory tract, systemic focal vasculitis of small- to medium-sized vessels, and glomerulonephritis, its underlying pathogenesis remains ill defined. Recent nomenclature identifies a "limited" form of the disease in patients with respiratory tract involvement without the renal disease that occurs in the more classic generalized form of the disorder. Some experts consider that limited WG actually represents an early stage of the disease before evidence of more widespread vasculitis becomes clinically apparent.

WG has a slight predilection for males and an age of presentation in the fifth decade of life. Symptoms due to sinus inflammation may be the presenting features in up to 70% of patients. Arthralgias, fever, weight loss, and anorexia are common. Although the lungs are eventually involved in greater than 90% of patients, initial complaints referable to the lower respiratory tract are less common than sinus symptoms. The chest radiograph, however, may be abnormal in as many as 70% of patients on initial evaluation.

When present, respiratory complaints include cough, chest discomfort, hemoptysis and pleuritic pain. Intense inflammation of the tracheobronchial tree may cause airway stenosis with atelectasis and lobar collapse. Involvement of the endolarynx may produce subglottic stenosis and a clinical presentation that mimics asthma. Massive pulmonary hemorrhage is an unusual presenting sign of WG but when present can result in respiratory failure.

Other presenting manifestations of WG include otitis media, rhinorrhea, and crusting or perforation of the nasal septum with resultant saddlenose deformity. Jaw pain, palate ulceration, and mulberry gingivitis are oral manifestations. Approximately one-half of patients will manifest some form of ocular inflammation. In 15% of patients, ocular symptoms may appear before clinical manifestations in other organ systems. When eye involvement is contiguous to sinus inflammation, proptosis may occur secondary to orbital pseudotumor, nasolacrimal duct obstruction or dysfunction of extraocular muscles. When unrelated to sinus inflammation, localized ocular granulomatous vasculitis clinically presents as conjunctivitis, episcleritis, corneoscleral ulceration, uveitis, or visual loss due to retinal vessel occlusion. Although lacrimal gland hypertrophy has been rarely reported in the literature, some authors suggest that previous reports of eyelid swelling in WG may have been actually due to lacrimal gland enlargement.

The typical radiographic features of WG are single or multiple parenchymal nodules with a tendency for central cavitation. The chest radiograph may also show alveolar infiltrates consistent with lung hemorrhage, as in the present patient. Pleural effusions due to subpleural infarction occur in about 10% of patients but are rarely clinically important.

The unequivocal diagnosis of WG requires histologic demonstration of a granulomatous vasculitis of small- and medium-sized vessels in involved organs. The nose and lung are the most frequent source of diagnostic tissue. Renal biopsies specimens are often nondiagnostic. Detection of antineutrophilic cytoplasmic antibodies (ANCA) represents a major advance in the diagnosis of WG. A cytoplasmic pattern of staining (c-ANCA) represents serum IgG antibodies against cytoplasmic proteinase 3 (anti-Pr3), which is highly specific (up to 90%) in patients with pulmonary involvement. Following the c-ANCA titer assists in monitoring of disease activity. Nonspecific laboratory findings include anemia, elevated ESR, and, in 50% of cases, a positive rheumatoid factor. When nephritis is present, urinalysis reveals proteinuria, leukocytes, red blood cells, and red blood cell casts.

Untreated patients with WG have limited survival, with greater than 90% mortality at 2 years. Combination therapy with high-dose corticosteroids and cyclophosphamide has markedly altered the course of the disease, producing remission rates as high as 93%. Early recognition of WG in patients with limited organ involvement is important to allow initiation of therapy before progression to multisystem organ failure occurs. Some centers have reported improvement in disease activity with the initiation of trimethoprim-sulfamethoxazole. The role of this antibiotic for limited disease and as an adjunct in the generalized form requires further definition. Secondary bacterial sinus infections are frequently superimposed on the vasculitic destruction of the sinus mucosa; some patients may require sinus drainage as an adjunct to therapy.

The present patient underwent a lacrimal gland biopsy that revealed nonspecific chronic inflammation. An open lung biopsy demonstrated necrotizing granulomatous inflammation of the arterioles and capillaritis in the alveolar septa. He was treated with high-dose corticosteroids, cyclophosphamide, and trimethoprim-sulfamethoxazole. The hemoptysis resolved and the lacrimal gland enlargement slowly improved.

Clinical Pearls

1. Ocular inflammation may herald the onset of generalized Wegener granulomatosis in 15% of patients.

2. Recurrent or severe pansinusitis should suggest the diagnosis of Wegener granulomatosis. Determination of a c-ANCA titer assists the initial evaluation.

3. Trimethoprim-sulfamethoxazole, in conjunction with high-dose corticosteroids and cyclophosphamide, may improve clinical disease activity and allow lowering of the dose of cytotoxic agents and corticosteroids.

4. Wegener granulomatosis may masquerade as asthma if the patient presents with complications secondary to subglottic stenosis.

REFERENCES

1. Haynes B, Fishman M, Fauci A, Wolff S. The ocular manifestations of Wegener's granulomatosis. Am J Med 1977;63:131–141.
2. Boukes BJ, De Vries-Knoppert WAEJ. Lacrimal gland enlargement as one of the ocular manifestations of Wegener granulomatosis. Doc Ophthalmol 1985;59:21–26.
3. Young KR. Pulmonary-renal syndromes. Clin Chest Med 1989;10:655–675.
4. Specks U, DeRemee R. Granulomatous vasculitis. Rheum Dis Clin North Am 1990;16:377–397.

PATIENT 35

A 32-year-old man with stridor and hypoxemia after laryngeal extubation

A 32-year-old comatose man was admitted to the ICU with head injuries after being struck by a car in a crosswalk. He required intubation in the field. A head CT scan demonstrated a small hematoma in the posterior fossa, and the neurologic examination revealed bilateral loss of function of cranial nerves VI, IX, and X. Three days after admission, the patient's mental status improved, allowing laryngeal extubation. Immediately after removal of the endotracheal tube, the patient developed severe restlessness and inspiratory stridor, requiring reintubation. Within 30 minutes of reintubation, mechanical ventilation was initiated because of progressive hypoxemia.

Physical Examination: Temperature 37°C; pulse 112/min; respirations 24/min; blood pressure 125/62 mmHg. Neck: no masses; normal neck veins. Chest: bilateral crackles. Cardiac: normal S1 and S2; positive S4; no murmurs. Abdomen: soft, normal bowel sounds. Neurologic: alert; bilateral paresis of cranial nerves VI, IX, X.

Laboratory Findings: Hct 32%; WBC 7,000/μl. ABG (FiO$_2$ 60%): pH 7.50; PCO$_2$ 30 mmHg; PO$_2$ 62 mmHg. Chest radiograph: shown below.

Question: What is the etiology of the patient's stridor and respiratory failure?

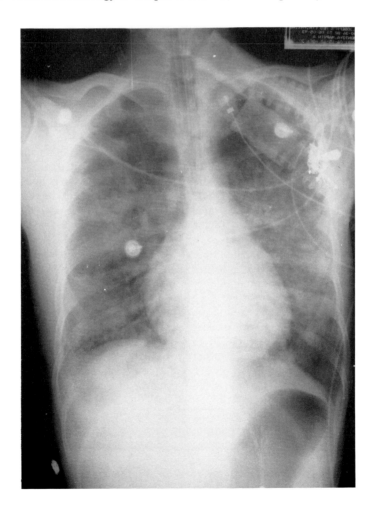

Answer: Acute pulmonary edema secondary to upper airway obstruction from bilateral vocal cord paralysis.

Discussion: Acute pulmonary edema subsequent to upper airway obstruction is a well-described clinical entity. Patients typically present with pulmonary edema minutes or as long as several hours after onset or relief of partial or complete airway obstruction. The reported conditions commonly associated with pulmonary edema include laryngeal tumors, hanging, strangulation, laryngeal hematomas, laryngospasm, laryngeal edema, epiglottitis, aspirated foreign bodies, goiters, and near drowning. Of these disorders, acute laryngospasm after removal of an endotracheal tube is presently the most common cause of obstruction-related pulmonary edema in adults. The incidence of pulmonary edema in patients requiring intubation or tracheotomy for relief of all causes of upper airway obstruction is reported to be as high as 11%.

The pathophysiology of pulmonary edema in this condition is unknown but may at least partially result from the marked negative intrapleural pressures that develop during attempts to inhale against an obstructed airway. Normal inspiratory intrapleural pressures range between -2 and -5 cm H_2O but may drop to as low as -50 to -100 cm H_2O during episodes of airway obstruction. These forces may decrease pulmonary perivascular pressures and initiate hydrostatic transudation of fluid into the lung interstitium. Negative intrathoracic pressure further promotes hydrostatic pulmonary edema by increasing both central venous return and transmyocardial wall pressure gradients, the latter of which depresses cardiac function by increasing myocardial afterload. It has also been suggested that hypoxic vasoconstriction during transient asphyxia may raise pulmonary capillary pressures.

Hydrostatic forces alone, however, do not adequately explain the onset of pulmonary edema after upper airway obstruction. Case reports exist of patients with obstruction-related pulmonary edema who had normal capillary wedge pressures and high protein contents in airway pulmonary edema fluid, both of which are consistent with increased membrane permeability edema. The etiology of altered capillary permeability is unclear but may result from shearing forces applied to capillary walls by the extreme negative intrathoracic pressures or endothelial cell disruption due to alveolar overdistension in patients with partial airway obstruction and hyperinflation. To date, none of the hydrostatic or membrane-permeability mechanisms suggested to underlie obstruction-related pulmonary edema has been validated in animal experimental models.

Young patients less than 40 years of age are at greatest risk for developing pulmonary edema after relief of upper airway obstruction. Young, relatively healthy patients have sufficiently well-developed thoracic musculature that enables them to generate profound intrathoracic negative pressures. Recent studies additionally report an increased risk after extubation for pulmonary edema in patients who undergo an anatomically difficult intubation or nasal, oral, or pharyngeal surgery, and in patients with short necks, sleep apnea syndrome, obesity, and acromegaly.

Bilateral vocal cord paralysis is an unusual cause of severe upper airway obstruction that rarely has been reported to cause pulmonary edema. Paralyzed vocal cords align in the paramedian, adducted position where positive airway pressure moves them apart during active expiration. During inspiration, however, negative airway pressure causes tight cord apposition and functional upper airway obstruction. Relief of obstruction by endotracheal intubation can then result in acute pulmonary edema. Bilateral vocal cord paralysis occurs in association with superior mediastinal tumors, neck injuries, cranial trauma to the posterior fossa, and central nervous system atrophy disorders.

The chest radiograph in patients with pulmonary edema after relief of airway obstruction demonstrates a symmetric and bilateral pulmonary edema pattern that is most pronounced centrally. The cardiothoracic ratio is normal in patients without underlying cardiac disease. A distinctive widening of the vascular pedicle is apparent in some patients. This finding may result from sudden redistribution of circulating blood volume to the systemic circulation in patients with intense hypoxic vasoconstriction of the pulmonary vasculature.

Most patients respond to supportive care with rapid resolution of pulmonary edema. The decision to intubate the patient depends on the nature of the upper airway obstruction and the results of emergency efforts to improve ventilation. Diuretic therapy should be guided by the patient's estimated intravascular volume since routine diuresis can result in hypotension in volume-depleted patients placed on positive pressure ventilation after relief of the airway obstruction.

The present patient had radiographic features of acute pulmonary edema after extubation and required urgent reintubation. On positive pressure ventilation, the pulmonary edema rapidly cleared over several hours. Subsequent evaluation determined that the patient had bilateral vocal cord paralysis due to the blunt head trauma and resulting injury to the vagus nerve (cranial nerve X) in the posterior fossa. He required a tracheotomy to allow removal of the endotracheal tube.

Clinical Pearls

1. Some degree of acute pulmonary edema will develop in up to 11% of adults undergoing intubation or tracheotomy for relief of upper airway obstruction.

2. Although extreme negative intrathoracic pressures generated during inspiratory efforts appear to be a likely hydrostatic cause of obstruction-related pulmonary edema, high protein content in edema fluid indicates a role for increased alveolar capillary permeability defect.

3. Patients less than 40 years of age are at greatest risk for developing pulmonary edema after relief of upper airway obstruction because they have well-developed thoracic musculature that enables the generation of profound intrathoracic negative pressures.

4. Blunt head trauma with posterior fossa injury is an unusual cause of bilateral vocal cord paralysis, which can cause upper airway obstruction and pulmonary edema.

REFERENCES

1. Lorch DG, Sahn SA. Post-extubation pulmonary edema following anesthesia induced by upper airway obstruction. Are certain patients at increased risk? Chest 1986;90:802–805.
2. Pfenninger J. Bilateral vocal cord paralysis after severe blunt head injury—a cause of failed extubation. Crit Care Med 1987;15:701–702.
3. Dohi S, Okubo N, Kondo Y. Pulmonary oedema after airway obstruction due to bilateral vocal cord paralysis. Can J Anaesth 1991;38:492–495.
4. Kollef MH, Pluss J. Noncardiogenic pulmonary edema following upper airway obstruction: seven cases and a review of the literature. Medicine 1991;70:91–98.
5. Cascade PN, Alexander GD, Mackie DS. Negative-pressure pulmonary edema after endotracheal intubation. Radiology 1993;186:671–675.

PATIENT 36

A 27-year-old woman with systemic lupus erythematosus and pulmonary infiltrates

A 27-year-old woman presented with a 5-month history of symmetric polyarthralgia, progressive dyspnea on exertion, pleuritic chest pain, and nonproductive cough. She also reported night sweats and a 26-pound weight loss. Several trials of oral antibiotics over the previous 2 months were not helpful.

Physical Examination: Skin: malar rash. Neck: subcutaneous emphysema. Nodes: normal. Chest: diffuse rales. Cardiac: normal. Extremities: no clubbing.

Laboratory Findings: Hct 30%; WBC 4100/μl with 58% neutrophils, 28% lymphocytes, 11% monocytes, 3% eosinophils; ESR = 56 mm/hr. ANA positive at 1:2,560 (homogeneous pattern). ABG (RA): pH 7.45; PCO_2 36 mmHg; PO_2 68 mmHg. PFTs: FVC 1.68 L (45% predicted): FEV_1 1.48 L (50% predicted). Chest radiograph (shown below): bilateral patchy alveolar infiltrates, pneumomediastinum, and subcutaneous emphysema.

Question: What diagnoses should be considered as a cause of this patient's pulmonary infiltrates?

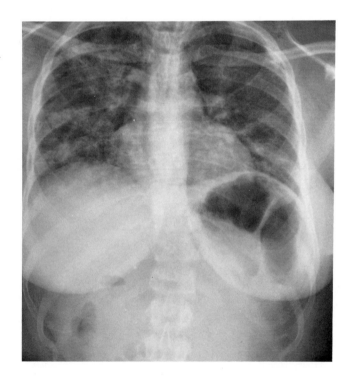

Diagnosis: Bronchiolitis obliterans organizing pneumonia (BOOP) as a manifestation of systemic lupus erythematosus (SLE).

Discussion: The respiratory system is affected more commonly in SLE than in any other collagen vascular disease, and respiratory symptoms may be the first clinical manifestation. Diagnoses to consider include lupus pleuritis, lupus pneumonitis, respiratory muscle dysfunction, pulmonary embolus, and, rarely, bronchiolitis obliterans or bronchiolitis obliterans with organizing pneumonia.

The pleura is the most common site of thoracic involvement in SLE, occurring in 60–75% of patients during the course of their illness. The usual clinical presentation is a small to moderate effusion with pleuritic pain. The pleural fluid is typically serous or serosanguinous, exudative, and with a variable cell count and differential. The presence of LE cells in the pleural fluid is highly specific but sensitivity is variable. Pleural fluid ANA greater than 1:160 or pleural fluid ANA:serum ANA of greater than 1.0 suggests lupus pleuritis. In contrast to rheumatoid pleurisy, lupus pleuritis is dramatically responsive to corticosteroids.

Lupus pneumonitis commonly presents with acute onset of dyspnea, fever, cough, hypoxemia, and sometimes hemoptysis. The chest radiograph shows bilateral or unilateral patchy, alveolar infiltrates, worse in the lower lung zones. Alveolar hemorrhage occurs in a subgroup of patients with lupus pneumonitis and may be subclinical or massive. The primary mechanism of injury is immune complex deposition, but vasculitis may also be present. Lupus pneumonitis may occur any time after the diagnosis of SLE is established; however, there appears to be an increased risk of lupus pneumonitis in the immediate postpartum period. Treatment of acute pneumonitis is high-dose corticosteroids (1–2 mg/kg/day). The addition of azathioprine (2–2.5 mg/kg), cyclophosphamide (1.5–2.0 mg/kg), and plasmapheresis have been used with variable success.

Some patients with SLE have an increased incidence of pulmonary thromboembolic disease due to the presence of lupus anticoagulant, which increases the risk of both arterial and venous thromboembolism. Pulmonary vasculitis is rarely the etiology for thromboembolism in SLE.

Respiratory muscle dysfunction related to SLE can lead to the "shrinking lung syndrome." Several studies have shown diaphragm and respiratory muscle weakness in at least 25% of patients who have normal phrenic nerve function and an absence of a generalized muscle disorder. There is a fall in forced vital capacity, which eventually tends to stabilize.

The risk of pulmonary infection is increased due to underlying immunologic abnormalities, immunosuppressive therapy, and respiratory muscle weakness. Bronchopneumonia is the cause of death in up to 15% of patients with SLE. Opportunistic pathogens, including *Nocardia, Aspergillus, Cryptococcus, Pneumocystis carinii,* and cytomegalovirus, are responsible for up to 7% of cases of pneumonia.

Obstructive pulmonary disease due to SLE is rare, occurring in only 5% of nonsmoking SLE patients. The mechanism of the obstruction is poorly understood, but there is a single report of bronchiolitis obliterans on lung biopsy. There are also reports of laryngeal inflammation with potential upper airway obstruction in the setting of an acute flareup of SLE.

BOOP is rarely associated with SLE and occurs anytime from initial presentation to 30 years after the diagnosis of SLE. BOOP may occur in the absence of other manifestations of active SLE. Treatment of SLE-associated BOOP has included high-dose corticosteroids and cyclophosphamide. Therapy is generally less successful in patients with lupus compared to those with other conditions complicated by BOOP.

The present patient underwent thoracoscopic lung biopsy that revealed BOOP. She was started on prednisone (1 mg/kg/day). Her cough and chest pain resolved, but her dyspnea and pulmonary function tests did not improve. Her pneumomediastinum, a result of severe cough, resolved spontaneously.

Clinical Pearls

1. Lupus pneumonitis is an acute disease caused by immune complex deposition in the lungs. There is an increased risk in the immediate postpartum period.

2. Bronchiolitis obliterans organizing pneumonia (BOOP) is a rare complication of SLE and tends to be less steroid-responsive than other forms of BOOP.

3. "Shrinking lung syndrome" is due to isolated respiratory muscle weakness and occurs in up to 25% of SLE patients; lung restriction usually stabilizes over time.

REFERENCES

1. Kinney WW, Angelillo VA. Bronchiolitis in systemic lupus erythematosus. Chest 1982;82:646–648.
2. Howe HS, Boey ML, Fong KY, et al. Pulmonary haemorrhage, pulmonary infarction, and the lupus anticoagulant. Ann Rheum Dis 1988;47:869–872.
3. Wiedemann HP, Matthay RA. Pulmonary manifestations of the collagen vascular diseases. Clin Chest Med 1989;10:677–722.
4. Godeau B, Cormier C, Menkes CJ. Bronchiolitis obliterans in systemic lupus erythematosus: beneficial effect of intravenous cyclophosphamide. Ann Rheum Dis 1991;50:956–958.
5. Gammon RB, Bridges TA, Al-Nezir H, et al. Bronchiolitis obliterans organizing pneumonia associated with systemic lupus erythematosus. Chest 1992;102:1171–1174.

PATIENT 37

A 69-year-old man with weight loss, dyspnea, and productive sputum

A 69-year-old man experienced a 3-month history of progressive dyspnea and a 20-pound weight loss. Several weeks before admission, a persistent dry cough became productive of a moderate volume of clear, watery sputum. Despite the administration of erythromycin for presumed pneumonia, the dyspnea and sputum production worsened. The patient denied occupational exposures, use of prescription or illicit drugs, a history of smoking, or extensive travel other than a recent move to Phoenix from San Francisco. He stated that previous HIV testing had been negative but refused to discuss his sexual history.

Physical Examination: Temperature 98°; pulse 110; respirations 26; blood pressure 128/89 mmHg. General: thin, chronically ill-appearing. Lymph nodes: scattered axillary nodes. Fundi: normal. Chest: scattered bilateral rhonchi and rales. Cardiac: Grade I/VI short systolic ejection murmur. Abdomen: no organomegaly.

Laboratory Findings: WBC 8,000/μl with a normal differential; Hct 41%. Electrolytes, BUN, creatinine, and liver function tests: normal. Urinalysis: no cells, 1+ protein. Sputum Gram stain: no WBC or bacteria. ABG (RA): PO$_2$ 66 mmHg; PCO$_2$ 32 mmHg: pH 7.47. Chest radiographs: shown below.

Question: Considering the patient's clinical presentation, what is the likely diagnosis?

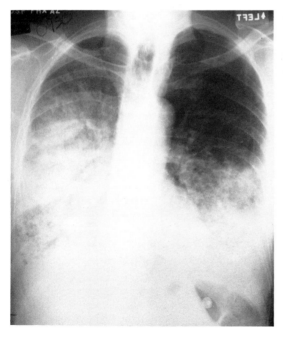 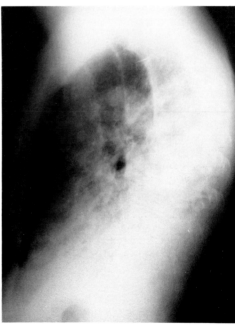

Diagnosis: Diffuse bronchoalveolar (alveolar cell) carcinoma with bronchorrhea.

Discussion: Bronchoalveolar carcinoma is a peculiar form of lung cancer with variable clinical, radiographic, and histologic presentations. Representing 2–6% of primary pulmonary malignancies, the relative rarity of bronchoalveolar carcinoma has delayed its accurate description by limiting the extent of clinical experience within individual institutions. Recent large patient series, however, have more clearly defined this cell type as a heterogeneous category of cancers that share similar epidemiologic and histologic features but differ in natural history and outcome.

Patients most commonly present between the fifth and eighth decades of life, although children as young as 12 years of age have been reported. Women have a high incidence of bronchoalveolar carcinoma compared to other forms of lung cancer, and represent 30–50% of patients. Causal linkage with cigarette use is not clearly established, as up to 25–50% of patients may be nonsmokers. Simultaneous development of bronchoalveolar carcinoma in adult identical twins suggests the importance of congenital factors in tumor growth and development. Underlying lung scars also appear important in tumorigenesis in that 13–60% of patients will have conditions that cause pulmonary fibrotic reactions, such as healed tuberculosis, pulmonary infarctions, bronchiectasis, lipoid pneumonia, idiopathic pulmonary fibrosis, or scleroderma.

The histologic appearance and manner of tissue spread of bronchoalveolar carcinoma represent unique features of the disorder. Arising in the peripheral lung beyond grossly recognizable airways, initial tumor growth occurs within alveolar or bronchiolar structures. Attempts to establish the specific cell of origin have fueled controversy in that different investigators using specialized histologic techniques have reached varying conclusions. In order to unify these observations, current concepts of pathogenesis accept a heterogeneous histogenesis of bronchoalveolar carcinoma from different cell lines that include type II cells, Clara cells, and bronchial mucus cells.

Once established, bronchoalveolar carcinoma presents a distinctive histologic appearance. Tumor cells line alveolar walls without disturbing the underlying pulmonary parenchyma. Well-differentiated tumors consist of tall columnar cells with vacuolated cytoplasm that use bronchoalveolar surfaces as supporting stroma and sources of nutrition. Nuclei are basally situated, cells in mitosis are rarely evident, and alveolar lumina are filled with mucin. Less well-differentiated tumors secrete less mucin and line the alveolar walls with low columnar or cuboidal cells that have bizarre nuclei. Alveolar walls may appear thickened by fibrous tissue in the poorly differentiated cell types.

Bronchoalveolar carcinoma subsequently spreads to adjacent alveolar units along the surfaces of peripheral airways. Central airways rarely become obstructed, remaining patent even when the lung regions they supply fill with tumor cells and mucin. Airway spread complemented by hematogenous and lymphatic routes of dissemination establishes multicentric deposits that simulate a synchronous onset of multiple primary tumors.

Primary and metastatic adenocarcinoma can simulate the histologic appearance of bronchoalveolar carcinoma, with tumor cells lining alveolar structures and mucin-filled alveolar lumina. Diagnostic criteria for bronchoalveolar carcinoma, therefore, require an absence of a known primary adenocarcinoma or central tumor of bronchogenic origin in addition to the peripheral tumor location, intact interstitial framework, and histologic appearance of cancer cells growing along alveolar walls.

Controversy has centered on the natural history of bronchoalveolar carcinoma, with some reports emphasizing the slow growth of tumors and others profiling patients as having a relentless cancer with rapid progression. At present, bronchoalveolar carcinoma appears to assume one of two different forms—localized and diffuse—each having different rates of progression, implications for management, and clinical presentations.

Patients with the localized form usually present with an asymptomatic solitary, peripheral pulmonary nodule 1–10 cm, but usually 2–4 cm, in diameter. The nodule has indistinct or spiculed borders because of the fibrotic reaction in surrounding pulmonary tissue. Prominent strands streaking to the pleural surface seen on tomography or CT ("tail sign") are commonly observed but also are found in patients with peripheral adenocarcinoma and granulomatous inflammation. The nodule may cavitate in 7% of patients but commonly contains an air bronchogram because of the tumor's mode of growth along the surface of airways that does not cause airway occlusion. Localized air bronchograms within lung nodules also occur in pulmonary lymphoma and round pneumonia. Mediastinal lymphadenopathy or pleural effusions rarely occur in the localized form of the disease.

Localized bronchoalveolar carcinoma may simulate benign pulmonary disorders because the tumor's slow growth can maintain radiographic stability for as long as 10 years. The preferred therapy is extirpation of the primary tumor whenever possible, which has a 70% rate of cure for tumors less than 3 cm in diameter. No apparent survival advantage has been demonstrated for lobectomy compared to wedge resection. Although solitary bronchoalveolar carcinoma appears not to progress to the diffuse form of the disease, preoperative lung CT is recommended to exclude multicentric tumors.

Diffuse bronchoalveolar carcinoma is defined by the presence of multiple nodules or consolidation within a single or multiple lobe. The nodules may appear radiographically well circumscribed, similar to those that occur in metastatic extrathoracic malignancies. Extensive lobar consolidation may simulate bacterial pneumonia or less commonly undergo lymphangitic spread and assume a more interstitial radiographic appearance, similar to interstitial pulmonary edema or idiopathic pulmonary fibrosis. Air bronchograms commonly occur because of the alveolar-filling nature of the disease.

Five to 30% of patients with diffuse disease have associated pleural effusions, and 15–30% have hilar or mediastinal adenopathy. Lobar or segmental atelectasis rarely occurs, although intra-airway spread can create a check valve obstruction, causing localized hyperinflation and pneumothorax. The CT appearance is unique, with homogeneously low attenuation within regions of tumor infiltration that allow enhanced pulmonary vessels to stand out after the intravenous infusion of contrast material ("CT angiogram sign"). This CT finding is caused by alveolar filling with mucin and the intact bronchovascular framework within the tumor.

Patients with the diffuse form of the disease commonly present with symptoms that include cough, weight loss, chest pain from pleural involvement, dyspnea, and increased sputum production. The severity of dyspnea and weight loss correlates with the extent of tumor spread.

Bronchorrhea is a classic but less common presentation that is characterized by copious watery sputum. Extreme volumes of airway secretions not only may cause respiratory embarrassment but also may produce electrolyte disturbances.

Diffuse bronchoalveolar carcinoma is an aggressive tumor that responds poorly to radiation and chemotherapy, and the 5-year survival is similar to that of other forms of lung cancer. Resectional surgery is rarely successful since even patients with apparent lobar localization of tumor have more widespread disease when examined by CT. Various therapies to manage bronchorrhea, such as atropine, stellate ganglion block, radiation therapy, and corticosteroids, have not had reproducible success.

Diagnosis of both localized and diffuse bronchoalveolar carcinoma depends on cytologic or tissue biopsy demonstration of malignant cells. Sputum cytology may be positive in 18–60% of patients, with the diffuse form of the disease having the higher yield. Cytologic examination cannot differentiate bronchoalveolar carcinoma from adenocarcinoma. Fiberoptic bronchoscopy detects an endobronchial lesion in less than one-third of patients, of whom 50% will have a positive tissue biopsy. Bronchoscopic washings are positive in 26% of patients. In diffuse bronchoalveolar carcinoma, transbronchial biopsies are more likely to demonstrate tumor than solitary nodules, which are diagnosed by percutaneous needle aspiration in 70 to 90% of patients. Thoracentesis and pleural fluid cytology are indicated in patients with pleural effusions.

The present patient had negative sputum cytologic examinations and underwent bronchoscopy, which demonstrated typical features of bronchoalveolar carcinoma in transbronchial biopsy specimens. He is undergoing radiation therapy in an attempt to control the severity of bronchorrhea.

Clinical Pearls

1. Bronchoalveolar carcinoma is characterized by tumor cells that line the alveolar surface without disrupting the underlying pulmonary parenchyma.

2. An intact pulmonary parenchyma and nonobstructed airways within regions of tumor infiltration produce air bronchograms on routine chest radiographs and the "angiogram sign" on CT thoracic examination.

3. The localized form of bronchoalveolar carcinoma may simulate benign disease with a slow rate of growth that maintains radiographic stability for many years.

4. Bronchoalveolar carcinoma appears less clearly linked to cigarette smoking than other forms of lung cancer, has a probable congenital basis of growth and development, and occurs more commonly in patients with underlying pulmonary scars.

5. Localized bronchoalveolar carcinoma may be a distinct entity since it rarely progresses to the diffuse form of the disease.

REFERENCES

1. Joishy SK, Cooper RA, Rowley PT. Alveolar cell carcinoma in identical twins: similarity in time of onset, histochemistry, and site of metastasis. Ann Intern Med 1977;87:447–450.
2. Harpole DH, Bigelow C, Young WG Jr, et al. Alveolar cell carcinoma of the lung: a retrospective analysis of 205 patients. Ann Thorac Surg 1988;46:502–507.
3. Im J-G, Han MC, Yu EJ, et al. Lobar bronchioalveolar carcinoma: "angiogram sign" on CT scans. Thorac Radiol 1990;176:749–753.
4. Epstein DM. Bronchioalveolar carcinoma. Semin Roentgenol 1990;24:105–111.

PATIENT 38

A 70-year-old man with a nonresolving pneumonia

A 70-year-old man was referred for evaluation of a nonresolving pneumonia. He reported a 4-month history of dyspnea, low-grade fevers, nightsweats, and nonproductive cough. There was no relief of symptoms or radiographic change in the infiltrate after 10 days of intravenous antibiotics. He reported a 15-pack-year history of smoking but denied exposure to tuberculosis or chronic use of nose drops or mineral oil. The patient had undergone a right lower lobe resection 20 years earlier for a necrotizing pneumonia.

Physical Examination: Temperature 100.3°; respirations 24; General: well nourished; in no acute distress. Chest: egophony over the left anterior and lateral thorax with bronchial breath sounds.

Laboratory Findings: Hct 38.6%; WBC 10,400/μl; platelets 308,000/μl. Electrolytes: normal; albumin 3.1 g/dl; LDH 186 IU/L. ABG (RA): pH 7.41; PCO_2 39 mmHg; PO_2 77 mmHg. Chest radiograph (shown below): lingular infiltrate with air bronchograms; volume loss on right with right hilar density.

Question: What should be included in the differential diagnosis of a nonresolving pneumonia in this patient?

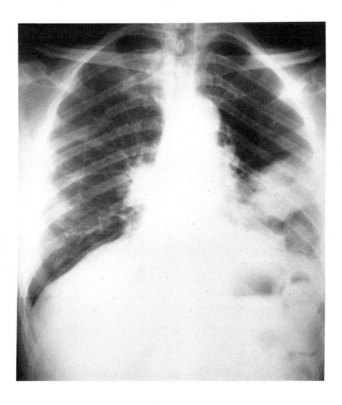

Diagnosis: Primary pulmonary lymphoma.

Discussion: Primary pulmonary lymphoma is a distinct entity that accounts for less than 5% of extranodal lymphomas. Arising de novo in lung tissue, a primary lymphoma is defined by the absence of other organ system or hilar/mediastinal lymph node involvement. Most of these tumors are small-cell lymphomas that follow an indolent course.

Symptoms commonly include nonproductive cough, chest pain, fever, hemoptysis, and dyspnea. Almost half of the patients with non-Hodgkin lymphoma confined to the thorax, however, are asymptomatic.

Three distinct radiologic patterns of parenchymal lymphoma have been described: nodular, bronchovascular, and pneumonic-alveolar. Nodular involvement, the most frequent radiographic pattern, is characterized by round or oval lesions with ill-defined edges that may have spicules or surrounding satellite nodules and air bronchograms with occasional cavitation. These solitary lesions are most commonly found in the lower lobes and frequently traverse lobar fissures.

Bronchovascular involvement, when central, presents with a reticulonodular pattern radiating from the hilum and is usually (86%) associated with mediastinal adenopathy. In large-cell lymphomas, diffuse lymphangitic infiltrates are the most common presentation and can be rapidly progressive.

A pneumonic-alveolar infiltrate, as seen in the present patient (figure, previous page), occurs in about 25% of patients and is indistinguishable from bacterial pneumonia. Consolidation is not accompanied by volume loss.

The differential diagnosis of a nonresolving pneumonia with any one of these radiographic patterns includes a postobstructive process (endobronchial foreign body or malignancy), an inflammatory or granulomatous process, bronchoalveolar cell carcinoma, lipoid pneumonia, and amyloidosis, in addition to pulmonary lymphoma.

Endobronchial lymphomas can present in one of two patterns. Type 1 pattern describes diffuse submucosal lesions that arise by hematogenous or lymphangitic spread. Type 2 pattern defines a solitary mass that causes respiratory symptoms and occurs by direct spread from adjacent lymph nodes. Both types are associated with mediastinal adenopathy and are, therefore, not considered true primary pulmonary lymphoma.

Diagnosis requires an understanding of the classification system. Histologic types include well-differentiated lymphocytic, lymphoplasmacytoid, small cleaved cell and large cell. Findings such as germinal centers and well-differentiated lymphocytes and plasma cells have been used as criteria to imply a more benign process. The use of in situ hybridization, immunohistochemistry, and gene rearrangement techniques has enabled the establishment of monoclonality of the involved lymphocytes by examining the light chains. The absence of cytoplasmic immunoglobulin staining should not be interpreted as absence of a neoplastic process, because it can occur in resting B-lymphocytes and in T-cell lesions.

Transbronchial biopsies, brushings, bronchoalveolar lavage, and transbronchial needle aspiration all may be diagnostic provided that cells are sent for cytoplasmic immunoglobulin studies when a preponderance of lymphocytes is found.

Treatment for primary pulmonary lymphoma is surgical resection. Radiation therapy is indicated for mediastinal disease (stages 1 and 2). Chemotherapy, combination or single drug, is reserved for pleural and widespread disease (stages 3 and 4).

The 5-year survival in patients with small-cell lymphoma of the lung is 70–88%, with recurrence a mean of 69 months following remission. Disseminated disease carries a median survival of 33 months.

The present patient underwent bronchoscopy with transbronchial biopsies that revealed a monomorphic lymphoid population suspicious for lymphoma. Immunochemistry demonstrated lambda light-chain monotypism consistent with a B-cell lymphoma. No hilar or mediastinal lymphadenopathy was found on CT scan of the chest. The patient was referred for surgical evaluation.

Clinical Pearls

1. A pneumonic-alveolar pattern of pulmonary lymphoma should be included in the differential diagnosis of nonresolving segmental or lobar consolidation on chest radiograph, particularly in the presence of air bronchograms without volume loss.

2. Immunohistochemistry of transbronchial biopsies, brushings, and BAL specimens can determine monoclonal proliferation, a diagnostic indicator of B-cell lymphoma.

3. Primary pulmonary lymphoma is an uncommon chest malignancy that can be cured by surgery.

REFERENCES

1. Balikian J, Herman P. Non-Hodgkin lymphoma of the lungs. Diagn Radiol 1979;132:569–576.
2. Peterson H, Snider H, Yam L, et al. Primary pulmonary lymphoma. Cancer 1985;56:805–808.
3. Yam L, Lin D, Janckila A, Li C. Immunocytochemical diagnosis of lymphoma in serous effusions. Acta Cytol 1985;29:5;833–841.
4. Breuer R, Berkman N. Pulmonary lymphoma. Pulmonary and Critical Care Update, Am Coll Chest Physicians 1993;8:1–7.
5. Koss MN. Pulmonary lymphoproliferative disorders. Monogr Pathol 1993;36:145–194.
6. Drent M, Wagenaar SS, Mulder PH, et al. Bronchoalveolar lavage fluid profiles in sarcoidosis, tuberculosis, and non-Hodgkin's and Hodgkin's disease: an evaluation of differences. Chest 1994;105:514–519.

PATIENT 39

A 34-year-old man with systemic lupus, chest pain, and hemoptysis

A 34-year-old man with systemic lupus erythematosus was admitted because of a 2-day history of pleuritic chest pain, dyspnea, moderate frank hemoptysis, and fever unresponsive to azithromycin. He denied recent travels, loss of consciousness, exposure to others with known respiratory infections, or contact with animals. His lupus had been well controlled until 1 month earlier when worsening thrombocytopenia had required 60 mg of prednisone a day. The patient did not drink or use illicit drugs.

Physical Examination: Temperature 40.1°C; pulse 120; respirations 22; blood pressure 120/75. Skin: truncal petechiae. Fundi: normal. Chest: dullness right posterior mid-chest with tubular breath sounds and pleural friction rub. Cardiac: S4 present without murmur. Abdomen: no hepatosplenomegaly.

Laboratory Findings: Hct 34%; WBC 13,500/μl with 85% polymorphonuclear cells and 10% bands. Electrolytes and renal indices: normal. ABG (RA): pH 7.48; PCO_2 28 mmHg; PO_2 62 mmHg. Sputum Gram stain: red blood cells mixed with leukocytes; no organisms. Sputum special stains: negative for *Legionella* species, fungi, and acid-fast organisms. Chest radiographs: shown below.

Question: Considering the patient's rapid progression of symptoms and underlying immuno-compromise, what diagnosis requires early exclusion?

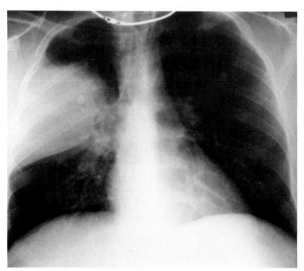
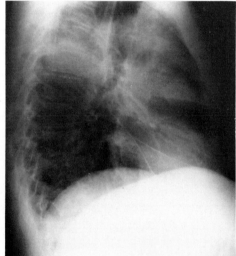

Diagnosis: Pulmonary mucormycosis.

Discussion: The rapid progression of respiratory symptoms suggestive of pulmonary infarction in a febrile, immunocompromised patient warrants urgent evaluation for mucormycosis. This highly lethal but relatively rare disorder has a predilection for vascular invasion and occurs as a result of infection with fungal pathogens from the order Mucorales. Within this order, 12 classes of fungi are considered pathogenic for man, with the most common infections caused by *Rhizopus, Rhizomucor, Absidia,* and *Mucor.*

Although ubiquitous in nature and easily isolated from decaying vegetation, soil, and air, these organisms are relatively avirulent and require an underlying immunocompromised state to initiate infection. Commonly associated underlying conditions include diabetes mellitus (especially with diabetic ketoacidosis), hyperglycemia, hematologic malignancies, neutropenia, immunosuppressive therapy, soft tissue trauma, and chronic renal failure. Of interest is an association of deferoxamine therapy with disseminated mucormycosis in patients with renal failure who are undergoing therapy for iron or aluminum overload. The conditions that predispose patients to mucormycosis share in common defects in either local or systemic neutrophilic and mononuclear phagocytic function. Rare reports exist of patients with pulmonary mucormycosis who do not have clinically apparent immunocompromise.

The five major clinical forms of mucormycosis include rhinocerebral, pulmonary, cutaneous, gastrointestinal, and disseminated disease. Pulmonary infection is initiated when sporangiospores are inhaled and deposited in alveolar structures. Spores germinate into hyphal elements that then penetrate bronchiole walls. Once within the lung interstitium, hyphae invade pulmonary blood vessels, causing vascular thrombosis with resultant necrosis and hemorrhagic infarction of distal lung parenchyma. Dissection of the vascular lamina away from the media by the invading fungi can result in vascular rupture and major hemoptysis. More proximal extension of fungal infection also may cause formation of pseudoaneurysms of the major pulmonary arteries. Additional complications include bronchial erosion, bronchopleural fistulas, granulomatous mediastinitis, and embolic dissemination.

Although rare instances of a chronic form of the disease have been reported, most patients have rapidly progressive, fulminant disease. Patients typically present with clinically apparent immunocompromise combined with fever, chills, dyspnea, and pleuritic chest pain that have failed to respond to antibiotic therapy. Because of the vascular tropism of Mucorales and resultant infarction of lung tissue, clinical manifestations commonly simulate those of pulmonary thromboembolic disease, including a pleural friction rub. Hemoptysis of varying degrees is a frequent finding.

The chest radiograph is variable in appearance, reflecting the presence of pulmonary hemorrhage, localized infection, and tissue gangrene with varying infiltrates with or without cavitation. Rounded infiltrates with ill-defined margins are the most common radiographic findings; nodular, lobar, wedge-shaped, and miliary pulmonary infiltrates also occur. Regions of atelectasis may represent airway plugging with thick purulent material. Mycotic aneurysms of the pulmonary arteries may appear as rapidly enlarging round or fusiform masses that may simulate neoplasms, lung abscesses, or regions of pneumonia. As in invasive aspergillosis, the chest CT scan may reveal target lesions with a surrounding "halo sign," which may represent a zone of hemorrhage or edema around a nidus of infection.

Pulmonary mucormycosis typically requires invasive procedures for diagnosis because Gram stains and cultures of expectorated sputum are rarely positive and serologic tests are unreliable. Recent reports indicate that fiberoptic bronchoscopy with bronchoalveolar lavage may demonstrate the characteristic nonsepte, broad, fungal hyphae that branch at a 90° angle. Tissue specimens from transbronchial or open lung biopsies are often required, however, to diagnose the disorder. The fungi stain most avidly with Grocott-Gomori methenamine-silver nitrate and frequently appear in tissue actively invading vessels surrounded by an inflammatory exudate of neutrophils. Cultures of lavage fluids are often negative, even in patients with tissue confirmation of large numbers of fungal elements. The diagnostic yield is enhanced if tissue is submitted to the microbiology laboratory for culture.

Although prospective studies of optimal therapy in pulmonary mucormycosis do not exist, clinical experience indicates that an aggressive, combined surgical and medical approach improves outcome. Any underlying immunocompromised state should be reversed as rapidly as possible. Patients with localized disease who are surgical candidates may be considered for removal of infected and necrotic lung tissue. Patients with pseudoaneurysms of the pulmonary arteries require vascular surgery with insertion of a graft before massive arterial rupture occurs. Amphotericin B should be initiated in doses of 1 mg/kg/day (1.5 mg/kg/day initially in severe cases) and tapered to a maintenance dose of 0.8 to 1 mg/kg/day after stabilization. Total duration of therapy is guided by the patient's clinical and radiographic response; some patients with pulmonary mucormycosis and localized disease have recovered with surgical resection alone without concomitant therapy with amphotericin B. Despite aggressive therapy, the mortality associated with pulmonary mucormycosis is as high as 80% in some clinical series.

The present patient had severe pneumonia with clinical features of pulmonary infarction that failed to respond to antibiotic therapy. The maintenance therapy with large doses of corticosteroids indicated a risk of opportunistic pathogens. He underwent fiberoptic bronchoscopy with bronchoalveolar lavage that identified Mucorales organisms. He was treated with intravenous amphotericin B followed by lobectomy, which resulted in full recovery.

Clinical Pearls

1. The rapid progression of respiratory symptoms suggestive of pulmonary infarction that fail to respond to antibiotics in an immunocompromised patient warrants evaluation for mucormycosis.

2. In addition to the usual immunocompromising conditions associated with fungal infection, patients with metabolic acidosis and patients treated with deferoxamine are at an increased risk for mucormycosis.

3. In addition to producing pulmonary parenchymal infection and tissue infarction, Mucorales organisms have a propensity to invade major pulmonary arteries and produce pseudoaneurysms.

4. Patients with pulmonary mucormycosis typically have a fulminant disease. Rare reports exist, however, of more indolent infections and pulmonary infections in patients without immunocompromising conditions.

REFERENCES

1. Bigby TD, Serota ML, Tierney LM, Matthay MA. Clinical spectrum of pulmonary mucormycosis. Chest 1986;89:435–439.
2. Potente G. CT findings in fungal opportunistic pneumonia: body and brain involvement. Comput Med Imaging and Graph 1989;13:423–428.
3. Coffey MJ, Fantone J III, Stirling MC, Lynch JP III. Pseudoaneurysm of pulmonary artery in mucormycosis: radiographic characteristics and management. Am Rev Respir Dis 1992;145:1487–1490.
4. Sugar AM. Mucormycosis. Clin Infect Dis 1992;14(Suppl 1):S126–S129.

PATIENT 40

A 27-year-old woman with chronic cough, wheezing, and hemoptysis

A 27-year-old woman who had maintained an active lifestyle of jogging, aerobics, and biking presented with a progressive cough. During the past several weeks she had also noted wheezing during exercise, decreased exercise tolerance, and a single episode of hemoptysis.

Physical Examination: Temperature 96.7°; pulse 80; respirations 18; blood pressure 100/60. Skin: no rash. Neck: no lymphadenopathy; normal thyroid gland. Lungs: localized wheezing over the right upper chest. Cardiac: no murmurs. Extremities: no clubbing or cyanosis.

Laboratory Findings: CBC: normal. Electrolytes and renal indices: normal. ECG: normal. FVC = 3.76 L (95% predicted). FEV$_1$ = 3.51 L (102% predicted). FEV$_1$/FVC = 93%. Cardiopulmonary exercise test: normal. Chest radiograph: below left. Chest CT: below right.

Question: Based on the presentation and subsequent work-up, what is the most likely diagnosis?

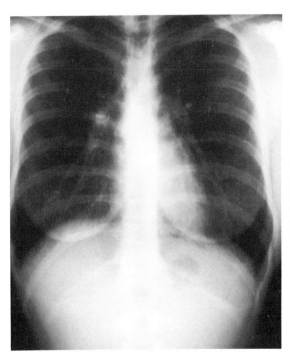
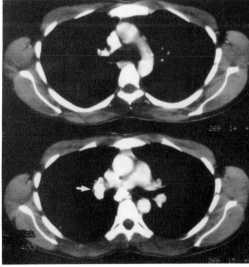

Diagnosis: Broncholithiasis.

Discussion: Broncholithiasis is an unusual condition that results from injury to the bronchial tree by the compressive or erosive effects of calcified mediastinal lymph nodes. Lymph node calcification results most commonly from infectious etiologies, with histoplasmosis being the most frequent underlying cause of broncholithiasis in the United States. Other causes include tuberculosis, coccidioidomycosis, actinomycosis, cryptococcosis, nocardiosis, and silicosis. Following a granulomatous infection, the alkaline pH of the healing lymph node promotes dystrophic calcification. Over time, constant cardiac and respiratory movements of the calcific node result in external compression or erosion of the adjacent airways and vascular structures, accounting for the clinical manifestations.

Broncholithiasis is found in equal frequency in males and females. Although any age group may be affected, the median age of onset is 50 years. In 60% of patients reported, the right lung is involved. Although lithoptysis (coughing up of "stones" or gritty material) is a diagnostic sign, it occurs in less than 20% of patients. The most common symptom is a nonspecific chronic cough. Other presenting features include hemoptysis, fevers and chills due to obstructive pneumonitis, pleuritic pain, wheezing, and dyspnea. Rarely, the chronic cough at presentation may be due to a bronchoesophageal fistula caused by the broncholith.

The expectoration of calcified gritty material or identification of a "stone" in the airways by radiographic studies or bronchoscopy establishes the diagnosis of broncholithiasis. The presence of hilar or carinal lymph node calcification with bronchoscopic evidence of distortion of the bronchial lumen in symptomatic patients can support the diagnosis. The mere presence of hilar calcification on a chest radiograph does not predict the subsequent development of broncholithiasis. Although most chest radiographs show lymph node calcification, the chest radiograph may be normal in some patients. Noncontrast CT scan of the chest will identify calcified lymph nodes in virtually every case, although peribronchial or endobronchial localization by this method is not 100% accurate.

Fiberoptic bronchoscopy can identify endobronchial broncholiths in 25–50% of patients. In one series, which retrospectively reviewed bronchoscopic findings, airway inspection was normal in 12% of patients who were eventually diagnosed with broncholithiasis. When attempted, bronchoscopic broncholithectomy is best done with a rigid bronchoscope for better stone mobilization and more secure management of the massive hemoptysis that may result from manipulation of the broncholith. Some experts advocate bronchoscopic removal only if the stone is loose and free, to avoid fistula formation or tearing of the adjacent pulmonary vasculature, or if the stone extends well into the lumen and is friable. Laser bronchoscopy has been reported in one patient to fracture a loose stone and allow its removal in fragments.

Surgical resection offers the most reliable therapy for a long-term, symptom-free result. Bronchotomy with sleeve resections may be technically possible to preserve lung function in patients with localized airway effects from the broncholith but no distal suppuration or bronchiectasis. Because of the attendant risks with any lung resection, such as bleeding and postoperative infection, surgery should be reserved for patients with severe symptoms or massive hemoptysis, or those who fail rigid bronchoscopy.

The present patient had a calcified lymph node in the right hilum that was apparent on the chest CT (arrow, previous page). The broncholith could not be removed by rigid bronchoscopy; thus she underwent a right upper lobectomy. It was noted intraoperatively that the perivascular structures of her right upper lobe were studded with calcified nodules. She recovered uneventfully and experienced no recurrence of symptoms.

Clinical Pearls

1. Chronic cough in the setting of hilar or carinal calcification on chest radiograph should alert the clinician to include broncholithiasis in the differential diagnosis.

2. Localized wheezing on physical examination warrants a close examination of the chest radiograph for evidence of hilar calcification.

3. Surgical resection may be indicated in patients with broncholithiasis who present with hemoptysis. Life-threatening hemoptysis may occur when a broncholith erodes into pulmonary vessels.

4. Forceful removal of broncholiths during fiberoptic bronchoscopy should not be attempted because of the possibility of life-threatening bleeding. Rigid bronchoscopy may be successful in 20% of patients.

REFERENCES

1. Arrigoni MG, Bernatz PE, Donoghue FE. Broncholithiasis. J Thorac Cardiovasc Surg 1971;62:231–237.
2. Faber LP, Jensik RJ, Chawla SK, et al. The surgical implication of broncholithiasis. J Thorac Cardiovasc Surg 1975;70:779–789.
3. Cole FH, Cole FH Jr, Khandekar A, et al. Management of broncholithiasis: is thoracotomy necessary? Ann Thorac Surg 1986;42:255–257.
4. Conces DJ. Broncholithiasis: CT features in 15 patients. Am J Radiol 1991;157:249–253.
5. McLean TR, Beall AC, Jones JW. Massive hemoptysis due to broncholithiasis. Ann Thorac Surg 1991;52:1173–1175.

PATIENT 41

A 20-year-old woman with respiratory failure and a swollen right arm

A 20-year-old woman with hypotension and a ruptured spleen was admitted to the hospital after being involved in an automobile accident. One day after emergency splenectomy, she developed the adult respiratory distress syndrome, which required ventilation with high airway pressures and high concentrations of oxygen. During the first week of care, she received bilateral chest tubes for management of pneumothoraces, total parenteral nutrition, and a tracheotomy. On the fifteenth hospital day, the patient complained of swelling and pain in her right arm.

Physical Examination: Temperature 38°; pulse 110; respirations 24; blood pressure 110/60. Neck: normal venous patterns. Chest: bilateral rhonchi and crackles; subcutaneous emphysema. Cardiac: increased S2. Abdomen: nontender; healing laparotomy incision. Extremities: mild swelling in the right arm with right upper arm and axillary tenderness.

Laboratory Findings: Hct 32%; WBC 12,000/μl; platelets 140,000/μl. Electrolytes and renal indices: normal. Prothrombin time: 12 sec. Partial thromboplastin time: 24 sec. Chest radiograph: shown below.

Question: What diagnostic studies should be pursued?

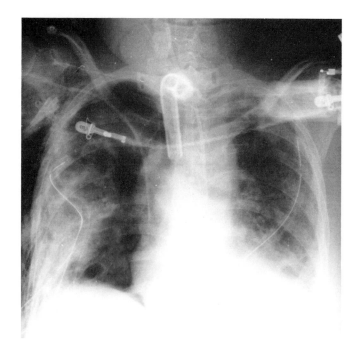

Answer: Ultrasonographic evaluation of the right arm followed by contrast venography if needed to exclude catheter-induced subclavian vein thrombosis.

Discussion: Symptomatic subclavian vein thrombosis is a relatively uncommon disorder, occurring with a frequency that is less than 3% of the reported incidence of lower extremity deep venous thrombosis. Several factors appear to protect the upper extremity from symptomatic thrombophlebitis. First, the effects of gravity maintain blood flow and prevent venous stasis. Second, the subclavian and axillary veins have fewer valves and no sinusoids, both of which tend to propagate clots in the lower extremity. Third, the arm and shoulder have extensive collateral venous networks that allow many instances of subclavian thrombosis to remain asymptomatic and undetected. Finally, the fibrinolytic system of the upper extremity vasculature appears to be more active than that in the lower extremity, as shown by high concentrations of plasminogen activator in endothelium of the subclavian vein.

Various clinical conditions, however, can promote an increased risk of subclavian vein thrombosis in individual patients. An underlying malignancy may directly compress thoracic vascular structures or generate a hypercoagulable state that predisposes to subclavian vein thrombosis. The combination of an intrathoracic malignancy and thoracic radiation presents a particularly high risk. Direct vascular trauma, septic thrombophlebitis as occurs in drug addicts, and the hypercoagulable states associated with congestive heart failure and nephrotic syndrome are additional predisposing conditions. Young patients may develop spontaneous subclavian thrombosis (Paget-Schroetter syndrome) subsequent to forceful upper extremity muscular contraction (effort thrombosis) or anatomic compression of venous structures by a first cervical rib, hypertrophied subclavian musculature, or the costocoracoid ligament.

Venous irritation from a central venous catheter has become a leading cause of subclavian vein thrombosis. Although catheter-induced thrombosis is considered to represent 30–40% of all instances of subclavian thrombosis, the exact incidence of this disorder is unclear because many patients remain asymptomatic and undiagnosed. Several studies indicate that only 3% of patients undergoing central venous catheterization experience clinically evident subclavian vein thrombosis. In contrast, other studies demonstrate a 33–60% incidence when all catheterized patients in an intensive care unit are screened with contrast venography. The etiology of this disorder appears to be multifactorial, as suggested by the low incidence of venous thrombosis in otherwise healthy patients with transvenous pacemakers (0.18%). Critically ill patients have multiple risk factors for subclavian thrombosis, such as low cardiac output, hypercoagulable state, sepsis, and underlying carcinomas, that contribute to the thrombogenic effects of central catheterization.

The frequency of clinically important consequences from catheter-induced subclavian vein thrombosis is difficult to define because of the high rate of subclinical disease. Furthermore, many reported clinical series tend to group patients with different causes of subclavian vein thrombosis together, even though prognosis appears to correlate with the nature of the underlying disease. Available data, however, indicate that symptomatic catheter-induced subclavian vein thrombosis may produce venous gangrene, pulmonary emboli, and postthrombotic syndrome.

Venous gangrene subsequent to subclavian vein thrombosis is presently rare since the advent of anticoagulant and fibrinolytic therapy. The incidence of pulmonary emboli in patients with catheter-induced thrombosis appears to be approximately 10%. Rare reports exist of lethal pulmonary embolic disease from upper extremity thrombophlebitis. Postthrombotic syndrome characterized by arm swelling, venous hypertension, and chronic pain occurs in 23% of patients with catheter-induced subclavian vein thrombosis, in contrast to a 40% incidence in patients with other underlying etiologic conditions.

Diagnosis of catheter-induced subclavian thrombosis depends on recognition of the clinical manifestations of pain, swelling, and venous engorgement in the affected arm. Because of the extensive venous network of shoulder collateral vessels, extensive thrombosis can occur with minimal or no signs or symptoms. Ultrasonography is the initial diagnostic study because of its acceptable patient tolerance and high specificity. Detection of venous thrombosis by duplex Doppler or color Doppler scans is sufficient evidence to initiate therapy. Unfortunately, the sensitivity of ultrasonography may be as low as 50% in patients with nonobstructing or short segments of thrombosis, possibly because of acoustic shadowing from the clavicle. Negative ultrasonographic studies, therefore, should be followed by contrast venography when clinical suspicion remains high.

Once diagnosed, patients with catheter-induced subclavian vein thrombosis require central catheter removal and initiation of anticoagulant therapy with intravenous heparin. Anticoagulant therapy has not been shown to decrease the incidence of pulmonary emboli in this condition, but the risk of postthrombotic syndrome can be lowered from 64% to 36%. No data exist to guide the duration of long-term anticoagulation with warfarin (Coumadin), but experiences with lower extremity deep venous thrombosis support recommendations of 6–12 weeks of anticoagulation with longer therapy in patients with persistent underlying thrombogenic risk factors.

The role of thrombolytic therapy in catheter-induced subclavian vein thrombosis is limited by concerns for breakaway thromboemboli, high cost, allergic reactions, and catastrophic complications. Thrombolytic agents are presently reserved for patients with extensive clot, severe symptoms, thrombosis within 6 and preferably 3 days, and low risk for hemorrhagic complications. Low-dose local infusion of thrombolytic drugs into the subclavian vein may be an additional therapeutic option. Preventive therapy has been investigated with 1 mg of Coumadin daily, which decreases the incidence of catheter-induced venous thrombosis from 37.5% to 9.5%.

The present patient was evaluated with duplex Doppler ultrasonography that detected extensive thrombosis of the right subclavian vein. The central catheter was removed and the patient was started on full systemic anticoagulation. She eventually recovered from respiratory failure and was discharged on warfarin therapy to complete a 3-month course.

Clinical Pearls

1. Subclavian vein thrombosis occurs less than 3% as often as deep venous thrombosis of the lower extremity.

2. Catheter-induced thrombosis contributes to 30% of all instances of subclavian vein thrombosis.

3. Although only 3% of patients undergoing central venous catheterization develop symptomatic subclavian vein thrombosis, as many as 33–66% of catheterized patients will have evidence of venous thrombosis when evaluated with screening contrast venography.

4. Postthrombotic syndrome occurs in 23% of patients with catheter-induced subclavian vein thrombosis compared to 40% in patients with other underlying etiologic conditions.

5. Duplex Doppler and color Doppler ultrasonography are highly specific for subclavian vein thrombosis. Because of a lower sensitivity, however, negative studies in high-risk patients require contrast venography to adequately exclude the diagnosis.

REFERENCES

1. Hill SL, Berry RE. Subclavian vein thrombosis: a continuing challenge. Surgery 1990;108:1–9.
2. Aburahma AF, Sadler DL, Robinson PA. Axillary-subclavian vein thrombosis: changing patterns of etiology, diagnostic, and therapeutic modalities. Am Surg 1991;57:101–107.
3. Baxter GM, Kincaid W, Jeffrey RF, et al. Comparison of colour Doppler ultrasound with venography in the diagnosis of axillary and subclavian vein thrombosis. Br J Radiol 1991;64:777–781.
4. Becker DM, Philbrick JT, Walker FB. Axillary and subclavian venous thrombosis. Arch Intern Med 1991;151:1934–1943.
5. Haire WD, Lynch TG, Lund GB, et al. Limitations of magnetic resonance imaging and ultrasound-directed (duplex) scanning in the diagnosis of subclavian vein thrombosis. J Vasc Surg 1991;13:391–397.
6. Wechsler RJ, Spirn PW, Steiner PW, et al. Thrombosis and infection caused by thoracic venous catheters: pathogenesis and imaging findings. AJR 1993;160:467–471.

PATIENT 42

A 58-year-old man with abdominal pain, skin lesions, pruritus, and wheezing

A 58-year-old retired coal miner was evaluated for pruritus, abdominal pain, intermittent wheezing, and fatigue of 2-months' duration. He had smoked one pack of cigarettes per day for 20 years. A benign bladder papilloma had been removed 8 years previously.

Physical Examination: Temperature 98.6°; pulse 82; respirations 22; blood pressure 140/78. Skin: several raised reddish-brown lesions on hands, axillae, anterior abdominal wall, and groin (shown below); a wheal and flare developed when the lesions were stroked. Chest: bilateral wheezes. Cardiac: normal. Abdomen: normal.

Laboratory Findings: Hct 40%; WBC 10,600/μl with a normal differential; platelets 206,000/μl; ESR 14 mm/h. Chest radiograph: minimal bilateral reticulonodular infiltrates. PFTs: FVC 1.90 L (49% of predicted); FEV$_1$ 0.98 L (34% of predicted); FEV$_1$/FVC 52%; RV 3.92 L (186% of predicted); TLC 5.95 L (98% of predicted).

Question: What diagnosis is most likely with this constellation of symptoms and signs?

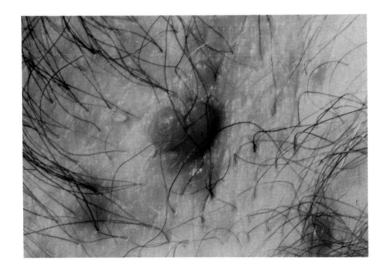

Diagnosis: Systemic mast cell disease.

Discussion: Systemic mast cell disease (SMCD) is an idiopathic disorder characterized by proliferation of mast cells in multiple extracutaneous tissues, including bone marrow, liver, spleen, and lymph nodes. Clinically, mastocytosis may be classified as cutaneous (urticaria pigmentosa), SMCD, mastocytoma presenting as isolated skin nodule, and mast cell leukemia.

Systemic symptoms are observed in 10% of all patients with mastocytosis and occur in the absence of skin lesions in less than 1% of patients. Common symptoms include nausea, vomiting, diarrhea, abdominal pain, weight loss, headache, fatigue, flushing, tachycardia, hypotension, dizziness, and syncope. A high level of circulating histamine/kinins is responsible for symptoms of abdominal pain, esophagitis, diarrhea, cramps, flushing, and syncope. In addition, fever, seizures, back and chest pain, paresthesias, and weakness may occur. Physical examination will show urticaria pigmentosa (small red-brown macules or papules) (see figure), Darier's sign (stroking the lesions causes pruritus and erythema), splenomegaly (50%), hepatomegaly (45%), and lymphadenopathy (40%). Anemia, leukocytosis, and thrombocytopenia are observed in over 30% of patients and eosinophilia in less than 20% of patients. Bone marrow involvement occurs in 70% of patients with this condition and is associated with an increased serum alkaline phosphatase. Radiographic abnormalities include osteoblastic and osteolytic lesions of the skull, vertebrae, ribs, and pelvis in 70%, interstitial fibrosis in 43% and pleural effusion in 10% of patients. Clinical involvement of the lung in SMCD is uncommon. Although some patients complain of dyspnea and rhinitis, wheezing is an unusual finding.

The criteria used for diagnosing SMCD are (1) clinical symptoms related to mast cell disease; (2) increased urinary excretion of histamine (>40 $\mu g/24$ hr); (3) increased urinary excretion of prostaglandin D_2 metabolite; and (4) histologic evidence of increased mast cell proliferation in skin biopsies (>10 mast cells/40 fields). In the absence of skin lesions, bone marrow or liver biopsy is often required to establish the diagnosis. Bone scan is useful in localizing the best site for obtaining a bone biopsy. When the patient has systemic symptoms caused by circulating histamines/kinins in the absence of urticaria pigmentosa, carcinoid syndrome should be considered in the differential diagnosis. Carcinoid syndrome can be excluded by the absence of an elevated 24-hour urine 5-hydroxyindoleacetic acid (5-HIAA). Furthermore, patients with SMCD usually have elevated serum and urinary methyl histamine levels.

Because no curative treatment exists for SMCD, patients are managed symptomatically. H_1 and H_2 antihistamines remain the primary drugs for symptom control. Oral disodium cromoglycate has been used in the management of gastrointestinal symptoms.

Following diagnosis, approximately one-half of patients are alive at the end of 3 years. Old age, absence of skin involvement, elevated serum LDH, hepatomegaly, and a hypercellular bone marrow indicate a poor prognosis, with death often occurring from a hematologic malignancy.

The present patient underwent a biopsy of one of the skin lesions that showed increased mast cells and an elevated urinary methyl histamine level was found. A trial of disodium chromoglycate inhaler alone failed to improve the wheezing. Addition of prednisone and β_2 agonists improved his respiratory symptoms. The skin lesions improved with topical application of corticosteroids.

Clinical Pearls

1. SMCD should be considered in a patient with skin lesions and vasoactive symptoms such as flushing, syncope, and hypotension.

2. In the absence of skin lesions, elevated urinary methyl histamines or the finding of increased mast cells in extracutaneous sites establishes the diagnosis.

3. Even though interstitial lung disease and pleural effusions are found in 40% and 10% of patients with SMCD, respectively, these findings are usually clinically unimportant.

4. Despite elevated serum histamine levels, wheezing is an uncommon finding.

REFERENCES

1. Roberts PL, McDonald HB, Wells RF. Systemic mast cell disease in a patient with unusual gastrointestinal and pulmonary abnormalities. Am J Med 1968;45:624–638.
2. Webb TA, Yanli C, Yam LT. Systemic mast cell disease: a clinical and histopathological study of 26 cases. Cancer 1982;49:927–938.
3. Huang TY, Yam LT, Li CY. Radiological features of systemic mast cell disease. Br J Radiol 1987;60:765–770.
4. Keyzer JJ, Monchy JG, Doormal JV, et al. Improved diagnosis of mastocytosis by measurement of urinary histamine metabolites. N Engl J Med 1988;309:1603–1605.
5. Travis WD, Li C, Bergstralh EJ, et al. Systemic mast cell disease: analysis of 58 cases and literature review. Medicine 1988;67:345–368.

PATIENT 43

An 82-year-old woman with mild dyspnea on exertion

An 82-year-old woman with moderate rheumatoid arthritis was referred for pulmonary evaluation of mild dyspnea on exertion that interfered with her active lifestyle. She had been previously evaluated by her primary physician with pulmonary function testing that revealed mild airway obstruction. The patient was started on inhalation bronchodilator therapy with beta-agonists and a sustained-release theophylline compound, which caused tremulousness and indigestion without improving her symptoms.

Physical Examination: Pulse 110; respirations 12; blood pressure 145/92. Chest: normal to percussion and auscultation. Cardiac: S4, no murmurs. Extremities: moderate ulnar deviation; mild swelling and moderate tenderness in both knees.

Laboratory Findings: Hct 40%; WBC 8,500/μl. Blood chemistry: normal. Chest radiograph: normal for age. ECG: normal. ABG (RA): pH 7.42; PCO_2 38 mmHg; PO_2 72 mmHg. Exercise pulse oximetry: blood oxygen saturation 93% without desaturation with walking. Pulmonary function tests: shown below.

Result	Measured	Predicted	% Predicted
FEV_1 (L)	1.25	1.54	81%
FVC (L)	1.98	2.31	86%
FEV_1/FVC (%)	63	70	

Question: On the basis of the laboratory results, what additional pulmonary function testing and treatment are indicated?

Answer: The patient's laboratory studies and pulmonary function results are normal for age; no further pulmonary evaluation is needed.

Discussion: Screening spirometry is a valuable tool for evaluating patients with suspected lung disease. Although microprocessor technology allows the immediate and routine generation of extensive spirometric data, the FEV_1, FVC, and FEV_1/FVC ratio ($\times$ 100%) are the most important and reliable of the measured tests. Other values, such as the FEFmax, FEF 200–1,200, FEF 25–75, FEF 50, FEF 75, and FEF 75–85, are frequently misleading, falsely positive indicators of lung disease when they are the only abnormalities observed.

In order to determine the clinical meaning of pulmonary function measurements, spirometric data from an individual patient must be compared to normative values derived from population studies. Most clinical pulmonary function laboratories use results from one of the three major studies that provide normal predicted values: Morris and coworkers, Crapo and coworkers, and Knudson and coworkers. These investigations conform to the American Thoracic Society's (ATS) recommendations that normative populations should comprise subjects from different communities with climatic, ethnic, and socioeconomic diversity and should not include hospitalized patients. Additionally, subjects with known lung disease or those with conditions that can alter pulmonary function, such as cigarette smoking, should be excluded. It is important in interpreting the pulmonary function of an individual patient to be certain that the normative population contained subjects with characteristics similar to those of the studied patient. For instance, normal blacks have lower FVC values than Caucasians and may appear to have lung restriction if compared to predicted values derived from healthy Caucasian populations.

The spirometric data collected from normal population studies are used to create normative equations that can calculate predicted spirometric values for the studied patient. Patient variables incorporated in these equations include standing height, which has been found by all recent studies to be a better predictor of spirometric values compared to other measurements of patient size such as body surface area. Age is an important factor in determining results from normative equations since most population studies show a linear age regression for FVC and FEV_1 of approximately 30 ml/yr. Although the ATS suggests that spirometric reference equations should not extrapolate for patients who are older than the subjects in the normative population, the three commonly used studies contain few subjects over the age of 70 years.

Recently, the Cardiovascular Health Study (CHS), which is a multicenter, prospective investigation of cardiovascular risk factors and disease in persons 65 years of age and older, provided data for the derivation of reference spirometric equations for elderly patients. These normative equations appear to give similar results for FEV_1 and FVC as the three commonly used reference equations now in clinical practice. The calculated FEV_1/FVC ratios for elderly patients derived from the CHS study, however, are lower than those previously reported. In the CHS study, FEV_1/FVC ratios ranged from 76% to 67% with advancing age, and had a lower limit of normal that ranged from 64% to 56%. These observations indicate that the commonly used "rule of thumb" that FEV_1/FVC ratio values below 70% indicate obstruction do not apply in elderly patients.

The equations derived from the CHS study shown below apply to patients 65–85 years of age between the heights of 145 and 175 cm for women and 160 and 185 cm for men. The lower limit of normal (LLN) is calculated by subtracting the value in the LLN column from the calculated predicted mean value.

	Equation	LLN
Men		
FVC	0.0567 Ht – 0.0206 Age – 4.37	–1.12
FEV_1	0.0378 Ht – 0.0271 Age – 1.73	–0.84
FEV_1/FVC%	–0.294 Age + 93.8	–11.7
Women		
FVC	0.0365 Ht – 0.0330 Age – 0.70	–0.64
FEV_1	0.0281 Ht – 0.0325 Age – 0.09	–0.48
FEV_1/FVC%	–0.242 Age + 92.3	–9.3

Abbreviations: Ht = height in cm; LLN = lower limit of the normal value (fifth percentile). Volumes in liters, BTPS.

Modified and reprinted with permission from Enright PL, Kronmal RA, Higgins M, et al. Spirometry reference values for women and men 65 to 85 years of age: Cardiovascular Health Study. Am Rev Respir Dis 1993;147:125–133.

The present patient's symptoms of indigestion and tremor improved with discontinuation of the inhaled beta-agonist and oral theophylline. It was determined that the patient's dyspnea on exertion resulted from worsening knee arthritis that caused increased effort of ambulation. Her exercise capacity improved with systemic and local management of her rheumatoid arthritis. It is important to recognize the normal alterations of spirometric values in the extremes of age to avoid exposing elderly patients to the complications of unnecessary diagnostic and therapeutic interventions.

Clinical Pearls

1. Reference equations used to derive predicted spirometric values should not be extrapolated for ages and heights not contained within the normal subject population that generated the equations.

2. Most reference equations used in clinical pulmonary function laboratories were derived from subject populations that had a small percentage of patients over 70 years of age.

3. Recent studies indicate that the FEV_1/FVC ratio decreases from 76% to 68% with advancing age and that the lower limit of normal ranges from 64% to 56% in elderly patients. The commonly accepted rule of thumb that a FEV_1/FVC ratio less than 70% indicates obstruction is invalid in elderly patient population.

REFERENCES

1. Gardner RM, Hankinson JL, Clausen JL, et al. Standardization of spirometry: 1987 update. Official statement of the American Thoracic Society. Am Rev Respir Dis 1987;136:1285–1298.
2. Ghio AJ, Crapo RO, Elliot CG. Reference equations used to predict pulmonary function: survey at institutions with respiratory disease training programs in the United States and Canada. Chest 1990;97:400–403.
3. Becklake M, Crapo RO, Buist AS, et al. Lung function testing: selection of reference values and interpretative strategies. An official statement of the American Thoracic Society. Am Rev Respir Dis 1991;144:1202–1218.
4. Enright PL, Kronmal RA, Higgins M, et al. Spirometry reference values for women and men 65 to 85 years of age. Cardiovascular health study. Am Rev Respir Dis 1993;147:125–133.

PATIENT 44

A 41-year-old woman with 1 year of progressive dyspnea, nonproductive cough, and dry eyes

A 41-year-old woman presented with a 1-year history of progressive dyspnea. At the time of presentation she was unable to perform simple household tasks or walk more than 50 feet. She noted a nonproductive cough that had developed over the previous 6 months. She denied fever, chills, or arthralgias but did note a minimal weight loss and dry eyes. The patient had no significant past medical, travel, or exposure histories.

Physical Examination: Temperature 100° F; pulse 88; respirations 18; blood pressure 106/66. General: thin. Head: normal. Lymphatics: no adenopathy. Chest: "Velcro" rales over the lower half of both lung fields. Cardiac: normal. Abdomen: normal. Extremities: clubbing without cyanosis.

Laboratory Findings: Hct 39%; WBC 9,300 cells/μl with a normal differential; platelets 426,000/μl; ESR 109 mm/hr. Urinalysis: normal. Serologies: ANA 1:160 (speckled); SSA 1:4; SSB negative; rheumatoid factor negative; HIV negative. Total protein 8.8 g/dl; albumin 3.3 g/dl. ABG (RA): pH 7.40; PCO_2 38 mmHg; PO_2 75 mmHg. Spirometry: FVC 0.99 L (38% of predicted): FEV_1 0.90 L (44% predicted). Chest radiographs: shown below.

Question: What is the most likely diagnosis? How would you proceed with your evaluation?

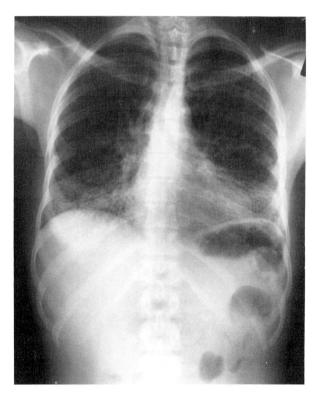
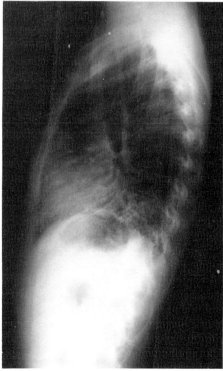

Diagnosis: Lymphocytic interstitial pneumonitis associated with Sjögren's syndrome.

Discussion: Lymphocytic interstitial pneumonitis (LIP) is an uncommon interstitial lung disease that is characterized by the presence of sheets of lymphocytes that expand the interstitium and fill the alveolar spaces. The infiltrates may represent either B- or T-lymphocytes. One factor that distinguishes LIP from pulmonary lymphoma is the polyclonal nature of the lymphocytes. Other histopathologic features include the formation of noncaseating granulomas, perivascular and paraseptal amyloid deposits, and well-formed germinal centers.

From 50–75% of individuals with LIP have an associated serum protein abnormality. While most patients commonly manifest as a polyclonal gammopathy, LIP has also been reported with agammaglobulinemia and hypogammaglobulinemia. Of non-HIV related cases, 25% of patients are found to have Sjögren's syndrome. Other associated autoimmune illnesses include chronic active hepatitis, myasthenia gravis, Hashimoto's thyroiditis, pernicious anemia, hemolytic anemia, and systemic lupus erythematosus. Allogenic bone marrow transplantation, AIDS, tuberculosis, celiac sprue, and phenytoin therapy have also been associated with LIP.

Non–AIDS-associated cases are more common in women between the ages of 30 and 60 years. Dyspnea and cough, which occur in over 70% of patients, are the most common presenting symptoms associated with LIP. Other symptoms, including weight loss, pleuritic chest pain, arthralgias, and fever, occur less frequently. While patients with Sjögren's may present with the classic triad of keratoconjunctivitis sicca, xerostomia, and collagen vascular disease, the pulmonary disease may precede these manifestations. Those with hypo- or agammaglobulinemia may have a history of recurrent pneumonia. Bibasilar rales are the most common physical finding. The prevalence of clubbing is much less frequent than in other forms of interstitial lung disease.

Basilar reticulonodular infiltrates are the most common chest radiographic finding. Infiltrates may coalesce as the lymphocytic infiltration progresses and produce nodular lesions. Honeycombing and changes consistent with pulmonary hypertension indicate chronic and progressive disease. Pleural effusions are infrequent. The presence of pleural effusions and hilar or mediastinal adenopathy is suggestive of lymphoma or other malignancy.

Prognosis in LIP is uncertain. Both progression of disease and resolution following therapy with corticosteroids and immunosuppressive drugs have been reported. While it has not been observed in larger series, there are well-documented cases of progression to lymphoma. In fact, it is the opinion of some that all cases of LIP represent an indolent malignant process. No clinical, pathologic, or laboratory parameters can predict therapeutic responsiveness or outcome.

HIV-associated LIP is much more common in the pediatric population than in adults. Children present with respiratory distress, pulmonary infiltrates, and failure to thrive, whereas adults usually present with insidious dyspnea and nonproductive cough. Because of the similarity of this presentation with other HIV-associated pulmonary illnesses, such as *Pneumocystis carinii* pneumonia, open lung biopsy is frequently required for diagnosis. Radiographic appearance in HIV-associated cases is similar to the early findings in non–HIV-associated cases. Basilar reticulonodular infiltrates with and without alveolar infiltrates are uniformly present. HIV-associated LIP rarely progresses to honeycombing, as patients invariably succumb to other AIDS-related illnesses. Patients have been treated with corticosteroids with variable success. Radiographic findings tend to remain unchanged throughout the course of the disease despite treatment.

In the present patient, the diagnosis was established by thoracoscopic lung biopsy. She was treated with prednisone (1 mg/kg) and at the end of 1 month had improvement in dyspnea, a reduction in cough frequency, an increase in FVC from 38% to 55% of predicted, and partial clearing of the chest radiograph. After 3 months of high-dose prednisone, no further improvement was noted in pulmonary function and azathioprine was added. Pulmonary function, chest radiograph, and symptoms have remained stable for 6 months following the addition of azathioprine and the reduction of prednisone. She has not developed any additional symptoms compatible with Sjögren's syndrome.

Clinical Pearls

1. LIP is an uncommon interstitial lung disease that is seen most often in women aged 30–60 years.

2. LIP is associated with a dysproteinemia in 50–75% of cases and may precede, coincide with, or follow the development of the protein abnormality. Over 25% of cases are associated with Sjögren's syndrome.

3. Over 70% of patients present with progressive dyspnea and cough. Bibasilar rales and reticulonodular infiltrates are the most common physical and chest radiographic findings, respectively.

4. HIV-associated LIP is more common in the pediatric population. The adult clinical and chest radiographic presentation of HIV-associated LIP is similar to non–HIV-associated disease with the exception of the rarity of progression to end-stage fibrosis.

5. Some investigators believe that LIP represents an early stage of lymphoma.

REFERENCES

1. Liebow AA, Carrington CB. Diffuse pulmonary lymphoreticular infiltrations associated with dysproteinemia. Med Clin North Am 1973;57:809–853.
2. Teirstein AS, Rosen MJ. Lymphocytic interstitial pneumonia. Clin Chest Med 1988;9:467–471.
3. Travis WD, Fox CH, Devaney KO, et al. Lymphoid pneumonitis in 50 adult patients infected with the human immunodeficiency virus: lymphocytic interstitial pneumonitis versus nonspecific interstitial pneumonitis. Hum Pathol 1992;23:529–541.

PATIENT 45

An 84-year-old woman with respiratory failure and a cystic mediastinal mass

An 84-year-old woman was admitted with postprandial back and lower substernal chest pain. She had previously experienced similar episodes lasting several hours, but the pain had never been so severe. The patient denied known cardiac or pulmonary disease but did take a diuretic for mild systolic hypertension.

Physical Examination: Temperature 99° F; pulse 110; respirations 22; blood pressure 150/80. General: moderate discomfort. Chest: few crackles over the right lower lung zone. Cardiac: I/VI systolic ejection murmur; normal S1. Abdomen: normal bowel sounds; moderate epigastrium tenderness. Extremities: equal pulses.

Laboratory Findings: Hct 39%; WBC 10,000/μl. Electrolytes, renal indices, and amylase: normal. Urinalysis: 1+ protein. ECG: sinus tachycardia.

Hospital Course: The patient improved with intravenous meperidine (Demerol), but 5 hours after admission she became stuporous with the following room air ABG: pH 7.01; PCO_2 92 mmHg; PO_2 45 mmHg. She was intubated and moved to the ICU. Her chest radiograph is shown below.

Question: What is the cause of the patient's radiographic abnormalities?

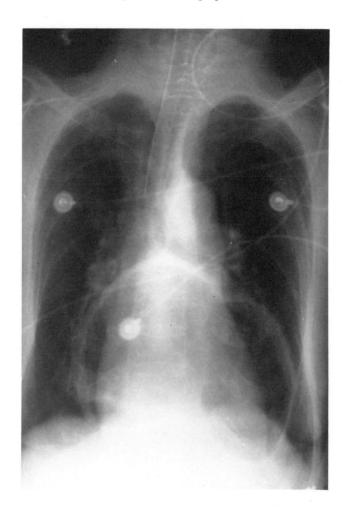

Diagnosis: Intrathoracic "upside-down" stomach.

Discussion: Hiatal hernias are the most common disorders of the upper gastrointestinal tract, occurring in up to 10% of all North Americans. Of the two major forms of the condition, "sliding" hiatal hernias are the more common and result from failure of the phrenoesophageal ligament to confine the esophagogastric junction in its normal position below the diaphragm. "Paraesophageal" hernias account for 5% of hiatal hernias treated surgically in most institutions. In this disorder, the esophagogastric junction remains below the diaphragm but a hiatal defect adjacent and anterior to the esophagus allows variable portions of the stomach to migrate into the chest.

Because the gastric cardia and pylorus are relatively secured by connecting intraabdominal structures, the more mobile portions of the greater curvature and body of the stomach are the first to migrate into the chest. Once within the thorax, the body of the stomach undergoes organoaxial rotation so that the greater curvature moves toward the right shoulder. Negative intrathoracic pressure and positive intraabdominal pressure eventually propel the stomach along with the greater omentum and transverse colon further into the chest and create traction that draws the pylorus toward the diaphragmatic hiatus. Completion of the process results in an intrathoracic hernia sac containing a gastric volvulus.

The underlying etiology of an intrathoracic "upside-down" stomach is incompletely defined. The rarity of the condition in children and young adults suggests the importance of acquired rather than congenital factors. Most patients with intrathoracic stomachs, however, do not report a history of major acute abdominal trauma. More long-term conditions such as chronic abdominal distension, pregnancy, and obesity may play an important role through effects on increasing intraabdominal pressure.

Intrathoracic stomachs are clinically important because of their inclination to incarcerate and produce obstructive symptoms. Because the gastric volvulus is angulated at its proximal and distal ends, incarceration compromises the vascular supply and may result in strangulation that can rapidly proceed to gastric gangrene and perforation. Additional complications include gastrointestinal hemorrhage and chronic aspiration with recurrent pulmonary infections and reactive airway disease. Bleeding appears to result from vascular engorgement of the gastric mucosa that causes small superficial erosions called Cameron's ulcers. Although up to 25% of patients with intrathoracic stomachs present with anemia or melena, massive acute hemorrhage rarely occurs.

Intrathoracic stomachs most commonly appear in patients during their sixth to seventh decades of life. Some patients have no symptoms and present after a routine chest radiograph detects a paraesophageal hernia. Others, however, report a long history of early satiety or postprandial, intermittent epigastric and substernal pain commonly misinterpreted as myocardial ischemia. Vomiting rarely occurs because of the proximal as well as distal location of the gastric obstruction. Occasional patients have combined elements of a paraesophageal and a sliding hernia, with the latter disorder contributing to symptoms of dyspepsia and reflux esophagitis. The classic triad of chest pain, retching without vomiting, and inability to pass a nasogastric tube identifies patients with early strangulation who can rapidly progress to vascular collapse.

The diagnosis can be confirmed by barium contrast studies. A chest CT scan provides an opportunity to identify the intrathoracic stomach in addition to accompanying misplaced structures such as the transverse colon. A single examination may underestimate the extent of gastric herniation in that the stomach may migrate in and out of the chest over time. Unfortunately, many clinicians fail to recognize the association of the paraesophageal hernia with the patient's presenting complaints of intermittent thoracoabdominal discomfort.

In contrast to sliding hiatal hernias, the mechanical nature of complications from paraesophageal hernia fail to respond to medical management. Symptomatic disease requires surgery, which is well tolerated and over 90% effective in improving the patient's condition. Either a transabdominal or transthoracic approach can reduce the gastric volvulus and repair the diaphragmatic defect. Because the stomach resumes its upside-down position when replaced in the abdomen, a gastric plication is commonly performed.

Patients with asymptomatic intrathoracic stomachs should be considered for elective surgical correction because of the risk for incarceration and the high operative mortality of emergency repairs. Present consensus recommends conservative observation only in asymptomatic patients who are poor operative candidates.

The present patient's admission symptoms resulted from postprandial engorgement of her intrathoracic stomach. Intravenous narcotic analgesia resulted in respiratory suppression that required intubation and mechanical ventilation. The preintubation positive-pressure face-mask ventilation caused insufflation of the stomach and the radiographic appearance of a cystic mediastinal mass. A chest CT scan (shown below) demonstrated the intrathoracic position of the stomach and transverse colon. The patient rapidly improved with extubation the following day and subsequently refused surgical repair.

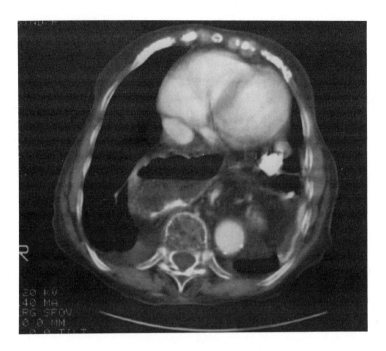

Clinical Pearls

1. An intrathoracic stomach is an extreme example of a paraesophageal hernia. The gastric body and fundus, frequently accompanied by the transverse colon, migrate through the diaphragmatic hiatus anterior to the esophagus and undergo organoaxial rotation to assume an "upside-down" position.

2. Most patients with intrathoracic stomachs do not have the reflux symptoms commonly associated with sliding hiatal hernias. Patients present with intermittent thoracoabdominal discomfort, which may simulate myocardial ischemia, and varying degrees of blood-loss anemia.

3. A single gastrointestinal contrast study may underestimate the degree of gastric herniation because the stomach may migrate to and fro through the diaphragmatic hiatus.

4. Symptomatic patients should undergo surgical reduction of intrathoracic stomachs because of the high mortality of sudden gastric strangulation. Asymptomatic patients without extreme operative risks should probably undergo surgery, although the long-term risks of gastric strangulation are not clearly defined.

REFERENCES
1. Hill LD. Incarcerated paraesophageal hernia: a surgical emergency. Am J Surg 1973;126:286–291.
2. Wichterman K, Geha AS, Cahow CE, Baue AE. Giant paraesophageal hiatus hernia with intrathoracic stomach and colon: the case for early repair. Surgery 1979;86:497–506.
3. Pearson FG, Cooper JD, Ilves R, et al. Massive hiatal hernia with incarceration: a report of 53 cases. Ann Thorac Surg 1983;35:45–51.
4. Ellis FH Jr, Crozier RE, Shea JA. Paraesophageal hiatus hernia. Arch Surg 1986;121:416–420.
5. Allen MS, Trastek VF, Deschamps C, Pairolero PC. Intrathoracic stomach: presentation and results of operation. J Thorac Cardiovasc Surg 1993;105:253–259.

PATIENT 46

A 33-year-old asymptomatic man with a left lower lobe infiltrate

A 33-year-old man with a history of a left lower lobe pneumonia 6 years earlier presented to the neurology service with symptoms of cervical stenosis. An abnormal preoperative chest radiograph prompted a pulmonary consultation. The patient denied any pulmonary or constitutional complaints. He did report a 40-pack-year history of cigarette smoking.

Physical Examination: Temperature 98.8° F; pulse 68; respirations 16; blood pressure 130/70. General: healthy appearing in no distress. Chest: mild dullness to percussion, increased fremitus, and decreased breath sounds over the left posterior chest.

Laboratory Findings: CBC: normal. Electrolytes and renal indices: normal. Chest radiographs: 4-cm opacity in the posterior basal segment of the left lower lobe (below).

Question: What is the diagnosis?

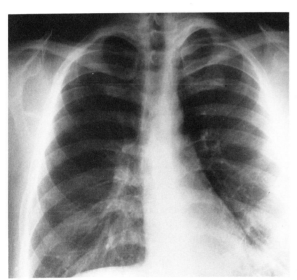 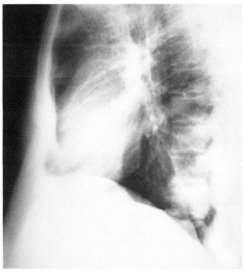

Diagnosis: Intralobar pulmonary sequestration.

Discussion: Bronchopulmonary sequestration is an uncommon developmental anomaly constituting only 0.15–6.4% of all congenital pulmonary malformations. It is characterized by abnormal, nonfunctioning pulmonary parenchyma that has no connection with the tracheobronchial tree and receives its blood supply from the systemic circulation. Two types of sequestration have been described: intralobar, in which the abnormal tissue is within the parenchyma of the normal lobe and does not have a separate visceral pleura, as in the present patient; and extralobar, in which the abnormal tissue is enclosed in its own visceral pleura separate from the adjacent normal lobe.

The most widely accepted theory considers that intralobar sequestration occurs during the early embryonic stages of lung development. As the bronchial tree undergoes formation of its branching elements, a branch fragment becomes separated from the remainder of the lung. This isolated lung tissue retains a systemic arterial blood supply because its pulmonary vasculature fails to develop. It has also been proposed that intralobar sequestration is an acquired lesion that results from focal bronchial obstruction caused by a foreign body or infection. This theory contends that the inflammatory process interrupts the pulmonary blood supply, resulting in hypertrophy of small systemic vessels that are normally present in the lung.

The intralobar variety accounts for 75% of all sequestrations. Two thirds of the time, the sequestration is located in the paravertebral gutter in the posterior segment of the left lower lobe. In most other instances, it occupies the same position in the right lower lobe. Unlike extralobar sequestration, it is rarely associated with other developmental abnormalities. It becomes manifest in adults after the age of 20 in 50% of cases and occurs equally in males and females. Patients present with signs and symptoms of pulmonary infection or a lower lobe mass is seen on a routine chest radiograph in an asymptomatic patient. It is believed that sequestrations become infected when bacteria migrate through the pores of Kohn or if the sequestration is incomplete.

Because pulmonary sequestration is an uncommon entity, it is not often considered in the differential diagnosis of a pulmonary mass in an adult. In a review of 540 cases of intralobar sequestration, the correct diagnosis was made or suspected in only 50% of the cases. Several fatal hemorrhages have occurred intraoperatively when aberrant vessels were transsected unknowingly because the diagnosis was not established and the vascular supply not delineated preoperatively.

The diagnosis is usually suspected on standard chest radiographs or CT scans when a lesion is detected in the characteristic location for a sequestration in the appropriate clinical setting. CT scans, however, do not reliably define the vascular anatomy. An arteriogram has been considered vital in documenting the systemic blood supply, allowing definitive diagnosis as well as preoperative planning. The advent of new noninvasive imaging techniques has changed this thinking. Magnetic resonance angiography (MRA) allows not only the definition of the systemic arterial supply but the precise localization, orientation, and even tissue composition of the sequestration. The main drawbacks of MRA are its cost and difficulties in obtaining static images within the thorax because of respiratory motion. Ultrasound with color Doppler and triplex Doppler have also been shown to be useful in documenting vascular anatomy due to the relatively solid nature of lung sequestrations.

Sequestrations should be resected. Surgery results in complete relief of symptoms and an excellent long-term outlook.

The present patient had a CT scan of the chest that demonstrated parenchymal consolidation in the posterior basal segment of the left lower lobe with a partially thrombosed vessel originating from the abdominal aorta supplying the segment. The vascular anatomy was confirmed with angiography, and the sequestration was resected. He had an uncomplicated postoperative course and is clinically well 1 year later.

Clinical Pearls

1. Intralobar sequestration may present as recurrent pneumonia or an asymptomatic left lower lobe mass on chest radiograph.

2. Intralobar sequestrations are almost always located in the posterior basilar segment of the left lower lobe, being left-sided in two-thirds of cases.

3. The diagnosis needs to be established preoperatively and the vascular supply delineated to avoid potentially life-threatening hemorrhage. Magnetic resonance angiography may replace standard angiography as a noninvasive procedure to define the vascular anatomy.

4. Surgical resection is curative.

REFERENCES

1. Doyle AJ. Demonstration of blood supply to pulmonary sequestration by MR angiography. AJR 1992;158:989–990.
2. Yuan A, Chang D, Kuo S, et al. Lung sequestration: diagnosis with ultrasound and triplex Doppler technique in an adult. Chest 1992;102:1880–1881.
3. Ke F, Chanq S, Su W, et al. Extralobar sequestration presenting as an anterior mediastinal tumor in an adult. Chest 1993;104:1:303–304.
4. Louie HW, Martin SM, Mulder DG. Pulmonary sequestration: 17-year experience at UCLA. Am Surg 1993;59:801–805.

PATIENT 47

A 49-year-old man with tachypnea and a rapidly enlarging pleural effusion

A 49-year-old man was admitted to the ICU after falling from a scaffold. His initial evaluation demonstrated a fractured pelvis and traumatic pancreatitis as shown by a serum amylase of 560 IU/L. He was stabilized with rapid fluid infusion and initiated on total parenteral nutrition with a glucose-containing solution. Five days later, the rapid onset of tachypnea prompted an urgent reevaluation.

Physical Examination: Temperature 100°; pulse 125; respirations 32; blood pressure 100/76. General: severe respiratory distress. Neck: elevated neck veins; trachea deviated to the left. Chest: dullness and decreased breath sounds on the right. Cardiac: grade II/VI systolic murmur. Abdomen: diffusely tender. Neurologic: alert.

Laboratory Findings: Hct 32%; WBC 11,000/μl; Na$^+$ 128 mEq/L; K$^+$ 3.5 mEq/L; Cl$^-$ 89; HCO$_3^-$ 22 mEq/L; glucose 238 mg/dl; amylase 235 IU/L. ABG (70% FiO$_2$ by face mask): pH 7.50; PCO$_2$ 30 mmHg; PO$_2$ 52 mmHg. ECG: sinus tachycardia. Chest radiograph: shown below (previous day's chest radiograph was normal).

Question: What is the likely cause of the patient's dyspnea and abnormal chest radiographic findings?

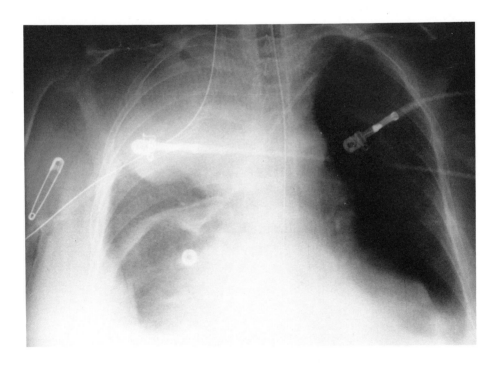

Diagnosis: Vascular erosion by a central catheter with right-sided hydrothorax.

Discussion: Insertion of central venous catheters is a valuable technique in the management of hospitalized patients. Unfortunately, complications of pneumothorax, line infection, and intravascular thrombosis occur in as many as 11% of all central venous catheter insertions.

Despite the advent of pliable catheters with tapered tips, catheter erosion through central venous structures is an additional potentially life-threatening complication of central venous access. Although the exact incidence of this complication is unknown, several reports indicate that as many as 0.5–1% of catheter insertions are associated with vascular perforation. Once catheters erode central venous structures, infusion of fluid results in collection of mediastinal fluid with eventual progression to unilateral or bilateral pleural effusions.

Mechanical forces appear to be the primary mechanism behind central venous catheter erosion. The superior vena cava and brachiocephalic veins are relatively thin structures that are subject to perforation when a catheter tip directly abuts the intima at or near a perpendicular angle. In this position, respiratory-related movement of mediastinal structures can abrade venous walls and promote venous erosion. Furthermore, catheters placed through the internal jugular vein may migrate to and fro as much as 3 cm with neck extension and flexion. The infusion of hypertonic solutions or irritative medications through a catheter tip that abuts the intima may contribute to vascular injury.

Placement of a catheter through a left-sided venous access appears to increase the risk of central venous erosion. Left-sided catheters orientate more toward a horizontal position as they pass through the left brachiocephaic vein into the superior vena cava. If the catheter is not inserted to a sufficient length, the catheter tip can abut the right laterosuperior wall of the superior vena cava at the level of the azygous arch. The catheter angle within 45° of horizontal promotes "catching" of the catheter within the ostium of the azygous vein and "pegging" of the intima. More than 70% of patients with central venous erosion reported in the literature had placement of left-sided catheters.

Chest pain and dyspnea are the most common symptoms of patients who experience venous erosion of a central catheter. The chest pain is central or precordial and may radiate to the shoulders because of stimulation of diaphragmatic nerve endings. Symptoms progress slowly or rapidly, depending on the rate of fluid infusion through the catheter. Eventual occurrence of a massive pleural effusion may result in cardiopulmonary arrest. Other signs and symptoms of central venous erosion include cough, physical findings of a pleural effusion, and Horner's syndrome. The onset of symptoms is usually within 1–7 days of catheter insertion but has been reported as long as 2 months later.

The diagnosis of central venous erosion requires a high clinical suspicion for this relatively rare disorder. Patients with a central catheter who develop new cardiopulmonary symptoms should be evaluated with a chest radiograph. Suggestive radiographic findings include widening of the mediastinum, most notably along the right paratracheal region, and unilateral or bilateral pleural effusions. Unilateral effusions may be ipsilateral or contralateral to the catheter insertion site. Additional clues include an extravascular location of the catheter tip or a gentle curve in the distal 3 cm of the catheter noted on the lateral chest radiograph. This latter sign results from "pegging" of the catheter at the site of an intimal perforation with bowing of the catheter by forward catheter migration.

Once the diagnosis is suspected, intravenous fluid should be discontinued until vascular erosion can be excluded. Inability to withdraw blood from the catheter suggests the presence of catheter erosion; however, the ability to withdraw blood freely does not exclude the diagnosis. Infusion of radioconstrast material through the distal catheter port followed by a plain chest radiograph can confirm the diagnosis. Perforating catheters should be removed immediately. When perforating catheters are removed, there is no risk of bleeding through the vascular erosion or creation of a hemothorax.

Occasionally, a characteristic pleural fluid profile suggests central catheter erosion when patients undergo thoracentesis before the diagnosis is considered. Pleural fluid is always a transudate, unless albumin is being infused through the catheter or low infusion rates instill small volumes of intravenous fluids into a preexisting exudative pleural effusion. The fluid appears straw-colored or serosanguinous, unless fat emulsions are infused, wherein the fluid is milky in nature. Pleural fluid glucoses range from 100 to 3,000 mg/dl but are always greater than a concomitantly measured serum glucose.

Previous reports indicate that the diagnosis of central venous erosion is often delayed for up to days or weeks after occurrence. Typically, the symptoms of chest pain and dyspnea and radiographic signs are ascribed to underlying conditions. Undue delays in diagnosis contribute to the reported 12% mortality of central venous catheter perforation.

The present patient was evaluated with efforts to draw blood from the catheter, which were unsuccessful, and infusion of radiocontrast material through the catheter, which demonstrated extravasation into the mediastinum. The catheter was removed and the patient recovered uneventfully after a therapeutic thoracentesis. The fluid was serosanguinous with a glucose content of 2,250 mg/dl.

Clinical Pearls

1. Central venous catheters erode through venous structures in as many as 0.5–1% of catheter insertions.

2. More than 70% of catheter erosions result from left-sided catheter insertions because of the relatively horizontal orientation of the left brachiocephalic vein that opposes the catheter tip against the intima of the superior vena cava.

3. The juncture of the superior vena cava and the brachiocephalic veins at the level of the azygous recess is a "danger zone." Catheter tips placed at this location result in "catching" of the tip within the azygous recess with a higher risk of vascular erosion.

4. Pleural fluid resulting from extravasation of a central venous catheter mirrors the infused fluid: low protein content with a pleural fluid/serum glucose ratio greater than 1.

5. A gentle curve of the distal 3 cm of a central venous catheter apparent on the lateral chest radiograph is a clue to the diagnosis.

REFERENCES

1. Criado A, Mena A, Figueredo R, et al. Late perforation of superior vena cava and effusion caused by central venous catheter. Anaesth Intens Care 1981;9:286–288.
2. Chute E, Cerra FB. Late development of hydrothorax and hydromediastinum in patients with central venous catheters. Crit Care Med 1982;10:868–869.
3. Tocino IM, Watanabe A. Impending catheter perforation of superior vena cava: radiographic recognition. AJR 1986;145:487–490.
4. Milam MG, Sahn SA. Horner's syndrome secondary to hydromediastinum: a complication of extravascular migration of central venous catheter. Chest 1988;94:1093–1095.
5. Duntley P, Siever J, Korwes ML, et al. Vascular erosion by central catheters: clinical features and outcome. Chest 1992;101:1633–1638.

PATIENT 48

A 31-year-old animal laboratory worker with fever, right lower lobe infiltrate, and right upper quadrant pain

A 31-year-old man presented with a 2-week history of fever, nonproductive cough, and abdominal pain. He smoked one pack of cigarettes per day for 10 years and consumed alcohol occasionally. The patient had spent 2 years in the navy aboard ship and presently worked as a research laboratory technician.

Physical Examination: Temperature 102.3°; pulse 104; respirations 22; blood pressure 120/80. General: mild respiratory distress. Chest: dullness to percussion, decreased fremitus, and crackles at the right base. Cardiac: normal. Abdomen: mild right upper quadrant tenderness.

Laboratory Findings: Hct 40%; WBC 8,300/μl, normal differential; platelets 214,000/μl; ESR 14 mm/hr. BUN 5 mg/dl; creatinine 0.9 mg/dl; AST 49 IU/L; ALP 395 IU/L; total bilirubin 2 mg/dl; total protein 6.6 g/dl; albumin 3.1 g/dl. HIV (ELISA): negative. Serum Mycoplasma, Legionella, Leptospira, and Brucella titers: nondiagnostic. Sputum Gram stain, AFB stain, and Legionella DFA: negative. Blood and sputum cultures: negative. Chest radiographs: shown below.

Question: How should the suspected diagnosis be confirmed?

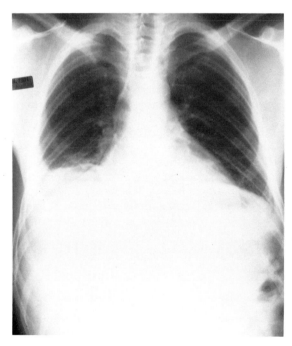 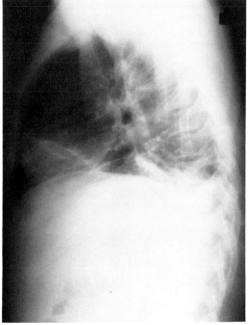

Diagnosis: Q fever confirmed by elevated serum acute and convalescent titer for antibodies to *Coxiella burnetii.*

Discussion: Q fever, a zoonosis with a worldwide distribution, is caused by the rickettsia *Coxiella burnetii.* First described in 1937 by Derrick in a group of abattoir workers in Queensland, Australia, the etiologic agent is a pleomorphic obligate intracellular bacteria that resides in phagolysosomes. *C. burnetii* is a hardy organism capable of producing spore-like structures that can survive for long periods in inanimate environments, resist desiccation, and travel wind-borne for long distances. The organism commonly infects the genital tract of wild and domestic animals, including cows, sheep, goats and cats. Spread to man usually occurs by inhalation of infectious particles or direct contact with purulent material. It is believed that a single inhaled organism is sufficient to initiate infection. In the United States, Q fever is an occupational hazard for persons working in animal research laboratories or slaughterhouses.

The incubation period varies from 14–39 days, after which the infection may be asymptomatic, acute, or chronic. The true incidence of Q fever is unknown, because most patients develop only mild symptoms. The common clinical presentations include a self-limited febrile illness that lasts 2–14 days. In severe disease, symptoms include high fever, (104–105° F), headache, retrobulbar pain, myalgia, neck stiffness, chest pain, and cough. Unlike other rickettsial diseases, Q fever rarely presents with skin rash. Other less common presentations include atypical pneumonia, rapidly progressive pneumonia, pneumonia as an incidental finding in a febrile patient, an infectious-hepatitis-like illness, fever of unknown origin, and endocarditis. Rarely, vertebral osteomyelitis, aseptic meningitis, and encephalitis occur. Clinical presentation varies from country to country. In France, the United States, and Australia, hepatitis is the most common presentation followed by pneumonia. In most other European countries and Canada, pneumonia is the most common presenting problem. The variation in clinical presentation is due to differences in clinical strains, the route of contamination (aerosol versus ingestion), and host resistance.

In a review of chest radiographs from 69 patients with Q fever, 10% were normal and 90% were observed to have multiple, round areas of "ground glass" consolidation situated in the lower lobes. Small pleural effusions were seen in three patients. Resolution of radiographic abnormalities occurred between 10 and 70 days. Rarely, pseudotumors (inflammatory masses) involving the upper lung zones have been reported.

The diagnosis is established by serologic testing because most laboratories do not have the facilities for isolating *C. burnetii.* In acute Q fever, complement-fixing antibodies to phase II antigen are elevated. Although a titer of 1:8 is considered diagnostic, confirmation of the diagnosis requires a fourfold rise in titer. In chronic Q fever, phase 1 complement-fixing antibody titer of greater than 200 is diagnostic.

Tetracycline, 500 mg orally every 6 hours for 2 weeks in adults, can be effective in decreasing the duration of fever if given within the first 3 days of the acute illness. For chronic Q fever, therapy with tetracycline alone or in combination with lincomycin or rifampin is recommended for 8–12 months. The prognosis for patients with pneumonia or hepatitis is excellent; however, mortality from endocarditis is estimated to be greater than 20%.

The present patient presented with a suggestive occupational history for Q fever with a compatable chest radiograph and laboratory findings. His complement-fixing antibodies to phase II antigen were elevated to 1:1024 and a convalescent titer was 1:4096. The illness responded well to a course of doxycycline. The abnormal liver function tests returned to normal on follow-up.

Clinical Pearls

1. Q fever should be considered in the differential diagnosis of patients with fever, pneumonia, or hepatitis who have been exposed to domestic or laboratory animals.

2. Unlike other rickettsial disease, Q fever rarely presents with skin rash.

3. The diagnosis is established by demonstrating antibodies against *C. burnetii.*

4. Although most cases of Q fever are self-limited illnesses, *C. burnetii* endocarditis carries a mortality of greater than 20%.

REFERENCES

1. Derrick EH. Q fever, a new entity: clinical features, diagnosis and laboratory investigations. Med J Aust 1937;2:281–299.
2. Sawyer LA, Fishbein DB, Mcdade JE. Q fever: current concepts. Rev Infect Dis 1987;9:935–946.
3. Harrison RJ, Vugia DJ, Ascher MS. Occupational health guidelines for control of Q fever in sheep research. Ann N Y Acad Sci 1990;590:283–290.
4. Smith DL, Wellings R, Walker C, et al. The chest x-ray in Q-fever: a report on 69 cases from the west midlands outbreak. Br J Radiol 1991;64:1101–1108.
5. Brouqui P, Dupont HT, Drancourt M, et al. Chronic Q fever: 92 cases from France, including 27 cases without endocarditis. Arch Intern Med 1993;153:642–648.

PATIENT 49

A 42-year-old woman with exertional dyspnea and systemic lupus erythematosus

A 42-year-old woman presented with exercise-induced dyspnea that had progressed during the past 1 year. She had a 20-year history of systemic lupus erythematosus (SLE) characterized by arthralgias, myalgias, Raynaud's phenomenon, and general malaise. The patient had discontinued her steroid therapy as well as medical follow-up 1 year earlier because of her frustration with "doctors and drugs."

Physical Examination: Temperature 98°; pulse 120; respirations 20; blood pressure 120/65. Skin: scattered petechiae; abnormal nailfold capillaries. Neck: venous distension. Chest: scattered basilar rales. Cardiac: parasternal heave; loud and widely split S2.

Laboratory Findings: Hct 30%; WBC 4,500/μl/L. Electrolytes and renal indices: normal. ANA: positive 1:320, anticardiolipin antibodies: positive. ECG: right ventricular enlargement. Chest radiograph: shown below.

Question: What etiologic possibilities exist for the patient's exertional symptoms?

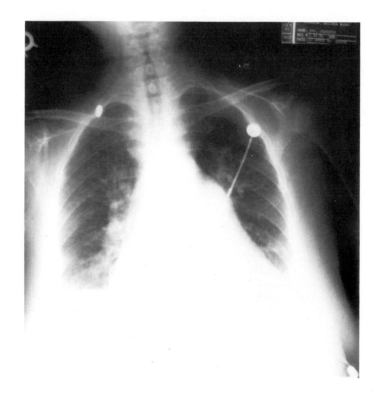

Diagnosis: Pulmonary hypertension associated with systemic lupus erythematosus (SLE).

Discussion: SLE is a multisystem disease characterized by chronic inflammation of fibroelastic connective tissues and an unpredictable and relapsing course. Since first described by Osler in 1904, pleuropulmonary complications have been recognized as a major manifestation of lupus, occurring in up to 50–70% of patients. Sterile pleural effusions represent the most common of these intrathoracic complications and may present as the initial manifestation of the underlying systemic disease. Patients with established lupus may also develop fibrosing alveolitis, atelectasis, recurrent bronchopneumonia, diaphragmatic weakness with decreased lung volumes ("shrinking lungs"), and intraalveolar hemorrhage. Many patients with lupus have measurable lung function abnormalities without clinically evident pulmonary disease. Commonly observed defects include pulmonary restriction, abnormal lung diffusion, decreased lung compliance, and hyperventilation with a widened alveolar to arterial oxygen gradient.

Pulmonary hypertension has been considered a rare complication of SLE that occurs more commonly in other connective tissue diseases such as scleroderma, particularly of the CREST variant, and mixed connective tissue disease. More recently, however, patient series using sensitive ultrasonographic Doppler techniques to determine pulmonary artery pressures have noted a 9–14% prevalence of pulmonary hypertension in SLE.

Lupus-related pulmonary hypertension commonly occurs in association with Raynaud's phenomenon and presents with progressive dyspnea, substernal chest discomfort, varying degrees of cor pulmonale, and limitations to exercise. The chest radiograph shows clear lung fields with enlarged pulmonary vasculature as observed in primary pulmonary hypertension. Serologic evaluation may detect the presence of anti-RNP antibodies, rheumatoid factors, and anticardiolipin (aCL) antibodies.

As with most of the manifestations of the disease, the pathophysiology of pulmonary hypertension in patients with SLE is unknown. The high incidence of Raynaud's phenomenon suggests that vasoconstriction of muscular pulmonary arteries may play a role. Other potential pathophysiologic factors include deposition of immune complexes, platelet abnormalities, and defective fibrinolysis with resulting thromboembolic disease. However, pulmonary vascular deposition of immune complexes may exist in patients with lupus who do not have pulmonary hypertension. Furthermore, thromboemboli are not a common pathologic finding in the pulmonary vasculature of patients who die with lupus-related pulmonary hypertension.

A perplexing association exists between pulmonary hypertension and aCL antibodies in patients with SLE. Up to 60% of patients with SLE-related pulmonary hypertension have aCL antibodies compared to 40% of lupus patients who do not have pulmonary vascular disease. The presence of aCL antibodies strongly correlates with large nonpulmonary vessel arterial and venous thromboses in SLE; 40% of patients with SLE who experience ocular thrombosis, Budd-Chiari syndrome, arterial gangrene, or thrombotic endocardial valvular disease have aCL antibodies compared to the 18% incidence of aCL antibodies in patients without thrombotic complications. It is attractive to consider that the procoagulant effects of aCL generate pulmonary hypertension through promotion of venous thromboembolic disease or in situ thrombosis of the pulmonary vasculature. Most pathologic studies, however, detect an early inflammatory stage consistent with a pulmonary vasculitis that progresses to irreversible fibrosis rather than evidence of intravascular thrombosis.

Unfortunately, pulmonary hypertension in patients with lupus usually has a rapid onset and follows an accelerated course, with death occurring within 2 years of presentation despite aggressive therapy with immunosuppressive agents, anticoagulants, and vasodilator drugs. Occasional patients may qualify for a heart–lung or lung transplantation. Possibly related to the presence of aCL antibodies, patients commonly experience wide fluctuations of anticoagulation requirements.

The present patient had clinical and radiographic features of pulmonary hypertension, which was confirmed by Doppler ultrasonography and cardiac catheterization. Despite therapy with corticosteroids and anticoagulation, she followed a rapidly downhill course and died 3 months later.

Clinical Pearls

1. Recent patient series using Doppler ultrasonography detects pulmonary hypertension in 9–14% of patients with SLE.

2. Common serologic accompaniments of lupus-related pulmonary hypertension include anti-RNP antibodies, rheumatoid factors, and anticardiolipin antibodies.

3. Anticardiolipin antibodies occur in 60% of patients with lupus-related pulmonary hypertension in contrast to a 40% incidence in patients with SLE who do not have pulmonary hypertension.

4. Although anticardiolipin antibodies are associated with large-vessel thrombosis in nonpulmonary vascular beds, the pathogenetic relationship of aCL with lupus-related pulmonary hypertension is unknown. Most lupus patients with pulmonary hypertension have evidence of pulmonary vasculitis with vascular fibrosis rather than intravascular thrombosis.

REFERENCES

1. Asherson RA, Oakley CM. Pulmonary hypertension and systemic lupus erythematosus. J Rheumatol 1986;13:1–5.
2. Asherson RA, Higenbottam TW, Xuan ATD, et al. Pulmonary hypertension in a lupus clinic: experience with twenty-four patients. J Rheumatol 1990;17:1292–1298.
3. De Clerck LS, Michielsen PP, Ramael MR, et al. Portal and pulmonary vessel thrombosis associated with systemic lupus erythematosus and anticardiolipin antibodies. J Rheumatol 1991;18:1919–1921.
4. Greisman SG, Thayaparan RS, Godwin TA, Lockshin MD. Occlusive vasculopathy in systemic lupus erythematosus: association with anticardiolipin antibody. Arch Intern Med 1991;151:389–392.
5. Wilson L, Tomita T, Braniecki M. Fatal pulmonary hypertension in identical twins with systemic lupus erythematosus. Hum Pathol 1991;22:295–297.

PATIENT 50

A 26-year-old HIV-positive man with apical infiltrates

A 26-year-old man with a history of remote intravenous drug abuse and HIV infection presented to the emergency department with a persistent productive cough and a 4-week history of fever, chills, and dyspnea at rest. Four months earlier, he had been evaluated by his personal physician for a cough and had undergone a chest radiograph (shown below left) and PPD with anergy skin test panel, which were all negative. His CD4 count at that time was 121/μl, and sputum samples were nondiagnostic. Bronchoscopy was recommended; however, the patient refused further work-up and received empirical antituberculous medications. He was lost to follow-up until the present illness. The patient was taking no medications.

Physical Examination: Temperature 101.9°; pulse 122; respirations 25; blood pressure 108/58. General: thin. Chest: minimal respiratory distress with use of accessory muscles; rare rales and rhonchi throughout both lung fields. Cardiovascular: no murmurs. Abdomen: normal. Lymphatics: shotty, nontender posterior cervical, axillary, and inguinal adenopathy.

Laboratory Findings: Hct 37%; WBC 8,900/μl with 62% PMNs, 17% lymphocytes, 19% monocytes, 2% bands; platelets 446,000/μl. Electrolytes and renal indices: normal. Liver function tests: total protein 5.9 gm/dl; albumin 1.3 gm/dl; LDH 460 IU/L. ABG (room air): pH 7.42; PCO_2 38 mmHg; PO_2 66 mmHg. Chest radiograph: shown below right.

Question: What is the differential diagnosis and the most likely cause of the patient's illness based on the clinical course and chest radiographs?

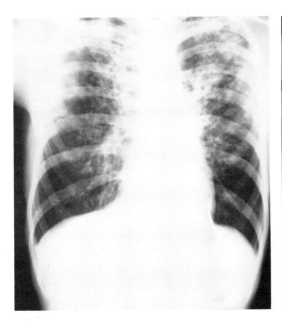 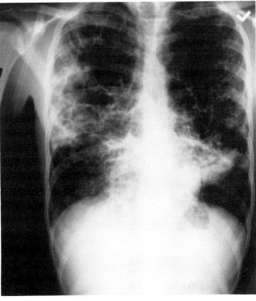

Diagnosis: *Pneumocystis carinii* pneumonia (PCP).

Discussion: The differential diagnosis of bilateral apical infiltrates in an HIV-positive patient is limited. The most common diagnosis by far is tuberculosis, especially in patients who have mild to moderate suppression of immune function. PCP also should be considered, particularly if the patient is receiving aerosolized pentamidine prophylaxis. Community-acquired pneumonia (including *Legionella* and *Mycoplasma*), *Cryptococcus neoformans, Toxoplasma gondii, Nocardia asteroides,* and *Rhodococcus equi* may present with focal infiltrates in any lobe, including the apices, but bilateral infiltrates are uncommon. Other organisms are known to cause pulmonary infections; however, apical infiltrates are extremely unusual in these disorders.

Excluding all causes of bacterial pneumonia, PCP is the most common pulmonary manifestation of AIDS. From 60–80% of patients will develop PCP during the course of their disease. Pneumocystis causes clinically significant infection when CD4 counts fall below $200/\mu l$. Patients present with slowly progressive dyspnea, nonproductive cough, fever, and chills. PCP may be mistaken for bronchitis or *Mycoplasma* pneumonia in the early stages, especially if infection with HIV is not suspected.

Laboratory examination often shows a normal leukocyte count with lymphopenia. Arterial hypoxemia is present in 75% of patients. An elevated serum LDH is found in > 90% of patients. A normal serum LDH suggests another process, and an LDH > 700 IU/L is highly predictive of a poor outcome.

The diagnosis of PCP is established by demonstrating the organism in an induced sputum specimen or pleural fluid, or at the time of bronchoscopy. In experienced laboratories, the sensitivity of induced sputum is as high as 75%. In institutions with less than full dedication to developing expertise with this technique, the diagnostic yield may plummet to 0%. The sensitivity of bronchoalveolar lavage (BAL) ranges from 84–97%. Transbronchial biopsy is not routinely recommended in some centers because it adds little diagnostically to BAL and because of the high (10%) risk of pneumothorax in these patients. In other AIDS centers, transbronchial biopsy is recommended to exclude additional pathogens that may be contributing to

pneumonia in patients with active PCP. Most agree that biopsies may be helpful in patients receiving aerosolized pentamidine prophylaxis or in the face of a negative BAL.

The radiographic manifestations of HIV-related PCP are variable. The most common appearance of diffuse, bilateral, perihilar interstitial infiltrates occurs in 80% of patients, whereas a normal chest radiograph may be found in 2–34% of patients. Upper lobe alveolar infiltrates mimicking tuberculosis occur more frequently in patients who are receiving aerosolized pentamidine prophylaxis (35% of patients) but also may be seen in those who are not (8%). Cysts, cavitation, pneumatoceles, honeycombing, blebs, bullae, and nodules have been reported but are much less common. Adenopathy is noted on as many as 20% of CT scans in patients with PCP. However, adenopathy is uncommon on the plain chest radiograph and is more suggestive of other processes such as tuberculosis, Kaposi sarcoma, and lymphoma. Adenopathy without other abnormalities on chest radiograph is rare in PCP.

Pleural effusions are uncommon in PCP; however, when present, pleural fluid analysis is remarkable for a pleural fluid to serum protein and LDH ratios of < 0.5 and > 1.0, respectively. Cytologic examination of the pleural fluid may reveal the organism. Pneumothorax is not uncommon in patients with PCP; the exact incidence is unknown. Spontaneous pneumothorax may occur more frequently in the patient who is receiving aerosolized pentamidine prophylaxis but also occurs in previously untreated patients or in those receiving trimethoprim-sulfamethoxazole (TMP-SMX). Disseminated *Pneumocystis* without lung involvement has been rarely reported.

TMP-SMX is the preferred drug for the treatment of PCP, with intravenous pentamidine being the alternative choice. Atovaquone is available for drug failures or for those who are unable to tolerate TMP-SMX or pentamidine. The addition of corticosteroids to the treatment of moderate PCP is recommended.

The present patient was treated with intravenous TMP-SMX and corticosteroids. His condition continued to deteriorate and he declined intubation and mechanical ventilation. He died of respiratory failure.

Clinical Pearls

1. The differential diagnosis of bilateral apical infiltrates in an HIV-positive patient is essentially limited to *Pneumocystis carinii* pneumonia and *Mycobacterium tuberculosis.* Community-acquired pneumonia, *Nocardia, Rhodococcus, Toxoplasma,* and *Cryptococcus* may produce apical infiltrates but are rarely bilateral.

2. The typical chest radiograph findings in PCP of bilateral, diffuse, perihilar infiltrates are seen in 80% of cases.

3. Upper lobe infiltrates mimicking tuberculosis are more common (35%) in patients receiving aerosolized pentamidine prophylaxis but may be observed in 8% of previously untreated patients.

4. Pleural effusions are rare with PCP. In the appropriate setting, pleural fluid to serum LDH ratios of > 1 with PF/S protein ratios of < 0.5 suggest PCP.

REFERENCES

1. Naidich DP, McGuinness G. Pulmonary manifestations of AIDS: CT and radiographic correlations. Radiol Clin North Am 1991;29:999–1017.
2. Kennedy CA, Goetz MB. Atypical roentgenographic manifestations of *Pneumocystis carinii* pneumonia. Arch Intern Med 1992;152:1390–1398.
3. Meduri GU, Stein DS. Pulmonary manifestations of acquired immunodeficiency syndrome. Clin Infect Dis 1992;14:98–113.
4. Horowitz ML, Schiff M, Samuels J, et al. *Pneumocystis carinii* pleural effusion. Pathogenesis and pleural fluid analysis. Am Rev Respir Dis 1993;148:232–234.

PATIENT 51

A 34-year-old man from India with cough, fever, and pleuritic pain

A 34-year-old man who had recently immigrated from India presented with cough, right chest pain, and fever. One week earlier, he was evaluated by his physician who noted a right lower lobe infiltrate and prescribed an oral cephalosporin for pneumonia. The cough productive of yellowish sputum progressively worsened with the onset of chills, fevers to 104°C, severe right-sided pleuritic chest pain, and discomfort in the right upper quadrant. There was no history of drug abuse, diarrhea, skin rash, previous illnesses, or use of medications.

Physical Examination: Temperature 103.5°; pulse 108; no paradox; respirations 28; blood pressure 130/80. General: moderate respiratory distress. Skin: normal. Chest: dullness to percussion, egophony, decreased fremitus, and decreased breath sounds over right posterior chest. Cardiac: grade I/VI systolic ejection murmur, normal neck veins. Abdomen: tender right upper quadrant; liver edge 7 cm below right costal margin. Extremities: no clubbing.

Laboratory Findings: Hct 42%, WBC 40,000/µl with 68% PMNs, 22% bands. Electrolytes and renal indices: normal. SGOT 2385 IU/L; SGPT 1855 IU/L; alkaline phosphatase 385 IU/L; bilirubin 1.2 mg/dl. Prothrombin time: 14.8 sec (control 11 sec). Sputum Gram stain: neutrophils without bacteria. Chest radiograph: shown below left. Abdominal CT: shown below right.

Questions: What is this patient's likely diagnosis? What is the best approach to diagnosis and management?

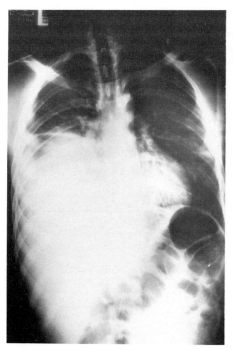
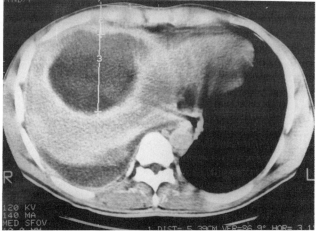

Diagnosis: Amebic liver abscess with an elevated right diaphragm and pleural effusion.

Discussion: *Entamoeba histolytica* is a protozoan that transmits to man through a fecal-oral route and causes an acute and chronic form of dysentery, which can progress to extraintestinal disease. Most common in underdeveloped regions of the world, amebiasis can occur anywhere in the United States because of increasing tourism to endemic areas and immigration from third-world nations.

Extraintestinal amebiasis most commonly affects the liver but may involve any region of the body, including the lung, pericardium, brain, peritoneal cavity, and genitourinary system. Hepatic infection results from spread of organisms through the mesenteric and portal venous radicals from a region of intestinal infection. Once established in the liver, amebic trophozoites lyse target hepatocytes through protease and calcium-dependent mechanisms. Destruction of liver tissue creates a hepatic abscess that involves the right lobe of the liver in 95% of instances. The abscess may enlarge to impressive dimensions, occasionally encompassing the entire hepatic lobe. The material from the abscess cavity is characteristically thick and brown in nature and variously described as "anchovy paste" or "chocolate" in quality.

Pleuropulmonary amebiasis—the second most common form of extraintestinal disease—nearly always occurs in patients with an underlying abscess in the right hepatic lobe and assumes at least three pathophysiologic forms. First, patients may develop a reactive inflammatory response of the lung or pleura that results in an exudative pleural effusion or localized region of pneumonitis. Second, frank rupture of a hepatic abscess into the pleural space may cause a pleural empyema. Third, erosion of a hepatic abscess into the bronchial airways may produce pulmonary consolidation, an intrapulmonary abscess, or a hepatobronchial fistula. The incidence of pleuropulmonary involvement in the setting of hepatic amebiasis is unknown but intrathoracic radiographic abnormalities may be present in 50% of patients.

In exceedingly rare instances, primary pleuropulmonary amebiasis may develop through hematogenous seeding from a colonic site of infection in the absence of an underlying liver abscess. Hematogenous spread is thought to occur when trophozoites enter hemorrhoidal or vertebral veins and pass through the inferior vena cava into the pulmonary circulation. The capacity of *E. histolytica* to spread through a hematogenous route is supported by the occurrence of amebic brain abscesses in patients with hepatic or intestinal

disease. Very rarely, primary pulmonary amebiasis may develop from the inhalation of dust particles laden with *E. histolytica* cysts.

Patients with pleuropulmonary amebiasis frequently present after a subacute course marked by persistent cough, dyspnea, fever, pleuritic chest pain, and hemoptysis. Occasionally, the hemoptysis is massive; only rarely do patients produce reddish-brown sputum from intrabronchial drainage of a hepatic abscess. Sudden rupture of a hepatic abscess into the pleural space may be associated with a dramatic onset of pleuritic pain and dyspnea. The degree of debilitation and associated weakness, weight loss, and anorexia may simulate lung cancer or pulmonary tuberculosis. The absence of abdominal symptoms in 10% of patients and the lack of diarrhea in 50% promote misdiagnosis of the pleuropulmonary form of the disease. Although typically moderately to massively enlarged, the liver in some patients with pleuropulmonary amebiasis may be nontender and normal in size.

The chest radiographic abnormalities observed in patients with pleuropulmonary amebiasis are right-sided and usually associated with pleural fluid formation. The diaphragm is typically elevated and may have a distinctive "tenting" contour called the "Mexican hat sign." Patients with rupture of a hepatic abscess into the pleural space may present with a massive pleural effusion and mediastinal shift. Other radiographic abnormalities include pulmonary consolidation and lung abscess formation. An enlarged cardiac silhouette may occur in patients with rupture of an abscess from the left lobe of the liver into the pericardial space. Patients commonly present with anemia and leukocytosis without eosinophilia. Most patients do not have jaundice or more than mild to moderate elevations of liver function tests.

The first consideration in diagnosing pleuropulmonary amebiasis begins with eliciting a history of travel through an endemic region. If diarrhea is present, stool examination may detect amebic trophozoites or cysts, but stools are usually negative in patients with pleuropulmonary disease. Proctoscopic examination may reveal mucosal changes consistent with amebiasis. Wet preparation sputum smears for ameba are usually negative in pleuropulmonary amebiasis, even in patients with hepatobronchial fistulas and "anchovy paste" sputum. Liver ultrasound or abdominal CT identifies the underlying amebic liver abscess; aspiration of abscess contents demonstrates the characteristic thick, brown material that contains identifiable ameba in only 2-10% of aspirates. Fine needle aspiration of the advancing edge of the abscess by ultrasound or CT guidance with cytologic examination of the aspirate increases diagnostic yield. Gallium scanning may assist the separation of bacterial from amebic liver abscesses because the latter have a cold central region that concentrates isotope only in the rim region where leukocytes are present.

Diagnosis of pleuropulmonary amebiasis, however, typically does not require identification of ameba. The distinctive clinical presentation in a patient with an underlying liver abscess combined with an exposure history, response to therapy, and positive antibody titer are sufficient diagnostic findings. The indirect hemagglutination assay (IHA) is the most commonly used serologic test. Patients with invasive amebiasis have an elevated test result in 85% of instances that is never falsely positive. The IHA remains positive, however, for up to several years after infection and requires the use of more specialized tests, such as counterimmunoelectrophoresis and gel diffusion, for the diagnosis of recurrent disease or initial episodes of clinically apparent active disease in patients from endemic regions.

The treatment of choice for patients with pleuropulmonary amebiasis is metronidazole for 5–10 days. Patients with reactive inflammatory pleural effusions recover with medical therapy alone. Patients with rupture of hepatic abscesses into the pleural space have a 14% mortality rate and are managed with chest tube drainage. Most patients do not require needle drainage of an underlying hepatic abscess unless they fail to respond to medical therapy within 5 or 6 days.

The present patient had radiographic evidence of a right-sided pleural effusion with elevation of the right diaphragm. The abdominal CT scan demonstrated a large liver abscess compatible with hepatic amebiasis. Refusing additional diagnostic studies, the patient was treated with 2 days of intravenous metronidazole followed by 5 days of oral metronidazole, which resulted in rapid resolution of his temperature and pain and normalization of his liver function tests within 3 weeks.

Clinical Pearls

1. Pleuropulmonary amebiasis is the second most common form of extraintestinal disease. Patients may present with reactive pleural and pulmonary inflammation, frank rupture of a hepatic abscess into the pleural space, or erosion of a hepatic abscess into a bronchial airway.

2. Rarely, patients may present with "primary" pleuropulmonary amebiasis defined by the presence of intrathoracic infection in the absence of an underlying hepatic abscess. Hematogenous spread through hemorrhoidal or vertebral veins from intestinal sites or inhalation of amebic cysts is considered the mechanism of pleuropulmonary infection in these patients.

3. Patients with pleuropulmonary amebiasis usually do not demonstrate ameba in sputum, stool, or pleural fluid. Sufficient clinical criteria for diagnosis are the typical clinical presentation, positive antibody titers to ameba, and clinical response to therapy.

4. Gallium scanning may distinguish bacterial from amebic liver abscesses in that an amebic abscess has a central "cold" region with radionuclide uptake only in the abscess rim where leukocytes are present.

REFERENCES

1. Walsh TJ, Berkman W, Brown NL, et al. Cytopathologic diagnosis of extracolonic amebiasis. Acta Cytol 1983;27:671–675.
2. Kubitschek KR, Peters J, Nickeson D, Musher DM. Amebiasis presenting as pleuropulmonary disease. West J Med 1985;142:203–207.
3. Lyche KD, Jensen WA, Kirsch CM, et al. Pleuropulmonary manifestations of hepatic amebiasis. West J Med 1990;153:275–278.
4. Sharma M, Mehta H, Sharma SK. Atrial septal defect presenting as recurrent primary amoebic lung abscess. Postgrad Med J 1991;67:474–475.

PATIENT 52

A 38-year-old man with fever, respiratory failure, and bilateral alveolar infiltrates following bone marrow transplantation

A 39-year-old man developed a cough productive of blood-tinged sputum 1 week after undergoing an allogeneic bone marrow transplantation for acute myelogenous leukemia. Over the next several days he experienced fever, progressive dyspnea, bilateral alveolar infiltrates, and hypoxic respiratory failure, necessitating mechanical ventilation.

Physical Examination: Temperature 102°; respirations 48; pulse 145; blood pressure 135/63. HEENT: severe mucositis. Neck: normal jugular venous distension. Chest: bilateral crackles. Cardiac: no murmurs or gallops. Extremities 1+ pedal edema.

Laboratory Findings: Hct 27%; WBC 600/μl; platelet count 62,000/μl. PT and PTT: normal. BUN 60 mg/dl, creatinine 1.8 mg/dl. ABG (60% FiO_2): pH 7.43; PCO_2 40 mmHg; PO_2 77 mmHg. Chest radiograph: bilateral diffuse alveolar infiltrates (shown below).

Questions: What diagnosis should be considered? How would you proceed with evaluation?

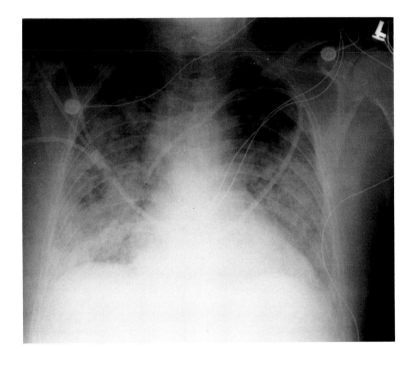

Diagnosis: Diffuse alveolar hemorrhage (DAH).

Discussion: Pulmonary complications occur commonly after bone marrow transplantation (BMT) and include pulmonary edema, infection, interstitial pneumonitis, and drug and radiation toxicity. Bronchoalveolar lavage (BAL) in the evaluation of these consequences has led to the recognition of DAH as an important and life-threatening pulmonary complication after BMT. The application of BAL is especially critical because hemoptysis is infrequent, radiographic findings are nonspecific, and noninvasive tests for pulmonary hemorrhage are often difficult to perform in this population of patients.

In contrast, when seen in idiopathic pulmonary hemosiderosis, collagen vascular disease, anti-basement membrane antibody disease, or rapidly progressive glomerulonephritis, pulmonary hemorrhage is manifested by a triad of hemoptysis, alveolar infiltrates on chest radiograph, and anemia. Also, nonimmune-mediated causes of DAH are often readily deduced from the clinical presentation or relatively straightforward diagnostic tests. Such etiologies include necrotizing infection (*Aspergillus, Pseudomonas,* and, occasionally, *Legionella* species), coagulopathy, high pulmonary venous pressure (mitral stenosis), drug or chemical exposure (D-penicillamine, lymphangiography, trimellitic anhydride), acute leukemia, and fat embolism.

Diffuse alveolar hemorrhage affects 10–35% of patients following autologous BMT, with a mortality ranging from 50–100%. The syndrome is characterized by fever, progressive dyspnea, nonproductive cough, hypoxemia, and diffuse infiltrates on chest radiograph. BAL fluid appears grossly bloody and reveals no underlying infectious pathogens. Hemorrhage is often not suspected because hemoptysis is absent and the clinical picture mimics infection. Onset of symptoms is usually within the first few weeks after transplantation and frequently coincides with leukocyte recovery.

Alveolar hemorrhage occurs more frequently in older patients who have autologous bone marrow transplantation for solid malignancies. These patients are more likely to have high fever, severe mucositis, and renal insufficiency than those who do not develop DAH. Although patients develop DAH during a period following transplantation when they are clearly thrombocytopenic, neither platelet counts nor coagulation parameters are significantly different from those of transplant patients without the syndrome. Furthermore, neither aggressive platelet transfusion nor correction of clotting abnormalities has been shown to alter the progression of hemorrhage.

Radiographic abnormalities are generally non-specific, although most patients initially exhibit a mild interstitial or alveolar pattern in the central and lower lung zones indistinguishable from edema or infection. Characteristically, the process is fulminant with rapid progression in 1 week to a diffuse, dense alveolar pattern.

BAL fluid should become progressively more hemorrhagic with sequential aspirations, since these later aliquots represent predominantly alveolar material. If local trauma to bronchial mucosa is induced during bronchoscopy, lavage fluid initially may appear bloody, reflecting bronchial sampling, but will clear with subsequent aspirations. In addition, numerous hemosiderin-laden macrophages are seen on cytologic iron stains, representing ingestion of alveolar erythrocytes and degradation to hemosiderin.

Several methods of quantitatively scoring the hemosiderin content of alveolar macrophages have been devised that correlate with histologic severity of hemorrhage. Some criteria for defining DAH rely solely on such quantitative macrophage hemosiderin scores, as elevated hemosiderin scores have been noted in lavage fluid that appeared grossly normal and contained a low number of red blood cells. As a result, the appearance of lavage fluid is sometimes considered to be an insensitive marker of alveolar hemorrhage. However, absence of hemosiderin-laden macrophages cannot exclude recent hemorrhage or remote alveolar bleeding, since alveolar macrophages may not demonstrate hemosiderin until a few days following exposure and can clear from the lungs within several weeks. Therefore, diagnosis of DAH requires a constellation of findings and a high index of suspicion.

The pathogenesis for DAH is most likely multifactorial, resulting in nonspecific injury to the lung endothelium. Chemotherapeutic conditioning regimen and use of the marrow preservative dimethyl sulfoxide have been suspected of inducing damage to alveoli. Chest irradiation prior to BMT has been associated with development of DAH. Meanwhile, the correlation observed between marrow recovery and development of DAH implicates a role for inflammatory cells as mediators of endothelial injury.

Therapy is generally not effective and mainly consists of supportive care. Treatment with high-dose corticosteroids has resulted in improved survival in recent studies. Unfortunately, the progression of hemorrhage and clinical decline is generally relentless despite maximal support.

The present patient underwent fiberoptic bronchoscopy with BAL, which revealed hemorrhagic fluid that contained numerous hemosiderin-laden macrophages and was negative for all stains and cultures. He received supportive care and subsequently recovered.

Clinical Pearls

1. Diffuse alveolar hemorrhage is a major pulmonary complication with a high mortality following autologous bone marrow transplantation.

2. The syndrome is manifested by fever, progressive dyspnea, cough, hypoxemia, and diffuse radiographic infiltrates, with onset in the first few weeks after transplant often coinciding with neutrophil recovery.

3. In contrast to other causes of alveolar hemorrhage, the presentation may be deceptive, as hemoptysis is rare, radiographic findings are often nonspecific, and diagnosis depends on characteristic bronchoalveolar lavage findings.

4. Bronchoalveolar lavage reveals fluid that appears more hemorrhagic with each aspirated aliquot, contains abundant hemosiderin-laden macrophages, and reveals no infectious pathogen.

REFERENCES

1. Kahn FW, Jones JM, England DM. Diagnosis of pulmonary hemorrhage in the immunocompromised host. Am Rev Respir Dis 1987;136:155–160.
2. Robbins RA, Linder J, Stahl MG, et al. Diffuse alveolar hemorrhage in autologous bone marrow transplant recipients. Am J Med 1989;87:511–518.
3. Ettinger NA, Trulock EP. Pulmonary considerations of organ transplantation. Am Rev Respir Dis 1991;144:213–223.
4. Witte RJ, Gurney JW, Robbins RA, et al. Diffuse pulmonary alveolar hemorhage after bone marrow transplantation. AJR 1991;157:461–464.
5. Grebski E, Hess T, Hold G, et al: Diagnostic value of hemosiderin-containing macrophages in bronchoalveolar lavage. Chest 1992;102:1794–1799.
6. Metcalf JP, Rennard SI, Reed EC, et al. Corticosteroids as adjunctive therapy for diffuse alveolar hemorrhage associated with bone marrow transplantation. Am J Med 1994;92:327–334.

PATIENT 53

A 23-year-old man with respiratory failure after a grand mal seizure

A 23-year-old man with a history of idiopathic epilepsy collapsed in a restaurant with a generalized grand mal seizure. The patient's family did not observe any emesis or aspiration during the 10 minutes of tonic clonic motor activity. When paramedics arrived, they found the patient in a postictal state with labored spontaneous respirations and transported him to the hospital emergency department. Otherwise in good health, the patient's only medication was phenytoin.

Physical Examination: Temperature 99.2°; pulse 118; respirations 28; blood pressure 162/92. General: severe dyspnea with generalized cyanosis. Head: no traumatic injury. Eyes: normally reactive pupils; no papilledema. Chest: bilateral crackles. Cardiac: normal heart tones without murmurs. Neurologic: stuporous; no focal deficits; negative Babinski sign.

Laboratory Findings: Hct 38.1%; WBC 13,900/μl with 78% granulocytes, 1% bands, 21% lymphocytes; electrolytes and renal indices: normal. ABG (face-mask high-flow O_2): pH 7.48; PCO_2 30 mmHg; PO_2 44 mmHg.

Hospital Course: The patient was intubated and transferred to the ICU. A postintubation chest radiograph is shown below.

Question: What is the probable explanation for the patient's initial hypoxemia and subsequent pulmonary infiltrates?

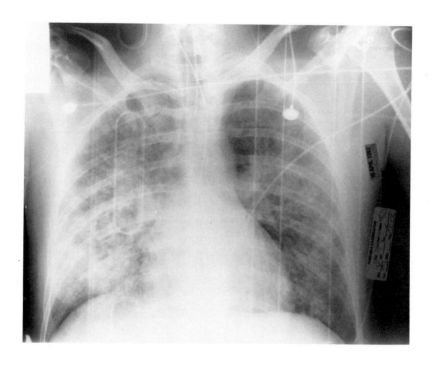

Diagnosis: Neurogenic pulmonary edema.

Discussion: Varied insults to the central nervous system (CNS) may produce the sudden onset of neurogenic pulmonary edema and respiratory failure. First described by Shanahan in 1908 in patients with epileptic seizures, neurogenic pulmonary edema also may occur in patients undergoing neurosurgical procedures, or in those with subarachnoid and intracerebral hemorrhages, head trauma, electroconvulsive therapy, trigeminal nerve blockade, or any condition that raises intracranial pressure.

The anatomic basis for neurogenic pulmonary edema is incompletely established in humans. Areas of the brain termed "edematogenic centers" have been suspected by clinicopathologic correlates to exist in the caudal hypothalamus and at the medullary Cushing receptor sites. More recent observations with magnetic resonance imaging (MRI) suggest the potential importance of edematogenic centers within the caudal brainstem at the medullary nucleus tractus solitarius. Independent stimulation of several regions within the hypothalamus and medulla appear capable of inducing pulmonary edema.

Regardless of their location, activation of these central edematogenic sites results in extravascular protein-rich fluid collections in the lungs and varying degrees of respiratory dysfunction. Although the mechanisms underlying the pulmonary edema are not clearly defined, experimental observations support the importance of a massive activation of the sympathetic nervous system, alterations of cardiovascular function, and enhanced pulmonary membrane permeability.

Evidence for this massive sympathetic discharge comes from animal studies wherein alpha-adrenergic blocking agents infused before head trauma prevents pulmonary edema. Adrenal catecholamines appear not to be the major source of adrenergic stimulation because adrenalectomized animals are not protected from neurogenic pulmonary edema. The sympathetic discharge in several animal models appears to mediate pulmonary edema by increasing venous return and pulmonary blood volume, raising systemic and pulmonary vascular resistance, and constricting pulmonary veins. These factors combine to elevate pulmonary capillary hydrostatic pressure and promote transudation of fluid into the pulmonary interstitium and alveolar space.

Most patients with neurogenic pulmonary edema do not demonstrate increased pulmonary capillary wedge pressures (P_{CW}) by the time a pulmonary artery catheter is placed because of the transient nature of the pulmonary pressor response. Reports exist, however, of transient increases in P_{CW} documented in patients sustaining insults to the CNS while a pulmonary artery catheter was already in place.

Several animal models further detect the presence of acute left ventricular dysfunction during the early phases of neurogenic pulmonary edema. Adrenergic-induced vasoconstriction may mediate decreased stroke volume by increasing left ventricular afterload, redistributing circulating blood volume to the thorax and thereby increasing preload, and decreasing ventricular compliance by shortening diastolic relaxation time. Increased vagal tone or inappropriately decreased beta responses may also hamper cardiac performance. Finally, neurogenic events may have direct negative effects on myocardial contractility through the effects of focal myocytolysis.

The hydrostatic cardiovascular alterations in animal models, however, do not explain the protein-rich nature of edema fluid observed in patients with neurogenic pulmonary edema that indicates the presence of increased pulmonary membrane permeability. The "blast theory" attempts to explain these findings by supposing that a transient and profound sympathetic-driven pulmonary hypertensive response leads to microvascular rupture with formation of exudative, hemorrhagic lung edema. This process is supported by autopsy studies in patients dying from neurogenic pulmonary edema that demonstrate hemorrhagic pulmonary edema with multiple parenchymal and pleural petechiae and histologic evidence of microvascular injury.

Countervailing experimental data exist to diminish the importance of the blast theory as the comprehensive pathophysiologic paradigm for understanding neurogenic pulmonary edema. Not all animal models clearly show protection from lung edema after prevention of the pulmonary pressor response. Furthermore, animal models of slowly progressive CNS injury demonstrate increased pulmonary vascular membrane permeability in the absence of pulmonary hypertension. These observations suggest the existence of alternative poorly defined mechanisms of neurogenic pulmonary edema, such as direct membrane effects of alpha-adrenergic stimulation, that increase membrane permeability and contribute in varying degrees to lung edema in different clinical settings.

In addition to pulmonary edema, patients with acute CNS disorders may develop hypoxemia in the absence of pulmonary radiographic abnormalities, as demonstrated by the present patient. Profound vasoconstriction and bronchospasm mediated through sympathetic discharge, increased vagal tone, and perhaps tissue or platelet release of vasoactive substances cause sudden mismatching of ventilation and perfusion. Sudden hypoxemia without pulmonary edema has been demonstrated in patients undergoing stereotaxic biopsy of localized CNS lesions.

Patients may present with neurogenic pulmonary edema within minutes or hours after a neurologic insult or delayed as long as 12–72 hours. Symptoms develop suddenly after onset characterized by dyspnea and rarely hemoptysis. Signs include tachypnea, tachycardia, rales, fever, and mild leukocytosis. The chest radiograph reveals a typical pattern of pulmonary edema, although focal or unilateral pulmonary infiltrates may occasionally occur. The severity of pulmonary dysfunction may be mildly symptomatic or severe, requiring intubation and mechanical ventilation. The incidence of neurogenic pulmonary edema may be much greater than previously suspected in that many patients may experience subclinical disease. Even in the presence of a fulminant course, patients usually recover rapidly, with normalization of the chest radiograph within 24–72 hours.

Neurogenic pulmonary edema is a diagnosis of exclusion that requires consideration of other conditions such as aspiration with chemical pneumonitis, primary pneumonia, and cardiogenic pulmonary edema secondary to volume overload or an acute myocardial event. The close temporal relationship of the CNS injury to the onset of the pulmonary edema and the absence of evidence for any of the alternative conditions warrant a presumptive diagnosis of neurogenic pulmonary edema.

Management is supportive with specific therapy directed against the underlying neurologic disorder. Patients require supplemental oxygen or intubation with positive-pressure ventilation in instances of severe respiratory failure. Physicians should recognize the potential of mechanical ventilation and the application of positive end-expiratory pressure to decrease cerebral venous drainage and aggravate raised intracranial pressure. The cerebral effects of positive pressure ventilation are difficult to predict without intracranial pressure monitoring. The role of continuous positive pressure breathing by face or nasal mask has not yet been reported for patients with postictal pulmonary edema. Introduction of mannitol, diuretics, or hypocarbia may be of value for patients with elevated intracranial pressure. Although the condition is usually self-limited with a rapid resolution, occasional sudden deaths from respiratory failure have been described.

The present patient was managed with mechanical ventilation and intravenous phenytoin. The hypoxemia and pulmonary edema resolved within 24 hours, allowing successful extubation the day after admission. The patient was subsequently discharged with normal mental status and pulmonary function.

Clinical Pearls

1. Although incompletely defined, "edematogenic centers" exist in the brain that produce pulmonary edema when stimulated. Recent MRI observations suggest that these centers may lie in the caudal brain stem at the nucleus tractus solitarius; other areas within the hypothalamus are probably also etiologically important.

2. In some models of neurogenic pulmonary edema, intense sympathetic discharge appears to mediate lung edema by increasing venous return and pulmonary blood volume, raising systemic and pulmonary vascular resistance, and constricting pulmonary veins. The resulting sudden increase in capillary hydrostatic pressure ("blast effect") ruptures the pulmonary microcirculation, causing exudative, hemorrhagic lung edema.

3. Other animal models demonstrate that CNS injury can directly damage pulmonary membranes without raising pulmonary artery pressures.

4. Although typically bilateral in distribution, radiographic infiltrates may be unilateral or focal in neurogenic pulmonary edema.

REFERENCES

1. Colice GL, Matthay MA, Bass E, Matthay RA. Neurogenic pulmonary edema. Am Rev Respir Dis 1984;130:941–948.
2. Minnear FL, Kite C, van der Zee H. Endothelial injury and pulmonary congestion characterize neurogenic pulmonary edema in rabbits. J Appl Physiol 1987;63:335–341.
3. Schell AR, Shenoy MM, Friedman SA, Patel AR. Pulmonary edema associated with subarachnoid hemorrhage: evidence for a cardiogenic origin. Arch Intern Med 1987;147:591–592.
4. Epstein FM, Cooper KR, Ward JD. Profound pulmonary shunting without edema following stereotaxic biopsy of hypothalamic germinoma: case report. J Neurosurg 1988;68:303–307.
5. Touho H, Karasawa J, Shishido H, et al. Neurogenic pulmonary edema in the acute stage of hemorrhagic cerebrovascular disease. Neurosurgery 1989;25:762–768.

PATIENT 54

A 47-year-old alcoholic man with cavitary pneumonia

A 47-year-old man presented with a 6-week history of fever, chills, cough productive of brown sputum, and a 20-pound weight loss. He had a long history of alcohol abuse.

Physical Examination: Temperature 102.1°; pulse 129; respirations 24; blood pressure 118/68. Mouth: poor dentition. Chest: coarse rhonchi over the left upper lung field. Cardiac: no heart murmurs. Abdomen: hepatomegaly with right upper quadrant tenderness to deep palpation.

Laboratory Findings: Hct 37%; WBC 12,900/μl with 62% neutrophils, 27% bands, 8% lymphocytes, 3% monocytes; platelets 564,000/μl. Na^+ 124 mEq/L; K^+ 4.2 mEq/L; Cl^- 87 mEq/L; HCO_3^- 24 mEq/L; BUN 26 mg/dl; creatinine 0.9 mg/dl; glucose 149 mg/dl. ABG (RA): pH 7.55; PCO_2 31 mmHg; PO_2 53 mmHg. PPD and controls: negative. Sputum AFB smear: negative. Sputum Gram stain: numerous neutrophils; 4+ gram positive bacilli. Chest radiographs: shown below.

Questions: What diagnoses should be considered? How should the patient be treated if the suspected diagnosis is confirmed?

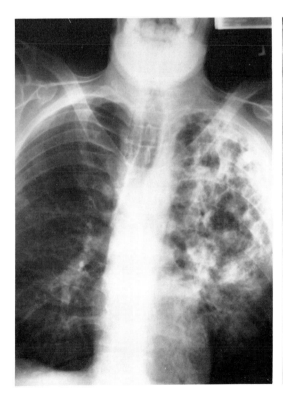 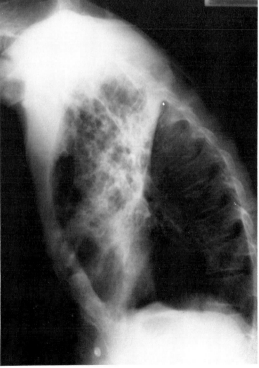

Diagnosis: *Corynebacterium* pneumonia.

Discussion: The differential diagnosis of a cavitary upper lobe infiltrate in an immunocompromised patient includes tuberculosis, atypical mycobacterial infection, aspiration pneumonia, or fungal infection. The presence of 4+ gram-positive bacilli on a good sputum sample suggests infection with anaerobic bacteria or *Corynebacterium*.

Corynebacteria are aerobic, gram-positive bacilli that are abundant saprophytes on skin and mucous membranes. They are usually judged to be contaminants when isolated in culture. In certain clinical settings, however, these bacteria are pathogenic deep-seated tissue infections.

Documented infections with Corynebacteria include pneumonia, empyema, bacteremia, endocarditis, shunt infection, abscess, and osteomyelitis. *Corynebacterium* pneumonia is usually insidious in onset, and is characterized by fatigue, weight loss, fever, and nonproductive cough. The chest radiograph usually reveals a unilateral cavitary infiltrate in either one of the upper lobes.

The usual patient with *Corynebacterium* infection is severely immunocompromised, most commonly from hematologic malignancy with neutropenia. A review of bone marrow transplant patients in Seattle over a 3-year period identified 32 cases of *Corynebacterium* bacteremia in 284 patients, with the most common site of infection being the lungs. The patients with *Corynebacterium* infections had a higher rate of marrow graft failure, more exposure to antibiotics, and more mucocutaneous defects than those without infection. Twenty-four of the 32 patients died during the initial hospitalization, with *Corynebacterium* infection being a major contributing factor in at least 10 of the 24 deaths. The *Corynebacterium* species associated with this outbreak was resistant to all antimicrobials except vancomycin.

Corynebacterium infection also has occurred in less severely immunocompromising conditions, including systemic lupus erythematosus, diabetes mellitus, and alcohol abuse. An increased incidence of *Corynebacterium equi* (renamed *Rhodococcus equi*) pneumonia has been reported in the AIDS population. There is a single report of *Corynebacterium* infection in an immunocompetent host.

Treatment of *Corynebacterium* infection is problematic because the organism is frequently resistant to multiple antibiotics. The drug of choice is vancomycin. Some investigators advocate two-drug therapy, with the addition of doxycycline, erythromycin, or rifampin.

The present patient was treated with intravenous vancomycin and doxycycline but had progressive respiratory failure and developed diffuse pulmonary infiltrates. His sputum cultures continued to grow a *Corynebacterium* species as a single isolate. He eventually died of massive pulmonary hemorrhage.

Clinical Pearls

1. *Corynebacterium* is a rare cause of bacterial pneumonia seen almost exclusively in immunosuppressed patients, most commonly neutropenic cancer patients. SLE, diabetes, and alcohol abuse are lesser risk factors.

2. *Corynebacterium* pneumonia is usually unilateral, cavitary, and upper-lobe predominant.

3. The drug of choice for *Corynebacterium* infection is vancomycin because of the high incidence of multiresistant strains. The addition of doxycycline, erythromycin, or rifampin may be efficacious.

REFERENCES

1. Stamm WE, Tompkins LS, Wagner KF, et al. Infection due to *Corynebacterium* species in marrow transplant patients. Ann Intern Med 1979;91:167–173.
2. Bowstead TT, Santiago SM. Pleuropulmonary infection due to *Corynebacterium striatum*. Br J Dis Chest 1980;74:198–200.
3. Donaghy M, Cohen J. Pulmonary infection with *Corynebacterium hofmannii* complicating systemic lupus erythematosus. J Infect Dis 1983;147:962.
4. Colt HG, Morris JF, Marston BJ, et al. Necrotizing tracheitis caused by *Corynebacterium pseudodiphtheriticum*: unique case and review. Rev Infect Dis 1991;13:73–76.
5. Williams EA, Green JD, Salazar S, et al. Pneumonia caused by *Corynebacterium pseudodiphtheriticum*. J Tenn Med Assoc 1991;84:223–224.

PATIENT 55

A 19-year-old woman with an acute exacerbation of asthma

A 19-year-old woman with a known history of asthma developed the sudden onset of wheezing 3 hours earlier. She had taken multiple inhalations of her albuterol metered-dose inhaler (MDI) but continued to cough and wheeze. During the last 1 year, asthma exacerbations had required one hospitalization and three evaluations in emergency departments. Her usual medications included an antihistamine and a sustained-release theophylline preparation in addition to her MDI.

Physical Examination: Temperature 37.8°C; pulse 130; respirations 28; blood pressure 135/90 with a 14 mmHg paradox. General: moderately severe respiratory distress. Chest: diffuse, high-pitched wheezes. Cardiac: no murmurs.

Laboratory Findings: Hct 40%; WBC 12,000/μl. ABG (RA): pH 7.38; PCO_2 38 mmHg; PO_2 62 mmHg. FEV_1: 1.0 L. Chest radiographs: shown below.

Question: What inhaled beta$_2$-agonist regimen would provide the most rapid initiation of bronchodilatory effect?

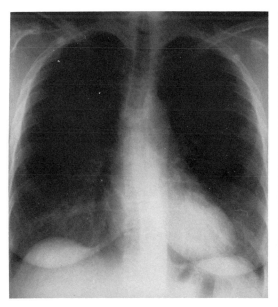
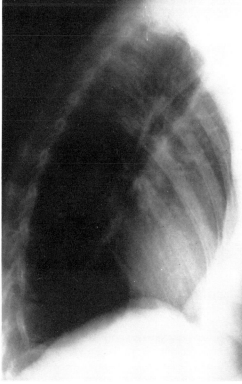

Answer: Initiate therapy with a metered-dose inhaler (MDI) combined with a spacer chamber.

Discussion: Inhaled beta-agonist drugs are the mainstay of therapy for patients with acute bronchospastic disease. Despite extensive clinical experience with these agents, however, investigators only recently have begun to define the most efficent methods in hospitalized patients for delivery of beta-agonist drugs to the airway. Traditionally, clinicians have reserved MDIs for ambulatory patients with clinically stable pulmonary disease. Patients with acute bronchospasm in the emergency department or inpatient services have been managed with powered handheld nebulizers (also called small-volume nebulizers [SVN] or jet nebulizers). This practice derives from the concepts that nebulizer therapy delivers a larger amount of drug and that acutely dyspneic patients cannot coordinate respiratory efforts to receive an effective MDI treatment. Recent experimental observations have largely dispelled these clinical impressions.

First, the inefficiency of handheld nebulizers reaches staggering proportions. Only 3–9% of a typically administered dose of 2.5 mg of albuterol reaches airway beta$_2$-receptor sites in the lung. The rest of the drug escapes into the atmosphere, remains in the handheld nebulizer, or deposits in the patient's oropharynx where mucosal absorption increases the incidence of adverse reactions but contributes little additional bronchodilator effect. Furthermore, recent data indicate that commercially available handheld nebulizers do not deliver reliable drug doses, which vary with small changes in technique and different device lots supplied from the same manufacturer.

At first consideration, aerosol treatments with MDIs may not appear much better. Only 6% of the administered dose reaches pulmonary beta$_2$-receptor sites, with the remainder being deposited on the oropharyngeal mucosa. Furthermore, patients with respiratory disorders often fail to coordinate inspiratory efforts with activation of the MDI, which is highly technique-dependent. The addition of a spacer chamber, however, drastically improves the efficiency of MDI therapy. A spacer allows dispersion of the aerosolized medication into smaller particles that are "respirable" deep into the lung's peripheral airways, increasing drug delivery from 6% to as high as 15–80% of administered dose. The amount of drug deposited ineffectively on oropharyngeal mucosal surfaces decreases from 86% to 10% with the addition of a spacer. Furthermore, a spacer decreases the importance of patient coordination with MDI activation.

In view of the MDI-spacer's greater efficiency, what evidence exists that patients with airway obstruction do as well with an MDI combined with a spacer as they do with a handheld nebulizer? So far, nearly all clinical studies demonstrate that MDI-spacer therapy is equivalent if not superior to SVN for patients with a broad array of respiratory conditions, including acute life-threatening asthma in the emergency department. Specifically, patients with acute exacerbations of asthma and severe airway obstruction experience a faster bronchodilatory response and a more prompt onset of peak bronchodilatory effect with MDI-spacer therapy. It appears well established that therapy with an MDI through ventilator tubing has greater effectiveness than nebulizer therapy in intubated patients with respiratory failure. These benefits are achieved with MDI regimens that deliver one-seventh the dose of total administered drug compared to nebulizer therapy.

The key to successful therapy with MDIs depends on recognizing that a puff of an albuterol MDI provides one-sixth to one-tenth of the amount of drug to the airway as delivered by SVN, even though MDI delivers the drug more efficiently and reliably. These data derive from titration dose studies of inhaled beta$_2$-agonists delivered by nebulizers or MDIs in patient volunteers with histamine-induced bronchospasm. Therefore, rather than using suboptimal, "routine" schedules of 2 puffs of MDI every 1–4 hours in acute bronchospasm, equivalent dosing of an MDI with a standard handheld nebulizer requires 6–10 puffs of MDI-spacer every 20–30 minutes for several doses until the goals of therapy are achieved. Some recent guidelines recommend up to 20 puffs from an MDI-spacer over a 10- to 20-minute treatment period initially every 20–30 minutes. The number of puffs and the frequency of therapy are then titrated against clinical effect. Patient series reported to date comparing the clinical response to 10 puffs of albuterol by MDI or 2.5 mg of albuterol by nebulizer demonstrate no differences in blood pressure or heart rate responses.

If an MDI-spacer provides effective hospital-based inhaled beta$_2$-agonist therapy, the question arises why most patients with reactive airway disease arrive at emergency departments after having failed intense usage of their MDIs at home. A partial explanation may lie in the observation that 90% of patients use incorrect technique. In an acute exacerbation, overly rapid inspiratory flow rates and underutilization of spacer chambers limit the efficacy of therapy. During the hospital phase, careful supervision of MDI-spacer treatments by a trained respiratory therapist, coaching inspiratory flow rates of no faster than 1 L/sec and postinhalation breathholding for 10 seconds, promotes adequate drug delivery even in severely dyspneic patients.

Several medical centers have reported their conversion to MDI-spacer therapy in up to 80% of inpatient treatments. This clinical approach not only maintains and in some instances improves therapeutic efficacy but also lowers the cost of respiratory care. Large tertiary care hospitals have demonstrated annual cost savings of $30,000 to $80,000, and $300,000 decreases in patient charges after limiting handheld nebulizer therapy. As recommended by a recent international consensus conference on aerosol therapy, an MDI with spacer should be the clinician's first choice for delivering aerosolized drugs to adult patients both during stable periods and acute exacerbations of bronchospastic disease.

The present patient was initiated on inhaled albuterol by MDI and a spacer chamber with 10 puffs every 20 minutes over 1 hour. After initial improvement in FEV_1 to 70% of predicted normal values, treatment intervals with 6–10 puffs of albuterol were extended to 1 hour. She was discharged with directions for using the spacer with home MDI therapy and for physician follow-up within 24 hours.

Clinical Pearls

1. During acute asthma exacerbations, patients become relatively resistant to beta$_2$-agonists and require higher drug doses for bronchodilatory effects.

2. By histamine challenge studies, approximately 10 puffs of albuterol by MDI are equivalent to one treatment with 2.5 mg of albuterol by handheld nebulizer.

3. A spacer chamber increases the portion of administered drug that reaches airway beta$_2$-receptor sites and decreases oropharyngeal drug deposition.

4. The flat portion of the dose response curve for albuterol by MDI-spacer in patients with acute asthma exacerbations typically ranges from 800–1600 μg.

5. MDI therapy in intubated, ventilated patients improves drug deposition and eliminates the use of wet nebulizers, which present a risk for nosocomial pneumonia.

REFERENCES

1. Fuller HD, Dolovich MB, Posmituck G, et al. Pressurized aerosol versus jet aerosol delivery to mechanically ventilated patients: comparison of dose to the lungs. Am Rev Respir Dis 1990;141:440–444.
2. Hollie MC, Malone RA, Skufca RM, Nelson HS. Extreme variability in aerosol output of the DeVilbiss 646 jet nebulizer. Chest 1991;100:1339–1344.
3. Pierson DJ. Toward international consensus on clinical aerosol administration. Chest 1991;100:1100–1101.
4. Blake KV, Hoppe M, Harman E, Hendeles L. Relative amount of albuterol delivered to lung receptors from a metered-dose inhaler and nebulizer solution: bioassay by histamine bronchoprovocation. Chest 1992;101:309–315.
5. Bowton DL, Goldsmith WM, Haponik EF. Substitution of metered-dose inhalers for hand-held nebulizers: success and cost savings in a large, acute-care hospital. Chest 1992;101:305–308.
6. Gay PC, Patel HG, Nelson SB, et al. Metered dose inhalers for bronchodilator delivery in intubated, mechanically ventilated patients. Chest 1991;66:66–71.

PATIENT 56

A 30-year-old woman with recurrent right-sided chest pain and dyspnea

A 30-year-old woman was admitted with right-sided pleuritic chest pain and dyspnea. During the past 6 years, she had experienced multiple similar events, two of which were associated with a pneumothorax. Despite several hospitalizations, her physicians had not established a specific diagnosis. A ventilation-perfusion lung scan done during a previous hospitalization was low probability for pulmonary embolism.

Physical Examination: Afebrile; pulse 88 and regular; respirations 14; blood pressure 120/80. General: no respiratory distress. Cardiac: normal. Chest: normal breath sounds; no clubbing. Extremities: no lymphadenopathy.

Laboratory Findings: Hct 30%; WBC 5,500/μl with a normal differential; platelets 343,000/μl. PT and PTT: normal. Electrolytes and renal indices: normal. Chest radiograph: shown below.

Question: What important information would aid in establishing the diagnosis?

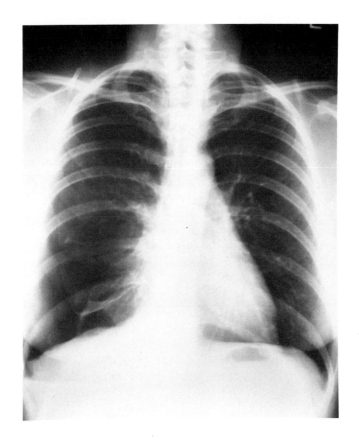

Diagnosis: Catamenial pneumothorax due to thoracic endometriosis. Noting the relationship of symptom onset with menstruation would aid in establishing the diagnosis.

Discussion: The term catamenial pneumothorax (CPT) describes a pneumothorax that occurs in temporal relationship to menstruation in a patient with underlying pelvic endometriosis. As a relatively unusual cause of secondary pneumothorax, only 96 patients with CPT have been reported in the English medical literature to date.

The disorder typically occurs in women older than 25–30 years of age, which is similar to the age of onset of pelvic endometriosis. Pneumothorax, manifested by pleuritic chest pain, varying degrees of dyspnea, or cough, develops within 48 hours of the onset of menstrual periods. Symptoms recur in the absence of therapeutic interventions. Many episodes may be mild, not prompting patients to obtain medical evaluation. Nearly 95% of the reported patients have had isolated right-sided pneumothoraces, with a presentation of simultaneous bilateral pneumothoraces reported in only two patients.

The pathogenesis of CPT is not well understood. One theory holds that endometrial tissue implants in the subpleural region of the lung and disrupts the pleura during menstruation, allowing air to enter the pleural space. The subpleural implants may occur either by microembolization of endometrial tissue via pelvic veins or transdiaphragmatic migration of shed pelvic endometrial tissue through diaphragmatic defects. A second theory suggests that air gains access to the peritoneum during menstruation and enters the pleural space through diaphragmatic defects. Any proposed theory for the pathogenesis of CPT would need to explain its nearly universal right-sided occurrence.

Most patients experience multiple episodes of pneumothorax before being correctly diagnosed as having CPT because clinicians fail to note the relationship of symptoms with menstruation.

Although some patients have associated pleural effusion, thoracentesis with pleural fluid cytologic analysis is seldom helpful in confirming the diagnosis, although benign, reactive, columnar-type epithelial cells may be noted. Thoracentesis may reveal a hemothorax, an infrequent manifestation of thoracic endometriosis. A chest CT scan, unless obtained during menses in the presence of intrapleural air, will be unremarkable.

The acute pneumothorax in patients with diagnosed CPT is treated symptomatically with analgesia and chest tube drainage. Suppression of ovulation with oral contraceptives is recommended to prevent recurrence; however, medical therapy is not universally effective. Danazol, a weak androgen, has been successful in some patients, but treatment failures have been reported.

Patients failing medical therapy or those wishing to become pregnant can undergo one of several surgical procedures. Thoracotomy with pleural abrasion or pleurectomy is definitive therapy that will prevent recurrent pneumothoraces. The diaphragm should be examined for defects, which can be oversewn at the time of surgery. Chemical pleurodesis, a relatively simple therapeutic alternative, has not been used widely in the management of catamenial pneumothorax or hemothorax. Talc insufflation at thoracoscopy or the instillation of talc slurry, minocycline, or doxycycline via a chest tube may be effective in inducing pleurodesis, thereby preventing further episodes of CPT.

The present patient had a classic presentation of CPT with recurrent chest symptoms at the onset of menstruation and a right-sided pneumothorax. She underwent thoracoscopy with talc insufflation and remains asymptomatic 1 year after pleurodesis.

Clinical Pearls

1. Thoracic endometriosis should be considered in the differential diagnosis of pneumothorax, hemothorax, hemoptysis, and chest pain in premenopausal women.
2. Catamenial pneumothoraces occur on the right side in 95% of patients.
3. Suppression of ovulation should be tried initially for CPT but may be ineffective.
4. Pleurodesis, either surgical or chemical, is recommended for recurrent pneumothorax or hemothorax.

REFERENCES
1. Lee CY, DiLoreto PC, Beaudoin J. Catamenial pneumothorax. Obstet Gynecol 1974;44:407–411.
2. Shearin RPN, Hepper NGG, Payne WS. Recurrent spontaneous pneumothorax concurrent with menses. Mayo Clin Proc 1974;49:98–101.
3. Wilhelm JL, Scommegna A. Catamenial pneumothorax: bilateral occurrence while on suppressive therapy. Obstet Gynecol 1977;50:227–231.
4. Nakmura H, Konishiike J, Sugamura A, et al. Epidemiology of spontaneous pneumothorax in women. Chest 1986;89:378–382.
5. Carter EJ, Ettenshom DB. Catamenial pneumothorax. Chest 1990;98;713–716.

PATIENT 57

A 35-year-old man with dyspnea on exertion and mild hemoptysis

A 35-year-old man presented with a 3-month history of progressive dyspnea on exertion and a nonproductive cough. He denied chest pain but noted blood-streaked sputum and intermittent low-grade fever during the previous 1 week. The patient smoked cigarettes for 15 years, worked as an air conditioning contractor, and denied use of illicit or prescription drugs, or homosexual activities.

Physical Examination: Temperature 37.8° C; pulse 89; respirations 20; blood pressure 125/65. General: well developed without lymphadenopathy. Eyes: normal fundi. Chest: scattered crackles at the lung bases. Cardiac: grade I/VI systolic murmur. Abdomen: no organomegaly. Extremities: digital clubbing.

Laboratory Findings: Hct 38%; WBC 8,900/μl with a normal differential. Electrolytes and renal indices: normal. Albumin 3.8 g/dl; bilirubin 0.9 mg/dl; LDH 450 IU/L; SGOT 25 IU/L; CPK 85 IU/L. Urinalysis: normal. ECG: normal. Chest radiographs: shown below.

Question: What condition is suggested by the patient's clinical presentation?

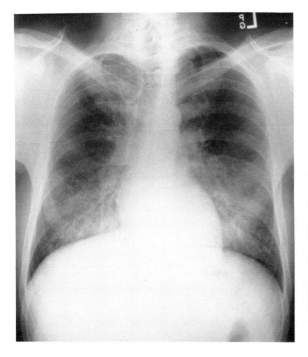
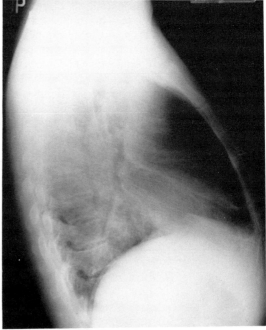

Diagnosis: Idiopathic pulmonary alveolar lipoproteinosis.

Discussion: Idiopathic pulmonary alveolar lipoproteinosis is a rare condition of unknown origin characterized by diffuse intra-alveolar deposits of periodic acid–Schiff (PAS)-positive proteinaceous phospholipids. Also termed "alveolar proteinosis" and "pulmonary alveolar phospholipoproteinosis," the intra-alveolar material largely comprises phospholipids with a small component of protein. Histologic sections demonstrate filling of the alveoli and distal airways with amorphous, eosinophilic material that contains within it needle-like clefts. A distinctive feature of the disorder is preservation of normal alveolar septal architecture, except for an occasional mild increase in septal cells. Diffuse alveolar damage or a marked influx of inflammatory cells is notably lacking.

The intra-alveolar phospholipid material appears to be similar in nature to surfactant, as shown by its positive staining with the immunoperoxidase method for identifying surfactant specific apoprotein. This observation suggests that abnormal accumulation of surfactant within the alveolus is an important mechanism of the disease. Mechanisms for increasing intra-alveolar surfactant include supranormal surfactant secretion by type II alveolar cells, increased sloughing into the alveolus and dissolution of type II cells with resultant intracellular surfactant release, and defective clearance of alveolar surfactant by alveolar macrophages. The latter mechanism may be particularly important, as indicated by the defects in macrophage function observed in patients with alveolar lipoproteinosis.

Exogenous inhalants may participate in the pathogenesis of pulmonary alveolar lipoproteinosis. Early reports observed that up to 50% of patients with this disorder had exposures to various dusts and chemicals before the onset of their disease. Subsequent studies have suggested a relationship with inhalational exposures to crystalline silica, fine particles of fiberglass, volcanic ash, and aluminum. Massive exposure to silica during sandblasting is a well-described condition (silicoproteinosis) that produces a pulmonary condition that shares clinical and pathologic features with alveolar lipoproteinosis. Reports of alveolar lipoproteinosis in siblings suggest a genetic predisposition, although environmental factors in such instances cannot be excluded. Additional associations with hematologic malignancies and lymphoma indicate that alveolar lipoproteinosis can occur as a reaction to an underlying neoplasm.

Although pulmonary alveolar lipoproteinosis occurs at any age, it most commonly affects patients between the ages of 20 and 50 years.

Patients typically present with a subacute prodrome characterized by cough, dyspnea on exertion, and occasional hemoptysis. The cough may be dry or productive of variable quantities of white sputum that may contain particulate matter. Weight loss, chest pain, low-grade fever, and progressive malaise may also develop. Clubbing may occur in 30% of patients, and a spontaneous pneumothorax occasionally develops secondary to air-trapping and rupture of blebs distal to airways partially obstructed with lipoprotein material. An elevated serum and alveolar concentration of lactic dehydrogenase and serum hypergammaglobulinemia are nonspecific findings.

Pulmonary function testing demonstrates a characteristic decrease in diffusion capacity. Lung volumes and spirometry may be normal or only mildly restricted early in the disease because of the preservation of the underlying pulmonary architecture. Patients with severe or long-term disease usually have more evidence of a restrictive defect and associated hypoxemia.

Early diagnosis of alveolar lipoproteinosis depends on considering the disorder in any patient with insidious effort-related dyspnea and a compatible chest radiograph. The chest radiograph characteristically demonstrates bilateral alveolar infiltrates in a symmetric, perihilar, "bat-wing" distribution. The infiltrates may also appear in an asymmetric and nodular pattern but never have associated mediastinal lymphadenopathy in uncomplicated instances of the disease. Segmental atelectasis may occur subsequent to bronchiolar occlusion by lipoproteinaceous material. Kerley B lines may result from lymphatic obstruction. No routine radiographic or CT finding, however, is unique to the disease.

Confirmation of the diagnosis depends on detection of PAS-positive intra-alveolar material in expectorated sputum, bronchoalveolar lavage (BAL) effluent, or tissue specimens. Unfortunately, PAS-positive material may be present in sputum from patients with other pulmonary conditions and in samples contaminated by mucus, desquamated cells, and food particles. Electron microscopic examination of sputum in patients with alveolar lipoproteinosis may demonstrate osmiophilic lamellar bodies. This finding, however, occurs in other disorders and presents logistical difficulties as a routine diagnostic study. Quantitation of sputum content of surfactant apoprotein A with monoclonal antibody techniques has recently been suggested as a valuable diagnostic study, although determination of the sensitivity and specificity of this test requires further experience.

Fiberoptic bronchoscopic BAL with or without transbronchial lung biopsy is sufficient for diagnosis in many patients. Demonstration of PAS-positive granules or electron microscopic evidence of osmiophilic granules with lamellar bodies within macrophages in the effluent from a patient with compatible clinical manifestations can confirm the diagnosis. Other features of the lavage specimen include a low number of macrophages, an increase in lymphocytes, and a variable CD4/CD8 ratio. Transbronchial lung biopsy samples may be normal because of a sampling error.

Open lung biopsy has been the definitive study that may still be necessary in some difficult instances but has been supplanted in most centers by bronchoalveolar lavage. Patients with the "secondary" form of the disease due to inhalational injury or underlying neoplasm usually have other clinical features of these disorders. Although *Pneumocystis carinii* pneumonia may present with a histologic pattern of alveolar lipoproteinosis, these patients have a more foamy intra-alveolar exudate, infiltration of alveolar septi with plasma cells and lymphocytes, and evidence of diffuse alveolar damage in contrast to the idiopathic form of the disease.

Whole-lung lavage is the only treatment for patients with alveolar lipoproteinosis. Because some patients with mild to moderate symptoms may remain stable or experience spontaneous remission, patients themselves may decide on the basis of symptoms and lifestyle limitations when to undergo therapy. Although most patients improve after lung lavage and may experience a remission, a progressive downhill course may occur despite repeated lavage. Patients with alveolar lipoproteinosis are also at increased risk for pulmonary infections from a variety of pathogens that include *Nocardia* species, *Cryptococcus neoformans, Mucor, Mycobacterium tuberculosis,* and *Histoplasmosis capsulatum.*

Alveolar lipoproteinosis was suspected in the present patient on the basis of the compatible chest radiograph showing diffuse alveolar infiltrates, elevated LDH, hemoptysis, and digital clubbing. Examination of the BAL effluent and the transbronchial biopsy specimens confirmed the diagnosis. The patient improved considerably after whole-lung lavage. It was speculated that his occupation in air conditioning exposed him to recurrent high concentrations of dust and fiberglass insulation particles while working in attics.

Clinical Pearls

1. Because of the preservation of normal underlying alveolar architecture, patients with alveolar lipoproteinosis may have normal spirometric and lung volume values early in their disease. Abnormally low measurements of lung diffusion, however, are hallmarks of the disorder.

2. The intra-alveolar phospholipid material appears to be surfactant, as indicated by its positive staining with immunoperoxidase methods for the detection of surfactant apoprotein.

3. Pulmonary alveolar lipoproteinosis may occur as a primary idiopathic form or secondary to other conditions such as *Pneumocystic carinii* pneumonia, silica inhalation, or underlying neoplasms. Secondary forms of the disorder may be distinguished by the clinical presentation, staining characteristics of the intra-alveolar material, and pathologic appearance of the underlying lung parenchyma.

4. Bronchoscopic BAL can confirm the diagnosis in most patients with a compatible clinical presentation by demonstrating PAS-positive granules or lamellar bodies within macrophages in the lavage effluent.

REFERENCES

1. Claypool WD, Rogers RM, Matusachak GM. Update on the clinical diagnosis and management of alveolar proteinosis (phospholipidosis). Chest 1984;85:550–558.
2. Gonzalez-Rothi RJ, Harris JO. Pulmonary alveolar proteinosis. Chest 1986;90:656–661.
3. Prakash UBS, Barham SS, Carpenter HA, et al. Pulmonary alveolar phospholipoproteinosis: experience with 34 cases and a review. Mayo Clin Proc 1987;62:499–518.
4. Rubinstein I, Mullen BM, Hoffstein V. Morphologic diagnosis of idiopathic pulmonary alveolar lipoproteinosis—revisited. Arch Intern Med 1988;148:813–816.
5. Milleron BJ, Costabel U, Teschler H, et al. Bronchoalveolar lavage cell data in alveolar proteinosis. Am Rev Respir Dis 1991;144:1330–1332.

PATIENT 58

A 19-year-old migrant farm worker with an acute febrile illness and a right middle lobe infiltrate

A 19-year-old migrant farm worker from Guatemala presented with a 1-week history of fever, chills, headache, myalgias, and intermittent abdominal discomfort. One day before admission, he had developed a sore throat and cough. He denied dyspnea, chest pain, nausea, vomiting, diarrhea, photophobia, or risk factors for HIV. A family member had similar complaints.

Physical Examination: Temperature 103.5°; pulse 88; respirations 13; blood pressure 112/78. Mouth: poor dentition. Chest: crackles and egophony in the right anterolateral lung field. Cardiac: normal. Abdomen: minimal tenderness to palpation; bowel sounds present. Neurologic: no meningismus.

Laboratory Findings: Hct 38%; WBC 3,800/μl with 66% neutrophils, 4% bands, 26% lymphocytes, 4% monocytes; platelets 49,000/μl. PT/PTT 13.9/32.2 sec. D-dimer > 8 μg/ml. Fibrinogen 366 mg/dl. Electrolytes and renal indices: normal. Liver function tests: AST 125 IU/L; ALT 88 IU/L; LDH 799 IU/L; total bilirubin 0.9 mg/dl. Chest radiograph: shown below left. Abdominal film: shown below right.

Question: Are there any other historical factors or physical findings that would help to establish the diagnosis?

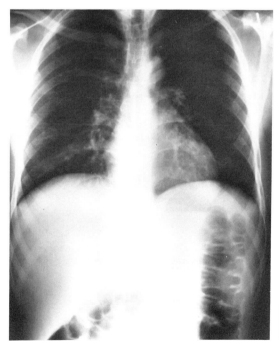 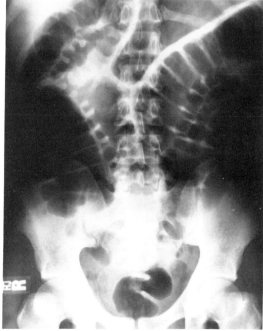

Diagnosis: *Salmonella typhi* bacteremia and pneumonia.

Discussion: *Salmonella* are non–spore-forming gram-negative rods of the family Enterobacteriaceae. In the vast majority of cases, *Salmonella* is acquired by the ingestion of contaminated food (primarily poultry) or water. Direct fecal-oral spread may occur, especially in children. Because humans are the only reservoir for *S. typhi,* direct or indirect contact with a carrier or currently ill person is necessary for infection to occur.

Risk factors for the development of *Salmonella* infection are primarily related to impairment of normal immune mechanisms and include gastrectomy, malignancy (especially hematopoietic), diabetes mellitus, systemic lupus erythematosus, HIV infection, renal transplantation, sickle cell disease, pregnancy, and cirrhosis.

Several clinical syndromes are associated with *Salmonella* infection, the most common of which is enterocolitis. This syndrome is usually self-limited and is characterized by a brief febrile illness with associated gastroenteritis that lasts less than 7 days. The most common causative organism is *S. typhimurium.* Enteric fever is produced classically by *S. typhi* and is the best studied enteric fever (typhoid fever). Bacteremia without manifestations of enterocolitis or enteric fever can cause a febrile illness. Localized infection may result following any of the clinical syndromes. A chronic carrier state also may exist in persons infected with *S. typhi* and is usually associated with disease of the biliary tract.

Although most strains of *Salmonella* cause illness in humans, the most widely studied organism is *S. typhi.* Typhoid fever typically presents with fever and headache. Faget's sign (elevated temperature without elevated pulse) is common with *Salmonella* infections. Cough, nausea, anorexia, diarrhea, abdominal pain, and vomiting are present in 30–50% of patients. Up to 30% of patients have no GI complaints at the time of presentation. Other prominent features include muscle aches, sore throat, and coryza. As many as 85% of patients present with some pulmonary complaint. Up to 65% of patients will have crackles or rhonchi on physical examination and 10% have evidence of lobar consolidation. *S. typhi* is demonstrated in sputum or pleural fluid cultures rarely (< 1% of cases).

Of the culture-positive pulmonary infections, 40% are empyemas, 40% pneumonias, 10% lung abscesses, and 10% pneumonias and empyemas. The most commonly reported causative organism is *S. typhimurium,* followed by *S. typhi* and *S. cholerasuis.* The pulmonary infection is likely the result of hematogenous spread in that 80% of patients have positive blood cultures in the first week of illness. Empyemas also result from direct extension from an abdominal focus to the thorax. The radiographic appearance of *Salmonella* pneumonia is not unlike other community-acquired pneumonias and is usually segmental, lobar, or multilobar. Cavitation and a miliary pattern have also been described.

Mortality associated with all *Salmonella* infections in the United States is < 1%, as is the case for most other localized *Salmonella* infections. The mortality associated with pulmonary disease is higher than in uncomplicated infections and may approach 25%. Significant antibiotic resistance to ampicillin, chloramphenicol, and trimethoprim-sulfamethoxazole has developed over recent years, and empirical treatment with third-generation cephalosporins is recommended until sensitivities can be obtained. As in all empyemas, tube thoracostomy drainage and/or decortication are recommended. *Salmonella* infections require prolonged periods of antibiotic treatment, and most authors recommend 3 weeks of therapy.

The present patient had a right middle-lobe infiltrate and extensive intestinal gas noted on the abdominal radiograph. He grew *Salmonella typhi* from blood and sputum. The patient received a 3-week course of ciprofloxacin. He remained febrile for 8 days but otherwise had an uncomplicated hospital course.

Clinical Pearls

1. *Salmonella* infections are associated with immunocompromised hosts, especially those with malignancy, gastrectomy, HIV, and sickle cell disease.

2. Respiratory complaints such as cough and coryza occur in up to 85% of patients with typhoid fever.

3. Although many patients with typhoid fever have rales or rhonchi on physical examination, most have a normal chest radiograph. Rarely are *Salmonella* organisms demonstrated in sputum and pleural fluid.

4. Pneumonia and empyema are the most common thoracic manifestations of *Salmonella* infection and are associated with a high mortality.

REFERENCES

1. Burney DP, Fisher RD, Schaffner W. Salmonella empyema: a review. South Med J 1977;70:375–377
2. Cohen JI, Bartlett JA, Corley GR. Extra-intestinal manifestations of salmonella infections. Medicine 1987;66:349–388.
3. Soe GB, Overturf GD. Treatment of typhoid fever and other systemic Salmonelloses with cefotaxime, ceftriaxone, and other newer cephalosporins. Rev Infect Dis 1987;9:719–736.
4. Ryan CA, Hargrett-Bean NT, Blake PA. *Salmonella typhi* infections in the United States, 1975–1984: increasing role of foreign travel. Rev Infect Dis 1989;11:1–8.

PATIENT 59

A 54-year-old man with cough and shortness of breath after a flu-like illness

A 54-year-old male farmer developed a flu-like illness with fever, cough, and myalgias. The myalgias remitted, but 5 weeks later he noted the onset of shortness of breath over several days. He denied sputum production, use of prescribed or illicit drugs, homosexual activities, or occupational exposure to inhaled toxins.

Physical Examination: Temperature 98.9°; pulse 92; respirations 24; blood pressure 135/85. Skin: normal. Neck: normal thyroid; right carotid bruit. Chest: bilateral fine crackles. Cardiac: S4; grade II/VI systolic ejection murmur. Abdomen: no organomegaly. Extremities: no clubbing.

Laboratory Findings: Hct 36%; WBC 11,000/µl. Electrolytes and renal indices: normal. LDH 220 IU/L (normal 95–180 IU/L). ABG (RA): pH 7.45; PCO_2 34 mmHg; PO_2 65 mmHg. FEV_1/FVC 78%; FVC 3.0 L (76% predicted); TLC 3.45 L (56% predicted). Chest radiographs: shown below.

Question: Although several conditions are compatible with the patient's presentation, which lung disorder should be listed high in the differential diagnosis?

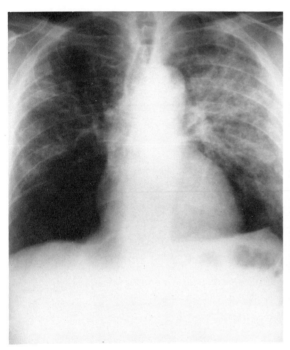
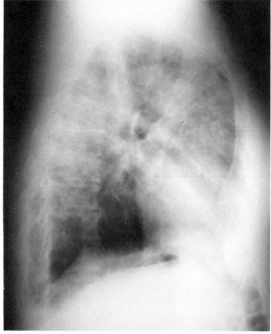

Diagnosis: Broncholitis obliterans with organizing pneumonia (BOOP).

Discussion: Intense interest has centered on the pulmonary disorder BOOP because of its unique clinical presentation, pathologic features, and responsiveness to therapy compared to other forms of interstitial lung disease. Also termed cryptogenic organizing pneumonitis by some investigators, BOOP is characterized by small airways and alveolar ducts that become filled with fibrous tissue, intraluminal polyps, and proliferating granulation tissue. The bronchioles undergo inflammatory changes that involve the surrounding interstitium with an influx of mononuclear cells. This "proliferative bronchiolitis" is commonly associated with foam cells in the alveolar space. In contrast to other forms of interstitial lung diseases, BOOP preserves the underlying pulmonary architecture and does not cause extensive interstitial fibrosis or honeycombing.

Multiple primary disorders have been associated with pulmonary reactions and pathologic features of BOOP. These disorders include lung infections with various bacterial and viral agents, inhalation of nitrogen dioxide, free-base cocaine, and plastic fumes, and ingestion of acebutolol, bleomycin, and amiodarone. BOOP also may occur secondary to pulmonary aspiration, eosinophilic pneumonia, malignancy, radiation therapy, and postobstructive pneumonitis. Additionally, BOOP has been reported in association with essentially all connective tissue diseases, including mixed connective tissue disease, lupus, polymyalgia rheumatica, dermatomyositis-polymyositis, and rheumatoid arthritis. In patients with systemic lupus erythematosus, BOOP may be the only manifestation of the underlying disease.

A large clinical category of BOOP, however, consists of patients with the idiopathic form of the disease. Idiopathic BOOP has a distinct clinical presentation that frequently suggests the diagnosis. Men and women between the ages of 20 and 70 years develop cough, mild dyspnea, and low-grade fever that progress in most patients in less than a 2-month period. Initial flu-like symptoms occur in 30% of instances. Patients rarely have hemoptysis or wheezing. The physical examination reveals fine end-inspiratory crackles in 60% of patients. The chest radiograph typically demonstrates bilateral patchy alveolar infiltrates with normal lung volumes. The infiltrates may have a peripheral distribution, as reported in eosinophilic pneumonia. Bilateral linear or nodular opacities occur in less than 20% of patients. Cavities, pleural thickening, and pleural effusions are rare radiographic findings. The chest CT shows regions of airspace consolidation in most patients that range from 2 cm to extensive bilateral disease.

Pulmonary function testing demonstrates a decreased vital capacity in 50% of patients, no evidence of airway obstruction in the absence of a smoking history, and depressed lung diffusion.

When clinically suspected, BOOP is initially managed with a course of antibiotics to exclude a responsive pulmonary infection. Patients who fail to respond or in whom recurrent disease develops are considered for lung biopsy. Recommendations for the method of lung biopsy vary. Some investigators emphasize the importance of open lung biopsy to obtain adequate tissue samples but will accept a transbronchial lung biopsy as confirmation of the disease if the specimen is sufficiently large to contain all elements of the pathologic lesion in a patient with characteristic clinical manifestations. Other investigators, however, strongly recommend an open lung biopsy—by thoracotomy or thoracostomy—in all patients to confirm the diagnosis and exclude other disorders. Unfortunately, although patients with BOOP commonly have more than 25% lymphocytes in bronchoalveolar lavage (BAL) fluid, this finding is not sufficiently specific to aid in diagnosis.

The differential diagnosis in patients with BOOP includes usual interstitial pneumonitis (UIP), pulmonary infections, eosinophilic pneumonia, organizing eosinophilic pneumonia, hypersensitivity pneumonitis, acute progressive interstitial pneumonitis (Hammond-Rich syndrome), and diffuse alveolar damage. Because the pathologic features of these conditions may overlap to some degree, pathologists should be alerted to the patient's clinical presentation to guide the search for the pathologic features of BOOP. The clinician usually can differentiate BOOP from UIP on the basis of the clinical presentation. Patients with UIP, compared to those with BOOP, typically experience more severe dyspnea, have a higher incidence of clubbing, demonstrate linear opacities and honeycombing on chest radiographs, have a longer course of symptoms at presentation usually greater than 2 months, and do not experience a viral-like prodrome. BOOP should also be separated from the related disorders termed "bronchiolitis obliterans without organizing pneumonia" and "constrictive bronchiolitis." These conditions do not have fibrous plugs within alveolar ducts and present with obstructive manifestations in patients with certain infections, toxic fume inhalations, underlying connective tissue diseases, and heart-lung transplantations.

Patients with idiopathic BOOP usually respond to corticosteroid therapy. Treatment is initiated with prednisone 1 mg/kg/day for 1–3 months and gradually tapered to 10–20 mg/day for 1 year.

Occasionally, the disease resolves spontaneously. More than 60% of patients treated with corticosteroids will have a complete normalization of the chest radiograph, rapidly responding over several days or weeks. Patients who fail to improve most often have diffuse linear or nodular infiltrates in the lower lung zones with reduced lung volumes or underlying collagen vascular diseases. Recurrence of symptoms during tapering or after the discontinuation of corticosteroids requires exclusion of infectious complications; most patients who relapse have the same clinical manifestations as occurred during the initial phases of the disease. Death from BOOP occurs in less than 5% of patients.

The present patient appeared to have BOOP on the basis of the flu-like illness, patchy alveolar infiltrates, restrictive pulmonary function tests, and duration of symptoms less than 2 months. He underwent a bronchoscopic transbronchial biopsy, which was nondiagnostic. An open lung biopsy revealed characteristic pathologic features of BOOP. The patient's symptoms and radiographic abnormalities resolved after a course of corticosteroid therapy.

Clinical Pearls

1. Patients with a flu-like prodrome followed within 2 months by progressive cough, mild dyspnea, and patchy alveolar infiltrates should be evaluated for BOOP.

2. Although both conditions occur in patients with collagen vascular diseases, BOOP is an "interstitial" lung disease, whereas "constrictive bronchiolitis" is an "airway" disease characterized by obstructive functional abnormalities.

3. The prognosis varies depending on the radiographic features; patients with patchy alveolar infiltrates are more responsive to corticosteroid therapy than patients with lower lung zone linear or nodular opacities.

4. When BOOP recurs during tapering or discontinuation of corticosteroid therapy, an opportunistic infection should be excluded. Patients with true relapses, however, usually experience identical symptoms as occurred during their initial illness.

REFERENCES

1. Epler GR, Colby TV, McCloud TC, et al: Bronchiolitis obliterans organizing pneumonia. N Engl J Med 1985;312:152–158.
2. Chandler PW, Shan MS, Friedman SE, et al: Radiographic manifestations of bronchiolitis obliterans with organizing pneumonia vs. usual interstitial pneumonia. AJR 1986;147;86:899–906.
3. Guerry-Force ML, Müller NL, Wright JL, et al. A comparison of bronchiolitis obliterans with organizing pneumonia, usual interstitial pneumonia, and small airways disease. Am Rev Respir Dis 1987;135:705–712.
4. Bellomo R, Finlay M, McLaughlin P, Tai E. Clinical spectrum of cryptogenic organising pneumonitis. Thorax 1991;46:554–558.
5. King TE Jr. Bronchiolitis obliterans. Lung 1991;169:S159–S183.

PATIENT 60

A 67-year-old man with myelodysplastic syndrome and hypoxemia

A 67-year-old man with myelodysplastic syndrome was admitted for treatment of a blast crisis. His myelodysplastic syndrome was diagnosed 6 months earlier when he was noted on a routine insurance examination to have thrombocytopenia. The patient had remained asymptomatic until 1 week previously when he developed anorexia, malaise, and easy bruising. He denied fever, chills, or dyspnea on exertion.

Physical Examination: Temperature 98.5°; pulse 135; respirations 18; blood pressure 146/91. General: no distress. Mouth: sublingual and soft palate petechial hemorrhages. Chest: clear. Abdomen: palpable spleen 5 cm below left costal margin.

Laboratory Findings: Hct 43%; WBC 93,000/μl with 76% blasts 20% lymphocytes, 3% PMNs, 1% monocytes; platelet count 15,000/μl. LDH 2168 IU/L; uric acid 17 mg/dl. ABG (RA): pH 7.47; PCO_2 38 mmHg; PO_2 53 mmHg; O_2 saturation 89%. Chest radiograph (shown below): normal.

Question: What is the explanation for this patient's hypoxemia?

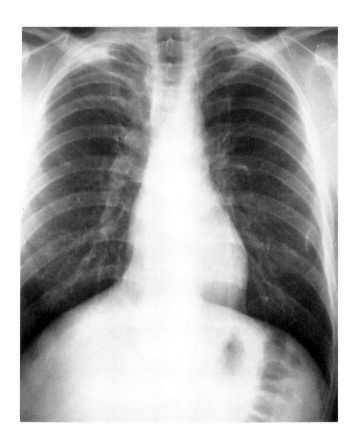

Diagnosis: Pseudohypoxemia secondary to extreme leukocytosis.

Discussion: Patients with hematologic malignancies frequently experience a wide array of pulmonary complications that may develop at their initial presentation or during therapy of their underlying disease. These complications may represent direct effects of the tumor, as occurs with pulmonary leukostasis syndrome, neoplastic invasion of the pulmonary parenchyma, and malignant pleural effusions. Hematologic malignancies also have the potential to indirectly cause pulmonary dysfunction, as occurs with acute lung injury from tumor lysis syndrome, toxicity of chemotherapeutic agents, and radiation pneumonitis. It is less well recognized that certain hematologic malignancies may alter measured arterial PO_2, even in the absence of pulmonary disease, which has been termed "pseudohypoxemia" and represents an instance of "leukocyte larceny."

Pseudohypoxemia occurs as a laboratory artifact in patients with normal or near-normal arterial blood oxygen tensions who develop profound leukocytosis. Leukocytes in a sampled specimen of arterial blood continue to consume oxygen in the syringe before the PO_2 is measured. The effects on blood oxygen tension, however, are usually negligible in patients with normal or moderately elevated peripheral leukocyte counts. Blood samples from patients with marked leukocytosis in excess of 10^5 cells/μl, however, may incorrectly indicate "hypoxemia," as leukocytes consume oxygen at a rate directly proportional to their blood concentration.

Several factors determine the degree of pseudohypoxemia in patients with leukocytosis. Cell type has an effect in that monocytes have a higher rate of oxygen consumption than lymphocytes and granulocytes. The degree of cell maturity also plays a role. Mature monocytes have an increased oxygen consumption compared to immature forms, whereas lymphocytes and granulocytes decrease their rates of oxygen consumption with maturation. Extreme reticulocytosis and thrombocytosis may also produce pseudohypoxemia. Because mature red blood cells have minimal oxygen consumptions, extreme polycythemia does not interfere with blood gas measurements. The temperature of the blood, the temperature at which the specimen is stored, and the time interval between obtaining the sample and PaO_2 are additional factors in determining the level of pseudohypoxemia.

Pseudohypoxemia secondary to leukocytosis should be considered in any patient with a peripheral leukocyte count in excess of 10^5 cells/μl, especially if the measured PO_2 appears disproportionately low compared to the patient's symptoms or clinical appearance. Although immediate placement of the arterial blood gas specimen in an ice bath may slow the fall in PaO_2, it will not negate the effect of extreme leukocytosis. When pseudohypoxemia is suspected, oxygen saturation by pulse oximetry may be a more accurate gauge of the patient's true oxygenation status than the measured PaO_2 or the calculated SaO_2.

The present patient demonstrated a marked discrepancy between the arterial oxygen saturation measured by pulse oximetry (96%) and the arterial PaO_2 and calculated SaO_2 determined by arterial blood gas analysis. With treatment of his blast crisis and reduction of the peripheral blood leukocyte count, the pseudohypoxemia resolved. Despite aggressive therapy, however, the patient failed to achieve a remission and died from an intracerebral hemorrhage secondary to thrombocytopenia.

Clinical Pearls

1. Extreme leukocytosis can cause pseudohypoxemia that is directly proportional to the peripheral leukocyte count. The maturity of the leukocytes has an additional effect that varies depending on the cell line.

2. The precipitous fall in vitro of the blood specimen's PaO_2 may be slowed but not eliminated with immediate placement of the sample on ice.

3. Pulse oximetry provides a more accurate measurement of arterial oxygen saturation in patients with profound leukocytosis than the directly measured or calculated SaO_2 determined by arterial blood gas analysis.

REFERENCES

1. Hess CE, Nichols AB, Hunt WB, Suratt PM. Pseudohypoxemia secondary to leukemia and thrombocytosis. N Engl J Med 1979;301:361–363.
2. Chillar RK, Belman MJ, Farbstein M. Explanation for apparent hypoxemia associated with extreme leukocytosis: leukocytic oxygen consumption. Blood 1980;55:922–924.
3. Loke J, Duffy TP. Normal arterial oxygen saturation with ear oximeter in patients with leukemia and leukocytosis. Cancer 1984;53:1767–1769.

PATIENT 61

A 54-year-old woman with dyspnea, hypoglycemia, and an abnormal chest radiograph

A 54-year-old woman presented with a 3-month history of recurrent dizziness and progressive dyspnea on exertion. Her "light-headedness" typically lasted 10 minutes, occurred most often in the morning or after missing meals, and improved with drinking orange juice. The shortness of breath limited the patient's ability to walk rapidly and occurred in association with right chest aching. Most recently, she had begun to notice painful shins and swelling of her fingertips. The patient denied smoking or occupational exposures to dusts or toxins, and took no medications.

Physical Examination: Temperature 98°; respirations 15; pulse 110; blood pressure 120/60. Head: normal. Neck: no lymphadenopathy. Chest: dullness and decreased breath sounds over the right upper thorax. Cardiac: normal. Abdomen: no organomegaly. Extremities: clubbed fingers; tenderness over both tibial ridges.

Laboratory Findings: Hct 38%; WBC 11,000/μl; Na$^+$ 135 mEq/L; K$^+$ 4.3 mEq/L; Cl$^-$ 102 mEq/L; HCO$_3^-$ 24 mEq/L; glucose 52 mg/dl; BUN 12 mg/dl, creatinine 1.1 mg/dl. Chest radiographs: shown below.

Question: What diagnosis could explain all of the features of the patient's presentation?

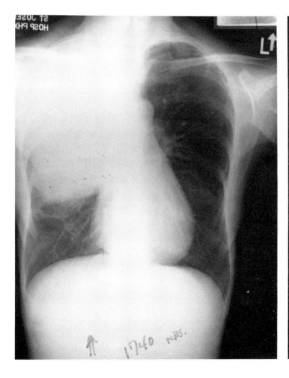 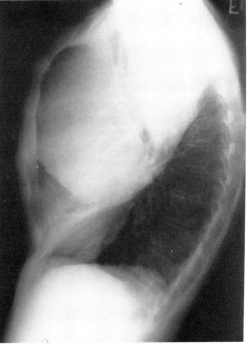

Answer: Localized fibrous tumor of the pleura.

Discussion: The traditional classification of pleural mesotheliomas into diffuse and localized forms is an incomplete description of these disorders. Diffuse mesotheliomas are spreading intrathoracic malignancies associated with asbestos exposure and a dismal prognosis. Localized mesotheliomas, although generally considered to be benign because of their more favorable course, actually range from benign, well-encapsulated neoplasms amenable to complete resection to aggressively invasive tumors with a grim clinical course. The absence of an association with asbestos exposure, lack of epithelial differentiation as seen in diffuse mesotheliomas, and a unique histogenesis have prompted recent investigators to reclassify localized mesotheliomas into a more distinct category termed "localized fibrous tumors of the pleura."

Although still open to debate, the histogenesis of localized fibrous tumors of the pleura appears to be related to mesenchymal submesothelial connective tissue cells that are also termed primitive fibroblasts, primitive multipotential cells, and primitive mesenchymal stem cells. The origin of diffuse mesotheliomas exists in malignant degeneration of mesothelial cells.

The most characteristic gross feature of localized fibrous tumors of the pleura is their encapsulation by a thin, translucent, glistening membrane that contains a network of vascular structures. Up to 60% of these tumors are attached to the visceral pleura by one or more pedicles through which courses feeding arteries. This gross feature is associated with a benign tumor and a favorable clinical course. Tumors also may have a broad-based ("sessile") attachment to the pleura or grow inward into the lung ("inverted") or into a pulmonary fissure. Tumors with the latter intrathoracic distribution are more commonly associated with a malignant progression. Attachment to the parietal pleural of the chest wall, diaphragm, or mediastinum are other common locations of tumor origin. Tumor size ranges from 1–39 cm, with the larger tumors more likely to be malignant. Tumor bulk may occasionally approach 4 kg in weight.

The histopathologic features of localized fibrous tumors of the pleura most often assume a "patternless pattern" in 60% of patients—fibroblast-like cells and connective tissue arranged in a random distribution. The remainder of patients have a "mixed pattern"—a patternless pattern mixed with a hemangiopericytoma-like appearance. The latter histologic appearance is made up of irregular, branching capillaries and larger vessels that can impart a hypervascular appearance to the tumor on CT scanning. The criteria for determining

malignancy in localized fibrous tumors of the pleura are the detection of high cellularity and mitotic activity, pleomorphism, hemorrhage, and necrosis. Although up to 50% of these tumors are initially misidentified by pathologists, the problem is largely semantic because the determination of malignancy is usually accurately established during the initial histologic evaluation. Immunochemistry and electron microscopy can exclude other sarcomas in localized fibrous tumors of the pleura presenting with complex histologic features.

Patients with localized fibrous tumors of the pleura typically present in the sixth or seventh decades of life with equal male and female distribution. Seventy-five percent of patients present with various combinations of chest symptoms that include thoracic pain, dyspnea, and cough. Particularly unique clinical features include hypoglycemia and acquired clubbing with or without hypertrophic osteoarthropathy, which occur in 25% of patients, as exemplified by the present patient. The pathogenesis of the hypoglycemia is unclear. Although hypoglycemia usually but not always remits after tumor resection, insulin-like compounds have not been isolated from tumor tissue. Women with localized fibrous tumors of the pleura are three times more likely than men to develop hypoglycemia, and the presence of hypoglycemia usually denotes a tumor size greater than 10 cm in diameter. Patients rarely present with hemoptysis, which is the only clinical feature that appears unique in the clinical presentation of the malignant versus the benign form of the disease.

The chest radiograph is often strikingly abnormal in patients with localized fibrous tumors of the pleura, because of the tumors' potential for impressive growth. More than 90% of patients have sharply circumscribed tumors, with 80% of the tumor contours being rounded and 16% lobulated. Thirty-five percent of tumors are 0–5 cm in diameter (some tumors are visualized only by CT), 43% are 6–10 cm, and 10% are larger than 10 cm. The tumor appears calcified in 7% of patients, and 17% have ipsilateral pleural effusions.

Diagnosis of localized fibrous tumors of the pleura depends on pathologic examination of biopsied or resected tumor tissue. Occasional patients with malignant tumors and associated pleural effusions may have positive pleural fluid cytologic examinations. Although frequently suggestive of the diagnosis, radiographic or CT findings are not sufficiently distinct to allow a noninvasive diagnosis.

Complete resection of tumor tissue is the foundation of effective therapy for localized fibrous tumors of the pleura. Pedunculated tumors, whether benign or malignant, usually are cured by resectional surgery. Nonpedunculated tumors also may be managed successfully if well encapsulated and removed en bloc. Simple excision with wedge resection of involved lung is usually adequate therapy, although more extensive pulmonary involvement may require a segmentectomy or lobectomy to remove all tumor tissue. Patients with localized extension into the chest wall may benefit from en bloc resection.

Over 95% of patients with benign tumors are successfully cured after complete surgical resection. Approximately 45% of patients with malignant localized fibrous tumors of the pleura are similarly cured without long-term recurrences. In the remaining 55% of patients with malignant disease, the tumors either are nonresectable (usually because of mediastinal invasion) or recur after surgery. They usually recur at the original site but contiguous spread or distant hematogenous metastases may occur.

The present patient was observed to have hypoglycemia during episodes of dizziness. Bronchoscopy revealed extrinsic airway compression and a CT scan demonstrated a homogeneous mass with increased vascularity. The patient underwent complete resection of a pedunculated, encapsulated tumor that proved to be a localized fibrous tumor of the pleura with hemangiopericytoma-like features. The patient is well 2 years after surgery with reversal of the hypoglycemia, digital clubbing, and pretibial tenderness from hypertrophic osteoarthropathy.

Clinical Pearls

1. Digital clubbing, hypoglycemia, and a large intrathoracic mass are suggestive of localized fibrous tumors of the pleura.

2. The term "localized fibrous tumor of the pleura" is preferred to "localized mesothelioma" because these tumors have no association with asbestos exposure, do not undergo epithelial differentiation, and probably arise from submesothelial rather than mesothelial cells.

3. Localized fibrous tumors of the pleura may be benign or malignant. The presence of histologic malignant features does not obviate the benefits of complete resection in that 45% of excised malignancies do not recur.

4. Although these tumors occur with equal frequency in men and women, women are three times more likely to present with hypoglycemia.

REFERENCES
1. Martini N, McCormack PM, Bains MS, et al. Pleural mesothelioma. Ann Thorac Surg 1987;43:113–120.
2. Bilbey JH, Müller NL, Miller RR, Nelems B. Localized fibrous mesothelioma of pleura following external ionizing radiation therapy. Chest 1988;94:1291–1292.
3. England DM, Hochholzer MD, McCarthy MJ. Localized benign and malignant fibrous tumors of the pleura: a clinicopathologic review of 223 cases. Am J Surg Pathol 1989;13:640–658.

PATIENT 62

A 71-year-old woman with chronic anemia, lymphadenopathy, and splenomegaly, and the recent onset of cough, dyspnea, and fever

A 71-year-old woman was evaluated for weight loss, fatigue, and lymphadenopathy of several months' duration. She recently had developed a nonproductive cough, increasing dyspnea, and a low-grade fever.

Physical Examination: Temperature 100°; respirations 20. Eyes: normal. Chest: normal. Lymph nodes: enlarged cervical and inguinal nodes. Spleen: palpable tip. Neurologic: intact.

Laboratory Findings: Hct 29%; WBC 5,500/μl with 57% PMNs, 30% lymphocytes; ESR 125 mm/hr. Chest radiographs: shown below. Serum immunoglobulins: IgA 369 mg/dl; IgM 2,700 mg/dl; IgG 429 mg/dl. Serum protein electrophoresis and immunoelectrophoresis: monoclonal band in the gamma region composed of IgM kappa. Bone marrow biopsy: infiltration by plasmacytoid lymphocytes. Bronchoalveolar lavage: abnormal population of lymphoplasmacytoid cells identical to those seen in the bone marrow that expressed IgM kappa by cytoplasmic immunoglobulin analysis.

Question: What is the etiology of this patient's systemic and respiratory complaints?

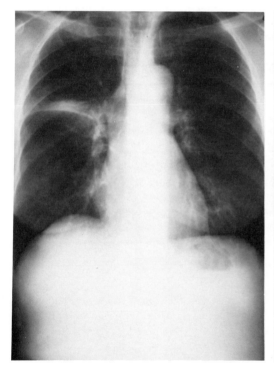 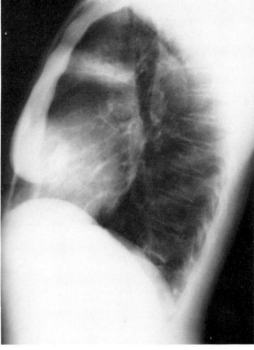

Diagnosis: Waldenström's macroglobulinemia (WMG) with pulmonary involvement.

Discussion: WMG is a rare disease characterized by malignant proliferation of plasmacytoid B-cell lymphocytes that secrete monoclonal IgM protein and typically infiltrate bone marrow, lymph nodes, liver, and spleen. It occurs most commonly in the elderly, and classically is associated with bleeding, anemia, and hyperviscosity.

The usual presenting symptoms are weakness, fatigue, weight loss, and hemorrhage. Epistaxis and gastrointestinal bleeding represent the most common form of hemorrhage and result from IgM protein coating on platelet surfaces that impairs platelet aggregation. Typical physical findings include adenopathy, hepatomegaly, splenomegaly, and ocular changes. Laboratory abnormalities of anemia and increased serum viscosity also may occur. Full-blown hyperviscosity syndrome manifests as hemorrhage, visual disturbances, neurologic symptoms, and congestive heart failure from hypervolemia. Cryoglobulinemia and Bence Jones proteinuria may be present but, as opposed to multiple myeloma, osteolytic lesions rarely occur. Treatment involves plasmapheresis for severe hyperviscosity and chemotherapy with alkylating agents, generally chlorambucil with or without prednisone, to control excessive IgM production.

Pleuropulmonary involvement with WMG has been reported to develop in 3% of patients with this disease, but recent observations suggest that WMG affects the lungs and pleura more commonly than was previously suspected. Patients with WMG have an increased risk of pulmonary infection both from the immunosuppressive effects of the disease and complications of chemotherapy. Noninfectious pulmonary complications also may occur, presenting with varying respiratory symptoms with or without associated pulmonary infiltrates.

Dyspnea, the most common symptom in patients with pulmonary involvement, occurs in over half of patients with WMG. A chronic, nonproductive cough may develop in a third of patients. Wheezing also may occur when airway narrowing results from diffuse endobronchial involvement. Many patients may remain asymptomatic despite pulmonary involvement.

Common chest radiographic manifestations of WMG include isolated or varying combinations of diffuse infiltrates involving multiple lobes, distinct parenchymal masses, pleural effusions, or hilar enlargement. Mediastinal adenopathy has been associated with pulmonary disease in a fourth of patients. Isolated pleural effusions without other chest involvement reportedly occur in 5–15% of patients. Pleural fluid typically is serosanguineous and exudative, but chylous effusions have been reported to occur. The latter have been attributed to compression and rupture of the thoracic duct by mediastinal lymph nodes. One case of transudative pleural effusion that developed after plasmapheresis was ascribed to rapid lowering of plasma colloid oncotic pressure.

Radiographic evidence of pulmonary involvement with WMG may be present on initial diagnosis of the disease, although pulmonary findings may also appear later during the course of the disease. Patients with WMG also may present with pulmonary manifestations in the absence of the more classic features of the disease.

The diagnosis of pulmonary involvement in WMG is made by immunologic studies of biopsied lung tissue, pleural fluid, or bronchoalveolar lavage fluid that demonstrate abnormal populations of plasmacytoid lymphocytes expressing monoclonal IgM. These proliferating cells occur in the lung as infiltrating lesions along the endobronchial mucosa, depositions on the pleural surface, and cohesive masses along interalveolar septa that obliterate the normal pulmonary architecture. Diagnostic techniques include thoracentesis, bronchoscopy with transbronchial biopsy or bronchoalveolar lavage, thoracoscopy, and open thoracotomy. Pulmonary involvement generally responds favorably to alkylating agents and does not appear to adversely affect prognosis.

The present patient appeared to have pulmonary involvement, as demonstrated by radiographic evidence of diffuse interstitial and patchy alveolar infiltrates. Demonstration by bronchoalveolar lavage of an abnormal population of lymphoplasmacytoid cells that expressed IgM kappa by cytoplasmic immunoglobulin analysis confirmed the diagnosis. After treatment with chlorambucil and prednisone, the patient's serum IgM concentration decreased, lymphadenopathy and splenomegaly diminished, respiratory symptoms resolved, and pulmonary infiltrates cleared.

Clinical Pearls

1. Pleuropulmonary involvement in WMG is an increasingly recognized manifestation of the disease that should be suspected when respiratory symptoms or radiographic abnormalities develop in these patients.

2. Pleuropulmonary involvement may appear at any time during the course of WMG and may precede other manifestations of the disease in some patients.

3. Radiographic manifestations of pleuropulmonary WMG include diffuse infiltrates, discrete masses, hilar adenopathy, and pleural effusions.

4. Diagnosis is established by immunologic studies that demonstrate malignant proliferation of monoclonal IgM-secreting plasmacytoid lymphocytes in lung tissue, bronchoalveolar lavage, or pleural fluid.

REFERENCES

1. Rausch PG, Herion JC. Pulmonary manifestations of Waldenström macroglobulinemia. Am J Hematol 1980;9:201–209.
2. Deuel TF, Davis P, Avioli LV. Waldenström's macroglobulinemia. Arch Intern Med 1983;143:986–988.
3. Filuk RB, Warren PW. Bronchoalveolar lavage in Waldenström's macroglobulinemia with pulmonary infiltrates. Thorax 1986;41:409–410.
4. Monteagudo M, Lima J, Garcia-Bragado F, et al. Chylous pleural effusion as the initial manifestation of Waldenström's macroglobulinemia. Eur J Respir Dis 1987;70:326–327.
5. Dimopoulos MA, Alexanian R. Waldenström's macroglobulinemia. Blood 1994;83:1452–1459.

PATIENT 63

A 76-year-old woman with hypotension and respiratory failure after total knee arthroplasty

A 76-year-old woman with rheumatoid arthritis developed sudden hypotension and hypoxemia 1 hour after undergoing a total left knee arthroplasty. No intraoperative difficulties occured during placement of the cemented condylar prosthesis except for a change in blood pressure from 120/90 to 100/70 after release of the thigh tourniquet (total tourniquet time, 1 hour and 30 minutes). In the recovery room, however, the patient complained of dyspnea and rapidly became obtunded and cyanotic, requiring intubation. No history existed of previous cardiac or pulmonary disease.

Physical Examination: Temperature 97°; pulse 135; respirations 32; blood pressure 85/60. General: unresponsive with severe respiratory distress. Skin: cyanotic. Neck: marked venous distension. Chest: scattered crackles. Cardiac: grade I/VI systolic ejection murmur; no gallop rhythm; loud S2. Abdomen: soft without organomegaly. Extremities: closed left knee surgical wound; no calf swelling.

Laboratory Findings: ABG (100% oxygen by Ambu bag): pH 7.51; PO_2 52 mmHg; PCO_2 28 mmHg. ECG: sinus tachycardia with ST-segment depressions consistent with myocardial ischemia. Chest radiograph: shown below.

Question: What is the probable cause of this patient's sudden cardiopulmonary event?

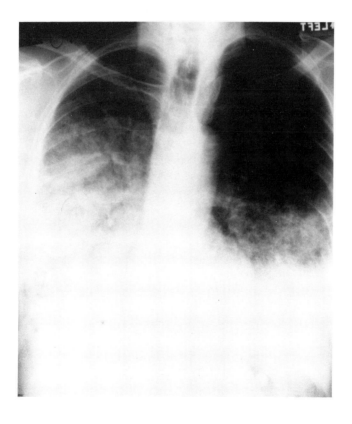

Diagnosis: Fat embolism during cemented total knee arthroplasty.

Discussion: Multiple reports document the occurrence of varying degrees of acute cardiopulmonary dysfunction during the intraoperative or immediate postoperative period in patients undergoing total hip arthroplasty with cemented prostheses. These episodes include transient hypotension in up to 80% of patients, hypoxemia, and occasional instances of unexplained cardiac arrest and sudden death. Although described since 1961 with the introduction of cemented hip arthroplasty, these cardiopulmonary events remain incompletely defined. The advent of total knee cemented arthroplasty, however, has renewed investigative interest in these complications since they appear to occur with greater frequency and severity in knee compared to hip replacement surgery.

The clinical events associated with these complications of knee arthroplasty follow a stereotypical course. Patients remain stable during the initial phase of surgery when the knee is prepared below a thigh tourniquet for prosthetic placement. Immediately or within 1 hour after insertion of the cemented prosthetic rod into the intramedullary space and deflation of the thigh tourniquet, patients rapidly deteriorate with varying degrees of dyspnea, confusion, hypotension, hypoxemia, and signs of pulmonary hypertension. Radiographic evidence of interstitial pulmonary edema that may progress in severity to the adult respiratory distress syndrome commonly develops. Although some patients may stabilize and survive after the initiation of pressor support and mechanical ventilation, others experience a progressive downhill course with intractable hypotension and profound respiratory failure that terminates in cardiac arrest and death.

The pathophysiology of these acute cardiopulmonary events appears to be unrelated to pulmonary thromboembolic disease or acute myocardial infarction. Although electrocardiographic features of myocardial ischemia frequently occur, cardiac enzyme confirmation of frank infarction or angiographic detection of pulmonary emboli are rarely observed. Previous investigators have suggested that systemic absorption of the methylmethacrylate glue used to cement the prosthesis in place may alter systemic and pulmonary vascular resistance. Recent clinical studies, however, indicate that blood levels of methylmethacrylate monomer achieved during surgery are insufficient to produce cardiovascular effects. Furthermore, the cardiopulmonary complications of knee arthroplasty can be reproduced in animal models without the application of intramedullary cement.

Autopsy studies of patients dying from cardiorespiratory failure after knee arthroplasty provide clues to a probable etiologic mechanism. In these studies, fat emboli lodged in the vascular beds of multiple organ systems are common pathologic findings. In some instances, up to 80% of the pulmonary microvasculature is occluded by fat particles, with emboli also noted in the cerebral, myocardial, and renal circulation. Presumably, insertion of the prosthetic rod causes high intramedullary pressure that forces bone marrow contents into the bloodstream. Once in the pulmonary and systemic circulation, the vasoactive properties of fat microemboli and other components of the bone marrow, including tissue thromboplastins, alter vascular tone and permeability, increase intrapulmonary shunting, and produce localized organ ischemia.

Fat embolism syndrome related to traumatic bony fractures is a paradigm for the events that follow knee arthroplasty. The majority of trauma victims seen at autopsy have detectable fat emboli, although most patients do not have clinically apparent antemortem disease. Less than 5% of patients with isolated fractures and 55% of patients with severe trauma have cardiopulmonary or cerebral manifestations of fat emboli syndrome. On the basis of these data, it is suspected that most patients undergoing hip or knee arthroplasty experience some degree of fat embolization. Only major extrusion of bone marrow contents into the systemic circulation, however, produces clinically important disease.

Once established, no specific therapy exists for fat emboli syndrome related to knee arthroplasty. Corticosteroids have an anecdotal rationale, having been used with variable success in trauma-related fat emboli syndrome. Otherwise, patients are managed with supportive care that includes intravascular volume expansion, pressor support, and mechanical ventilation.

Preventive surgical techniques and anticipatory monitoring are the most important measures. Patients undergoing knee arthroplasty should be closely observed for arterial oxygen desaturation with pulse oximetry during and after surgery. During placement of the prosthesis, excessive manipulation and compression of the intramedullary canal should be avoided. Animal studies indicate that only 150 torr of intramedullary pressure is required to introduce fat from the bone marrow into the femoral veins. In humans during knee arthroplasty, up to 1,000 torr of pressure may develop during insertion and cementing of the prosthetic rod. Therefore, venting of the intramedullary canal, elimination of intramedullary debris by meticulous intraoperative lavage, and gradual insertion of the prosthesis are critical measures to maintain low bone marrow pressures.

Placement of a thigh tourniquet during the medullary reaming maneuver and prosthetic placement has not been clearly established as a valuable adjunct; the tourniquet may delay the onset of cardiopulmonary complications but create a bolus effect during tourniquet deflation.

The present patient was treated with intravenous pressor agents, intravascular volume expansion, and mechanical ventilation. Despite these measures, hypotension and hypoxemia persisted and the chest radiograph progressed from an initial interstitial pattern of pulmonary edema to frank ARDS. The patient expired 2 hours later of a cardiac arrest. The autopsy demonstrated multiple fat emboli throughout the pulmonary microcirculation.

Clinical Pearls

1. Acute cardiopulmonary dysfunction from fat emboli may occur in patients undergoing total knee cemented arthroplasty.

2. Fat emboli in this clinical setting cause systemic hypotension, hypoxemia, pulmonary hypertension, and pulmonary edema.

3. Fat and other bone marrow contents are extruded into the bloodstream during insertion of the prosthetic intramedullary rod, which may cause intramedullary pressures as high as 1,000 torr.

4. No specific therapy exists for fat emboli syndrome after knee arthroplasty. Intraoperative preventive techniques to maintain low bone marrow pressures include venting of the intramedullary canal, elimination of intramedullary debris by meticulous intraoperative lavage, and gradual insertion of the prosthesis.

REFERENCES
1. Orsini EC, Richards RR, Mullen JMB. Fatal fat embolism during cemented total knee arthroplasty: a case report. Can J Surg 1986;29:385–386.
2. Orsini EC, Byrick RJ, Mullen JBM, et al. Cardiopulmonary function and pulmonary microemboli during arthroplasty using cemented or noncemented components. J Bone Joint Surg 1987;69A:822–832.
3. Monto RR, Garcia J, Callaghan JJ. Fatal fat embolism following total condylar knee arthroplasty. J Arthroplasty 1990;5:291–299.
4. Pell AC, Christie J, Keating JF, Sutherland GR. The detection of fat embolism by transoesophageal echocardiography during reamed intramedullary nailing: a study of 24 patients with femoral and tibial fractures. J Bone Joint Surg 1993;75B:921–925.

PATIENT 64

A 68-year-old woman with progressive dyspnea and cough 6 months after a hip fracture

A 68-year-old woman was referred by her local physician for evaluation of a 6-month history of progressive dyspnea and a nonproductive cough. Her past medical history was significant for mild hypertension, osteoporosis, and no use of tobacco. She had sustained a hip fracture 1 year earlier and was begun on estrogen replacement therapy.

Physical Examination: Temperature 98.8°; pulse 80 and regular; respirations 26. General: minimal respiratory distress. Chest: bilateral basilar inspiratory crackles. Cardiac: normal. Extremities: no clubbing, cyanosis, or edema.

Laboratory Findings: Hct 36%; WBC 8,000/μl with a normal differential. Sputum culture: normal flora. PPD negative with positive controls. FEV$_1$/FVC 59%; TLC 115% of predicted; DLCO 24% of predicted. ABG (RA): pH 7.42; PCO$_2$ 38 mmHg; PO$_2$ 52 mmHg. Chest radiograph: shown below.

Question: What is the differential diagnosis and most likely cause of the patient's interstitial lung disease?

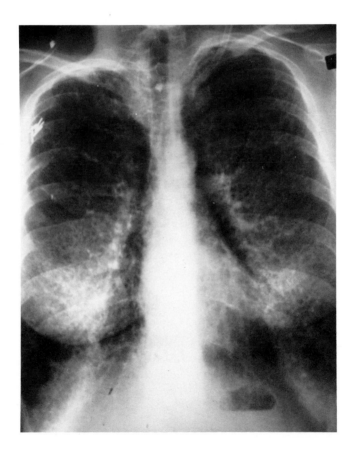

Diagnosis: Lymphangiomyomatosis (LAM).

Discussion: LAM is an unusual pulmonary condition that results from hamartomatous proliferation of smooth muscle in the peribronchial, perivascular, and perilymphatic regions of the lung, as well as within the abdomen. Because of its rarity, LAM is often not diagnosed until well after the initial manifestations of the disease. The condition occurs almost exclusively in women of child-bearing years (average age 43 years, range 12–89). Older women presenting with LAM have taken exogenous estrogens, and a single case report exists of the disease in a child. Other risk factors for LAM include oral contraceptive use, previous treatment with gonadotropin, early menarche, and pregnancy.

Most patients with LAM present with exertional dyspnea. Less common presentations include chest pain, cough, and hemoptysis. Resting dyspnea and chyloptysis rarely occur at presentation of the disease.

At the onset of the disease, the chest radiograph most commonly shows reticulonodular infiltrates with or without an accompanying pneumothorax. At some time during the course of the disease, reticulonodular infiltrates develop in 95% of patients, pneumothorax in 80%, chylothorax in 30%, cysts or bullae in 40%, and hyperinflation in 25%. As the disease progresses, small cystic changes may appear predominantly in the lower lung zones; hilar adenopathy may also be present. The chest radiograph occasionally may be normal in that symptoms may precede radiographic evidence of disease.

Spirometry shows a reduced FEV_1/FVC ratio, which may lead to an incorrect diagnosis of emphysema, asthma, or chronic bronchitis. Restrictive findings may be observed following tube thoracostomy, pleurodesis, or open lung biopsy. The diffusion capacity is decreased in most patients out of proportion to spirometric abnormalities. The pulmonary function abnormalities seen in patients with LAM contrast to those observed in patients with idiopathic pulmonary fibrosis. In this latter condition, a restrictive defect occurs with reduction of residual volume, vital capacity, total lung capacity, and diffusion capacity.

The gross pathology of LAM demonstrates diffuse effacement by cystic spaces separated by thickened interstitial tissue. Microscopy shows a proliferation of bronchial smooth muscle cells that result in narrowing of the conducting airways, leading to air trapping and the development of bullae and pneumothorax. Proliferation of venular and lymphatic smooth muscle resulting in obstruction and rupture of these structures underlies the hemoptysis and chylothoraces experienced by these patients.

LAM should be included in the differential diagnosis of interstitial lung disease in patients with normal to increased lung volumes. Other disorders that cause this pattern include sarcoidosis, cystic fibrosis, proliferative bronchiolitis, tuberous sclerosis, histiocytosis X, and chronic obstructive pulmonary disease with associated interstitial lung disease. The gold standard for diagnosis is open lung biopsy, although a diagnosis by lymph node biopsy has been reported. Typical findings on high-resolution CT scan when coupled with a clear clinical history can be considered diagnostic. The high-resolution CT demonstrates thin-walled, round cysts less than 10 mm in diameter distributed evenly throughout all lung zones with apical sparing. Other abnormalities that may be present on CT scan include pneumothorax, pleural effusion, and mediastinal or intraabdominal lymph node enlargement due to smooth muscle proliferation. Gallium 67 scintigraphy, SPECT imaging, and measurement of HMB45, a melanoma-related marker, have shown promise in assisting the diagnosis.

No clinical trials exist to support any specific therapy for LAM. Tamoxifen therapy has been disappointing, leading to the impression that estrogen sensitivity alone is not causative of the disease. Oophorectomy appears to have limited success, probably secondary to peripheral estrogen synthesis. Oophorectomy combined with medroxyprogesterone therapy has yielded the most promising results, with improvement of dyspnea, chylous effusions, and ascites. No apparent correlation exists between the status of progesterone and estrogen receptors and the response to hormone manipulation. Le Veen shunts and pleurodesis have been used for symptomatic treatment of chylothorax. Lung transplantation has been successful in some patients with progressive disease.

Survival averages 10 years after the diagnosis of LAM, although some patients may survive for many decades. Marked individual variation occurs in the course of the disease, which complicates interpretation of therapeutic trials in small patient populations.

The present patient's risk factor for development of LAM was the introduction of exogenous estrogens for treatment of osteoporosis. Tissue specimens from her open lung biopsy were diagnostic for lymphangiomyomatosis. Estrogen therapy was discontinued, and she has shown clinical improvement.

Clinical Pearls

1. Chylothorax, pneumothorax, or hemoptysis in a woman of child-bearing age should raise the possibility of LAM.

2. LAM should be suspected in a young woman with exertional dyspnea and a diffusion capacity decreased out of proportion to abnormalities of measured lung volume.

3. The clinical syndrome of LAM may develop in postmenopausal women who receive estrogen therapy.

4. Symptoms may appear before standard chest radiograph changes; high-resolution CT scans may assist in earlier detection and establish the diagnosis in the appropriate clinical setting.

5. Aggressive early treatment with oophorectomy and medroxyprogesterone may preserve lung function. Lung transplantation has been successful in patients with progressive disease.

REFERENCES

1. Miller WT, Cornog JL Jr, Sullivan MA. Lymphangiomyomatosis: a clinical-roentgenologic pathologic syndrome. Am J Roentgenol Radium Ther Nucl Med 1971;111:565–572.
2. Dishner W, Cordaaco EM, Blackburn J, et al. Pulmonary lymphangiomyomatosis. Chest 1984;85:796–799.
3. Shen A, Iseman MD, Waldron JA, et al. Exacerbation of pulmonary lymphangiomyomatosis by exogenous steroids. Chest 1987;91:782–785.
4. Taylor JR, Ryu J, Colby TV, et al. Lymphangioleiomyomatosis. N Engl J Med 1990;232:1254–1260.
5. Bonetti F, Chiodera PL, Pea M, et al. Transbronchial biopsy in lymphangiomyomatosis of the lung. HMB45 for diagnosis. Am J Surg Pathol 1993;17:1092–1102.
6. Case Records of the Massachusetts General Hospital. Weekly clinicopathological exercises. Case 18-1994: a 37-year-old woman with interstitial lung disease, renal masses, and a previous spontaneous pneumothorax [clinical conference]. N Engl J Med 1994;330:1300–1306.

PATIENT 65

A 73-year-old man with fever and chest pain

A 73-year-old man was admitted for evaluation of a 2-month history of a constant precordial aching that worsened with deep inspiration. He also noted a persistent fever that ranged between 100° and 102° F. There were no symptoms of rigors, cough, or dysphagia but mild dyspnea on exertion had recently developed. One month before the onset of symptoms, an extraction of his left lower second molar was complicated by a severe oral infection. After drainage of a submandibular abscess and a 2-week course of oral antibiotics, the dental symptoms resolved.

Physical Examination: Temperature 100.3°; pulse 92; respirations 15; blood pressure 132/80. General: no apparent distress. Mouth: normal. Neck: well-healed 1-cm left submandibular incision without swelling or erythema; normal neck veins. Chest: decreased breath sounds at both bases. Cardiac: grade I/VI systolic ejection murmur without a friction rub. Abdomen: normal bowel sounds. Extremities: no clubbing or edema.

Laboratory Findings: Hct 39.6%; WBC 12,400/µl with 90% granulocytes. Electrolytes and renal indices normal. Chest radiograph: shown below top. A left thoracentesis revealed serous pleural fluid with the following characteristics: protein 4.0 g/dl; LDH 350 IU/L; glucose 100 mg/dl; pH 7.42; white cell count 1,500/µl with 75% granulocytes. Gram stain: negative. Subsequent pleural fluid cultures were negative. A thoracic CT is shown below bottom.

Question: What is the likely diagnosis and how would you pursue it?

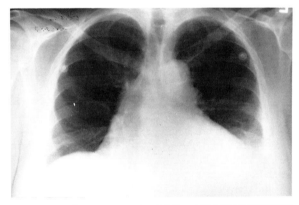

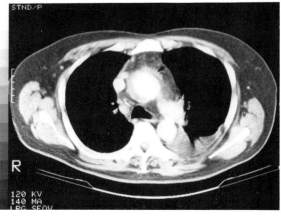

Diagnosis: A thoracic CT scan demonstrated radiographic evidence of bacterial mediastinitis.

Discussion: Acute bacterial mediastinitis represents a rapidly progressive and highly lethal condition that requires prompt diagnosis and aggressive therapy. In the preantibiotic era, mediastinitis was a relatively common problem that resulted from progressive infections of the head and neck, pleuropulmonary suppuration, vertebral osteomyelitis, and retroperitoneal abscesses. In the postantibiotic era, series of patients with acute mediastinitis unrelated to thoracic surgery or trauma indicate that over 90% of instances result from esophageal perforation subsequent to Boerhaave's syndrome, mediastinal malignancies, or endoscopic esophageal instrumentation.

Although presently rare, spread of bacteria from infections of the head and neck remains an additional clinically important cause of mediastinitis. Termed descending necrotizing mediastinitis, the primary site of infection may be pharyngeal, as occurs in pharyngitis, epiglottitis, tonsillitis, parotitis, and Ludwig's angina, or odontogenic, as demonstrated by the present patient.

Patients with odontogenic-related mediastinitis typically experience serious dental infections—most commonly of the lower second or third molars—that spread into the submandibular space. Once suppuration becomes established in the neck, cervical fascial planes composed of loose areolar tissue present a negligible barrier against extension into the mediastinum. The route of mediastinal infection typically occurs from the submandibular space into the parapharyngeal space, which then seeds the retropharyngeal fascial planes. The retropharyngeal space is continuous below the sixth cervical vertebra with the retrovisceral space, which enters the mediastinum below the third thoracic vertebra. Pus in the retrovisceral region of the mediastinum can then rupture into the loose connective tissue between alar fascia anteriorly and paravertebral fascia posteriorly; this space extends inferiorly to the diaphragm and can readily rupture into the pleural space, causing a thoracic empyema.

The onset of symptoms from descending necrotizing mediastinitis may occur dramatically within hours or days of a head and neck infection or several weeks after a drainage procedure promotes local recovery from a cervical abscess. Symptoms typically include fever, dysphagia, chills, increasing respiratory distress, and chest pain. The description of pain is nonspecific but often has a pleuritic component and centers in the upper anterior chest or precordium. Left untreated, bacteremia and ultimately shock may rapidly ensue. The 50% mortality rate of bacterial mediastinitis in the preantibiotic era has improved to only 40% since the availability of broad-spectrum antimicrobial therapy. The mortality increases further to 80% if the diagnosis is delayed for more than 24 hours. This latter point indicates the value of a thoracic CT scan to exclude mediastinitis in any patient with a serious cervical infection.

A high clinical suspicion in the appropriate clinical setting assists in the diagnosis of mediastinitis. Conventional chest radiographs may demonstrate a widened mediastinum with blurring of mediastinal contours, unilateral or bilateral pleural effusions, and rarely the presence of mediastinal air-fluid levels. The present patient's chest radiograph demonstrated a left pleural effusion with mediastinal widening at the level of the hilae. Thoracic CT scanning, however, is a more sensitive and specific examination. The presence of soft tissue attenuation within mediastinal fat, obliteration of normal mediastinal fat planes that surround brachiocephalic vessels, displacement of mediastinal structures, or the presence of frank mediastinal gas or abscesses may confirm the diagnosis. Results of pleural fluid analysis may demonstrate an empyema or a sterile, "sympathetic" inflammatory exudate. Blood cultures are usually negative in the absence of septic thrombophlebitis of a major cervical or mediastinal vein.

Specific therapy depends on the underlying etiology, duration, and extent of the mediastinal infection. In severely ill patients, initial medical management includes stabilization with intravascular fluids and evaluation for intubation to prevent upper airway obstruction. Broad-spectrum antibiotics are directed against the usual pathogens involved in odontogenic mediastinitis, which include a polymicrobial flora of beta-hemolytic streptococci, *Staphylococcus, aureus, Streptococcus pneumoniae, Bacteroides fragilis,* peptostreptococci, and other oropharyngeal anaerobic organisms. Immediate surgical evaluation for drainage of mediastinal pus and debridement of necrotic tissue remains the cardinal therapeutic principle in most patients with necrotizing mediastinitis. The traditional approach through the neck limits drainage to the superior mediastinum, which may be inadequate in many patients. If thoracic CT shows evidence of infection below the fourth thoracic vertebra, a transthoracic incision allows more effective mediastinal drainage. Recent reports indicate that CT-guided percutaneous catheter drainage in selected patients may obviate the need for thoracotomy.

The present patient demonstrated CT attenuation of mediastinal soft tissue densities and contrast enhancement surrounding the aorta (arrow) consistent with a spreading cellulitis in the mediastinum (figure, previous page). The patient's subacute presentation was unusual for bacterial mediastinitis and was attributed to either partial treatment by the earlier course of antibiotics or infection with a pathogen of low virulence. Twenty-four hours after initiation of broad-spectrum antibiotics, the fever and chest pain resolved and the patient remained well after long-term follow-up.

Clinical Pearls

1. Over 90% of patients with acute bacterial mediastinitis unrelated to surgery or trauma will have esophageal perforation.

2. Descending necrotizing mediastinitis may occur several weeks after apparent recovery from a cervical abscess. All patients with serious cervical infections, therefore, should undergo thoracic CT to exclude early mediastinitis.

3. The 50% mortality of bacterial mediastinitis in the preantibiotic era has decreased to only 40% since the advent of broad-spectrum antimicrobial therapy. Mortality increases to 80% if diagnosis and effective therapy are delayed for more than 24 hours.

4. Thoracic CT is the most sensitive diagnostic study for patients with suspected bacterial mediastinitis.

REFERENCES

1. de Marie S, Tjon RTO, Tham TA, et al. Clinical infections and nonsurgical treatment of parapharyngeal space infections complicating throat infections. Rev Infect Dis 1989;11:975–982.
2. Musgrove BT, Malden NJ. Mediastinitis and pericarditis caused by dental infection. Br J Oral Maxillofac Surg 1989;27:423–428.
3. Wheatley MJ, Stirling MC, Kirsh MM, et al. Descending necrotizing mediastinitis: transcervical drainage is not enough. Ann Thorac Surg 1990;49:780–784.

PATIENT 66

A 35-year-old man with right-sided chest pain and dyspnea

A 35-year-old man presented with an 8-hour history of right-sided chest pain and progressively severe shortness of breath. His symptoms began after he was hit in the right side of his chest during a fist fight.

Physical Examination: Temperature 98.7°; pulse 103; respirations 26; blood pressure 145/87. Chest: no crepitance: clear to auscultation. Cardiac: regular rhythm; no murmurs. Abdomen: normal. Neurologic: normal.

Laboratory Findings: Hct 38%, WBC 12,000/μl with 65% neutrophils and 30% lymphocytes. Electrolytes: normal. ABG (RA): pH 7.48; PCO_2 29 mmHg; PO_2 68 mmHg. Chest radiograph: shown below.

Question: What is the most likely diagnosis?

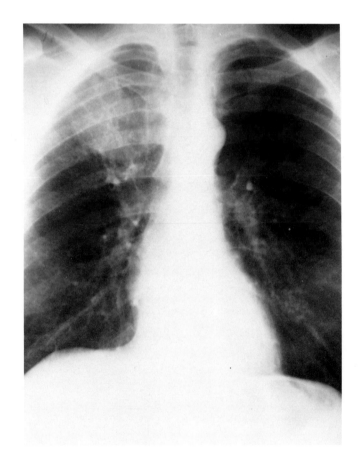

Diagnosis: Pulmonary contusion.

Discussion: Pulmonary contusions are the most common thoracic complications of nonpenetrating thoracic trauma, being even more common than rib fractures. Their impact on health is highlighted by the observation that trauma is the third leading cause of death in the United States and blunt chest wall injury accounts for 25% of those deaths. Approximately 90% of nonpenetrating chest trauma is caused by motor vehicle accidents, whereas blast injuries, falls, and altercations account for the remaining 10%. Rare causes of lung contusions include renal lithotripsy, which has been reported to cause life-threatening pulmonary contusion in a single patient.

The diagnosis of pulmonary contusion is suspected when an alveolar parenchymal infiltrate is noted in the setting of blunt chest wall trauma. Patients may be asymptomatic, although 50% of patients with lung contusions may experience minimal hemoptysis. Other symptoms and signs include chest pain, low-grade fever, and dyspnea that may progress to acute respiratory insufficiency. Often, other physical signs of associated injuries, such as rib fractures or head injury, may be present. An increased alveolar-to-arterial oxygen gradient is usually present and may be the first clue to the presence of pulmonary contusion if the initial chest radiograph is obtained before the onset of the pulmonary infiltrate.

The radiographic infiltrate associated with lung contusions usually develops within the first 6 hours of injury and resolves within the following 72 hours. The pattern of infiltrates varies between nodular alveolar densities with smooth or irregular borders, dense homogeneous consolidations, and multiple areas of patchy infiltrates. The infiltrates often extend beyond the confines of a lung segment or lobe. Persistence or progression of the infiltrates after the first 3 or 4 days from onset should raise the possibility of complications, such as pneumonia, lung laceration with hematoma, or ongoing pulmonary hemorrhage.

Evaluation of patients with pulmonary contusions with computed tomography (CT) has demonstrated that many patients have associated lung lacerations. Furthermore, histologic evaluation of contused lung specimens removed from trauma patients who require thoracotomy for other reasons has shown that some contusions represent lung lacerations with alveolar hemorrhage without evidence of interstitial damage. These observations have led some investigators to propose that lung contusion is a pulmonary laceration surrounded by alveolar hemorrhage rather than a true contusion with simple alveolar and interstitial edema. The consolidation seen on CT scan may reflect blood from torn vessels spilling into the dependent regions.

With this enhanced understanding of lung contusions, a new classification system has been proposed for this condition on the basis of the mechanism of injury, CT scan pattern, surgical findings, and presence of rib fractures. This system consists of four patterns of lung contusions. Type 1 laceration appears as a parenchymal cavity that is air-filled or contains an air-fluid level. This pattern is produced by a localized parenchymal rupture that develops when the severe chest wall compression occurs. Pneumothorax may develop if the laceration ruptures through the visceral pleura. Type 2 lacerations result from shearing of lung tissue across the vertebral body during rapid compression. The laceration commonly appears as a vertical tear within the paravertebral regions of the lung. Type 3 lacerations appear as small peripheral cavities due to parenchymal damage by fractured ribs. Type 4 lacerations, the least common, occur in lung regions that were adherent to the chest wall; type 4 lacerations may be confirmed to exist only at surgery or autopsy.

Chest CT scans are more sensitive than routine standard chest radiographs for demonstrating lung contusions and lacerations. The clinical importance of this improved sensitivity is uncertain, however, considering that most lung contusions resolve without specific therapy.

The management of pulmonary contusion is supportive. In minimally injured patients, observation, chest physiotherapy, and pain control usually suffice. Lung contusions can progress to respiratory failure, however, necessitating intubation and mechanical ventilation. Routine use of Swan-Ganz catheters, cardiotonic drugs, and diuretics in the absence of intravascular volume overload serves no useful purpose. Age greater than 60 years, severity of the sustained trauma, and concurrent shock or head trauma are risk factors for increased mortality in patients with pulmonary contusion.

Some animal models of lung contusion demonstrate that infusion of colloids may result in less lung edema and hemorrhage, and that high-dose corticosteroids cause reduction of the size of the contusion. Clinical trials have not yet established the value of colloid therapy in this setting. Some patients with severe lung contusions associated with lacerations require surgery. Indications for surgery include persistent large air leaks and continued lung hemorrhage.

The present patient responded well to supportive therapy with improvement of his symptoms and resolution of the right upper lobe alveolar infiltrates within 96 hours.

Clinical Pearls

1. Pulmonary contusion is the most common thoracic injury associated with blunt chest trauma.

2. Pulmonary lacerations may be the basis of lung injury in patients with pulmonary contusion.

3. CT of the chest is more sensitive than standard radiographs in detecting tissue injury in trauma patients. This enhanced sensitivity is of limited clinical value because most contusions resolve without complications.

4. Failure of pulmonary contusion to resolve within a few days should raise the suspicion of complications such as infection or continued bleeding.

5. Therapeutic benefits of fluid restriction, systemic corticosteroids, and colloids in the management of pulmonary contusion are unproved.

REFERENCES

1. Wagner RB, Jamieson PM. Pulmonary contusion: evaluation and classification by computed tomography. Surg Clin North Am 1989;69:31–40.
2. Malhotra V, Rosen RJ, Slepian RL. Life-threatening hypoxemia after lithotripsy in an adult due to shock-wave-induced pulmonary contusion. Anesthesiology 1991;75:529–531.
3. Stellin G. Survival in trauma victims with pulmonary contusion. Am Surg 1991;7:71–84.
4. Wagner RB, Slivko B, Jamieson PM, et al. Effect of lung contusion on pulmonary hemodynamics. Soc Thorac Surg 1991;52:51–58.

PATIENT 67

A 27-year-old man with recurrent bronchitis and pneumonia

A 27-year-old man was admitted for evaluation of productive cough, fever, and weight loss. Five years earlier, he had begun experiencing recurrent episodes of bronchitis with purulent sputum that responded to oral antibiotics. During the past 6 months, the cough and copious sputum became intractable, and four episodes of pneumonia required hospitalization. The patient smoked cigarettes but denied sinus disease, childhood respiratory infections, or known cardiac disorders.

Physical Examination: Temperature 101°; pulse 110; respirations 22; blood pressure 120/80. Chest: bronchial breath sounds over the left upper lobe with bibasilar wheezes and rhonchi. Cardiac: normal. Extremities: no clubbing, cyanosis, or joint laxity.

Laboratory Findings: Hct 41%; WBC 11,000/μl with 90% PMNs. Sputum: purulent with normal flora on culture. Serum immunoglobulins: slight polyclonal increase in gamma fraction. Sweat chloride: 51 mEq/L (normal). Chest radiographs: shown below.

Questions: What is the most probable diagnosis? How would you confirm the underlying condition?

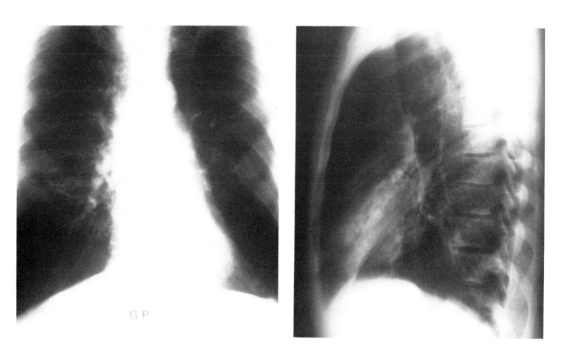

Diagnosis: Tracheobronchomegaly (Mounier-Kuhn syndrome).

Discussion: The onset in early adulthood of recurrent airway suppuration compatible with bronchiectasis warrants consideration of such underlying conditions as cystic fibrosis, dysgammaglobulinemia, immotile cilia syndrome, and sequelae of early childhood respiratory infections. The present patient's admission lateral chest radiograph, however, revealed a dilated tracheal air column that suggested the diagnosis of tracheobronchomegaly (Mounier-Kuhn syndrome).

Abnormal dilatation of the trachea and proximal bronchi was originally noted as an autopsy finding by Czyhlarz in 1897. Mounier-Kuhn in 1932, however, was the first to establish the clinical features and definition of tracheobronchomegaly, which is characterized by dilated, thin-walled trachea and bronchi that collapse on forced expiration. Atrophy of elastic and muscular tissue allows airway membranes to bulge between cartilaginous rings with formation of tracheal diverticulae—a commonly associated finding. Previously described by the alternative terms tracheal diverticulosis, tracheobronchiectasis, tracheocele, tracheomalacia, and tracheobronchopathia malacia, tracheobronchomegaly has been detected in 1% of patients undergoing bronchography and may be an underrecognized disorder.

Expiratory collapse of airways interferes with cough mechanisms and predisposes patients to chronic recurrent pulmonary infections. Most common in males, tracheobronchomegaly typically presents in the third or fourth decade with nonspecific symptoms of bronchitis. Eventually, airway suppuration worsens and patients develop bronchiectasis with copious sputum production and repeated episodes of pneumonia.

The etiology of tracheobronchomegaly is unclear. The late onset in early adulthood may seem to imply an acquired disorder possibly resulting from airway inflammation or inhaled irritants. Infants with tracheobronchomegaly clearly develop the condition as a result of barotrauma from mechanical ventilation for neonatal respiratory failure. Conversely, however, instances of Mounier-Kuhn syndrome clustered within families, associations with adult Ehlers-Danlos syndrome and childhood cutis laxa, and histologic abscence of myenteric plexus in the tracheal walls suggest a congenitally based pathophysiology.

Diagnosis depends on careful consideration of tracheobronchomegaly in the appropriate clinical setting and pursuit of radiographic documentation of airway dilatation. The routine chest radiograph may be normal or palpably diagnostic with tracheal dimensions extending beyond the vertebral bodies on the frontal view. Many patients, however, have abnormalities limited to the lateral radiograph (as occurred in the present patient). To fulfill the arbitrary definition of Mounier-Kuhn syndrome, the tracheal diameter should be ≥ 3.0 at a level 2 cm above the aortic arch, or the right or left mainstem bronchi should be ≥ 2.4 or 2.3 cm in caliber, respectively. The presence of tracheal diverticulae may impart a corrugated configuration to the tracheal air column. If routine radiography is nondiagnostic, CT scanning can document tracheal and bronchial dilatation and the characteristic thinning of airway walls. Pulmonary function studies typically demonstrate airway obstruction with increased residual volumes.

The risk of recurrent infection with ensuing bronchiectasis, lung scarring, cor pulmonale, and respiratory failure mandates aggressive therapeutic measures that include antibiotics and pulmonary hygiene to clear airway secretions. Intractable secretions may require bronchoscopy or tracheotomy. Segmental tracheal resection may transiently improve symptoms until the inevitable progression of airway enlargement. Endotracheal tube cuffs in patients requiring mechanical ventilation may promote sudden worsening of tracheomegaly that rapidly cicatrizes to tracheal stenosis within 48 hours of extubation.

The present patient underwent thoracic CT scanning that demonstrated a thin-walled, dilated trachea (figure on facing page, top) and enlargement of both mainstem bronchi (figure on facing page, bottom). He recovered from bronchopneumonia with parenteral antibiotics but resumed a course marked by recurrent airway suppuration.

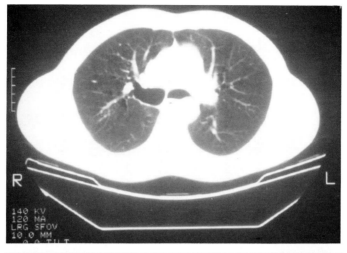

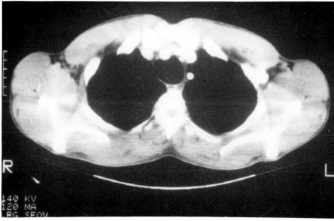

Clinical Pearls

1. When routine chest radiography fails to detect tracheobronchomegaly in young adults with recurrent pulmonary infections, thoracic CT scanning should be performed to exclude the diagnosis.

2. The arbitrary diagnostic criteria for tracheobronchomegaly are tracheal dilatation ≥ 3 cm measured 2 cm above the aortic arch, or enlargement of the right or left mainstem bronchi to ≥ 2.4 and 2.3 cm, respectively.

3. Tracheal diverticulae are associated findings that may be large enough to allow cannulation with a bronchoscope.

REFERENCES

1. Bateson EM, Woo-Ming M. Tracheobronchomegaly. Clin Radiol 1973;24:354–358.
2. Himalstein MR, Gallagher FC. Tracheobronchomegaly. Ann Otol Rhinol Laryngol 1973;82:223–227.
3. Shin MS, Jackson RM, Ho K-J. Tracheobronchomegaly (Mounier-Kuhn syndrome): CT diagnosis. AJR 1988;150:777–779.

PATIENT 68

A 61-year-old woman with progressive dyspnea

A 61-year-old woman noted a several-month history of dyspnea on exertion that had progressed to resting dyspnea during the preceding 1 week. She had been previously healthy except for an episode of acute dyspnea 5 years earlier that had resolved over 1–2 days without specific therapy.

Physical Examination: Temperature 97.9°; pulse 92; respirations 24; blood pressure 142/94. General: obese woman in mild respiratory distress. Chest: normal breath sounds; continuous murmur over the right midlung area. Cardiac: no jugular venous distention; regular rhythm; no gallop.

Laboratory Findings: Hct 38%; electrolytes, BUN, and creatinine: normal. ECG: normal. ABG (RA): pH 7.45; PCO_2 32 mmHg; PO_2 63 mmHg. Ventilation lung scan: normal. Chest radiograph: shown below left. Perfusion lung scan: shown below right.

Question: What condition should be considered as a cause of the patient's dyspnea?

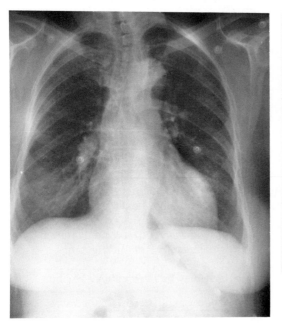 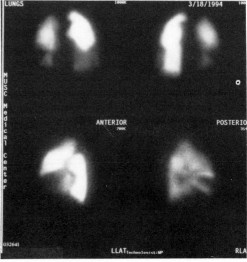

Diagnosis: Chronic thromboembolic pulmonary hypertension (CTEPH).

Discussion: Chronic pulmonary thromboembolism has been increasingly recognized since the first reported successful thromboendarterectomy in 1963. It is estimated that 450,000–500,000 persons a year develop acute pulmonary embolism, but only 35% of thromboembolic events are clinically recognized and appropriately treated. By conservative estimates, in about 0.1% of patients with acute pulmonary embolism (PE), the intravascular clot fails to resolve. Therefore, about 450–500 patients per year are at risk for CTEPH.

CTEPH appears to arise from recurrent, unrecognized pulmonary thromboemboli that occur over months to years. For unknown reasons, the emboli fail to resolve, resulting in propagation of intravascular clot in a retrograde direction toward the proximal pulmonary vasculature. Observations at surgery support this pathogenesis, reporting white distal emboli with reddish, proximal extensions that appear more recently formed. Approximately 35–50% of patients with CTEPH do not give a history of a previous PE or episode of venous thrombosis. Careful patient interviews, however, often reveal a history of a "pulled muscle" in the lower extremities, unexplained "asthma" episodes, or a previous diagnosis of "pneumonia" that caused shortness of breath. Patients commonly remain asymptomatic after these events, which most likely represent thromboembolic episodes, until marked pulmonary hypertension or overt cor pulmonale develops. This asymptomatic stage has been called the "honeymoon period," which may last months to years before the progressive decline of functional status.

Patients with established CTEPH present with dyspnea on exertion. The dyspnea progresses over months to years until patients are severely limited. Physical findings may be normal until pulmonary hypertension is severe. High-pitched, continuous murmurs that exentuate with inspiration represent partial pulmonary artery obstruction and assist the clinical diagnosis. This type of murmur has not been reported in patients with pulmonary artery agenesis or primary pulmonary hypertension. The cardiac exam is normal until later in the course of the disease when evidence of cor pulmonale develops.

A high clinical suspicion is essential for diagnosis. The ECG is often normal at initial presentation, eventually demonstrating right-axis deviation later in the course of the disease. The chest radiograph may appear normal during the patient's initial symptoms but eventually shows unilateral engorgement of the pulmonary arteries (as in the present patient), zones of avascularity, and cardiomegaly with filling of the retrosternal space on the lateral view. Doppler echocardiography demonstrates increased pulmonary artery pressure. Although spirometric lung function measurements are usually normal, 20% of patients demonstrate a restrictive ventilatory defect that may suggest an incorrect diagnosis of interstitial lung disease. Interestingly, the DLCO is normal in CTEPH, perhaps reflecting extensive bronchial arterial collateral flow with back perfusion into the capillary bed. Early in the course of the disease, oxygenation abnormalities are limited to exercise desaturation. With disease progression, resting hypoxemia can become severe.

The ventilation-perfusion lung scan is the most important evaluative test in patients with pulmonary hypertension in whom CTEPH is a diagnostic consideration. A normal perfusion scan essentially excludes recurrent pulmonary emboli and warrants consideration of other conditions associated with pulmonary hypertension, such as interstitial lung disease or primary pulmonary hypertension. Abnormal perfusion scans indicate a need to further evaluate patients for CTEPH. The extent of perfusion defects often underestimates the degree of central vascular obstruction. Right heart catheterization establishes the severity of pulmonary hypertension and usually determines that the pulmonary artery occlusion pressure (PAOP) is normal. False elevation of PAOP may result when the catheter wedges into the region of the intravascular clot. The presence of a mean pulmonary arterial pressure greater than 30 mmHg is associated with a 30% 5-year survival. The pulmonary angiogram confirms the diagnosis and establishes surgical feasibility for thromboendarterectomy. Even after extensive clinical evaluations, some patients with pulmonary hypertension still elude a specific diagnosis. In such instances, pulmonary artery angioscopy can determine the location and extent of intravascular clot.

Medical management of CTEPH is entirely unsuccessful. Anticoagulants and thrombolytics provide no benefit because the intravascular clot is organized and not amenable to lysis. Surgery offers the only opportunity for cure and resolution of right-sided heart failure. To be approachable by surgery, however, the thrombi must be centrally located in the pulmonary vasculature at the level of or proximal to the segmental arteries. Additional criteria for surgery include willingness to accept the surgical risks, a pulmonary vascular resistance greater than 4 Wood units or mean pulmonary arterial pressure > 30 mmHg, and an absence of comorbid medical conditions that would complicate surgery or jeopardize the prognosis. With careful patient selection, centers with extensive experience with thromboendarterectomy now report an operative mortality of less than 13%.

Reperfusion pulmonary edema, which occurs after a successful thromboendarterectomy reestablishes pulmonary arterial blood flow to regions of lung that were previously ischemic, represents an important cause of postoperative mortality. The pathogenesis of this complication appears to depend on the generation of oxidants in the pulmonary microvasculature and leukosequestration. After thromboendarterectomy, some patients demonstrate new lung scan perfusion defects in vascular distributions not supplied by the pulmonary arteries that were surgically repaired. It is speculated that these nonembolic, nonocclusive defects result from a redistribution of vascular resistance after reestablishment of more normal pulmonary artery flow. Patients who survive surgery usually show significant hemodynamic and functional improvement.

The present patient's lung scan showed multiple segmental and subsegmental perfusion defects. The presence of these findings with a normal ventilation scan indicated a high probability of thromboembolic disease. After initiation of anticoagulant therapy, a subsequent evaluation confirmed the presence of CTEPH. She is now awaiting evaluation for thromboendarterectomy.

Clinical Pearls

1. Unexplained pulmonary hypertension or right-sided heart failure should raise the suspicion of chronic pulmonary thromboembolism.

2. Patients with CTEPH may have falsely elevated pulmonary artery occlusion pressure measured during right heart catheterization if the catheter wedges into the region of intravascular clot.

3. The presence of a high-pitched, continuous murmur over the chest that accentuates with inspiration strongly favors the diagnosis of CTEPH over primary pulmonary hypertension.

4. Up to 20% of patients with CTEPH demonstrate a restrictive ventilatory defect that may suggest an incorrect diagnosis of interstitial lung disease.

REFERENCES

1. Rich S, Levitsky S, Brundage BH. Pulmonary hypertension from chronic pulmonary thromboembolism. Ann Intern Med 1988;108:425–434.
2. Kapitan KS, Clausen JL, Moser KM. Gas exchange in chronic thromboembolism after pulmonary thromboendarterectomy. Chest 1990;98:14–19.
3. Olman MA, Auger WR, Fedullo PF, et al. Pulmonary vascular steal in chronic thromboembolic pulmonary hypertension. Chest 1990;98:1430–1434.
4. Buchalter SE, Groves RH, Zom GL. Surgical management of chronic pulmonary thromboembolic disease. Clin Chest Med 1992;13:17–22.

PATIENT 69

A 25-year-old man with chest discomfort after weightlifting

A 25-year-old man experienced the sudden onset of an aching, lower substernal chest pain at the end of a weightlifting training session. During the ensuing 4 hours, the discomfort persisted with only brief periods of relief provided by the ingestion of iced water. When the patient noted extension of the pain through to the back with mild dyspnea 6 hours after onset of symptoms, he sought evaluation in the emergency department.

Physical Examination: Temperature 37.2°C; respirations 27; pulse 112; blood pressure 127/68. General: uncomfortable patient shifting frequently on the gurney. Thorax: crepitance in the left subclavicular and lower cervical region. Chest: clear lung fields without wheezes. Cardiac: "crunching" sound during cardiac systole that increased in intensity during expiration. Abdomen: epigastric tenderness; no organomegaly.

Laboratory Findings: Hct 42%; WBC 12,000 cells/μl. Na$^+$ 134 mEq/L; K$^+$ 4.2 mEq/L; Cl$^-$ 90 mEq/L; HCO$_3^-$ 24 mEq/L; BUN 15 mEq/L; Cr 1.2 mEq/L. ABG (RA): pH 7.55; PCO$_2$ 27 mmHg, PO$_2$ 100 mmHg. ECG: sinus tachycardia. Chest radiograph: subcutaneous (black arrow) and mediastinal (white arrows) emphysema.

Questions: What is the suspected diagnosis? How would you initiate the diagnostic evaluation?

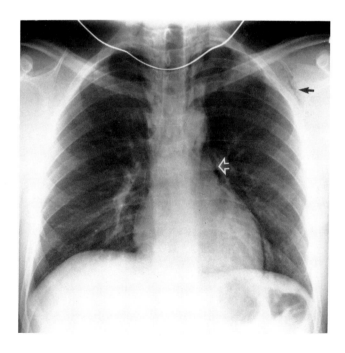

Answer: Esophageal rupture (Boerhaave's syndrome).

Discussion: Spontaneous transmural rupture of the esophagus (Boerhaave's syndrome) is a rare but clinically important condition because of its nearly universal fatality when left unrecognized and untreated. The diagnosis usually receives sufficient consideration when patients present with classic manifestations of overindulgence in food and alcohol, repeated emesis, and sudden onset of retrosternal or upper abdominal pain with eventual vascular collapse. This picture may occur in only two-thirds of patients, with the remainder experiencing atypical manifestations after a variety of clinical events not usually associated with esophageal injury. Such events include weightlifting, parturition, straining at defecation, seizures, severe asthma, coughing or hiccuping, and other activities that generate a Valsalva maneuver. Patients with emesis may present with symptoms of esophageal rupture unrelated temporally to the vomiting episodes. These varied clinical manifestations complicate patient evaluation and underlie the low 20% frequency of correct diagnosis within the first 12 hours after esophageal rupture.

The onset of symptoms of esophageal rupture may be dramatic or insidious, with pain varying in location and quality. Typically, patients experience substernal pleuritic chest pain, although a dull or aching discomfort may also occur. The pain often radiates to the back and left shoulder, simulating myocardial infarction or aortic dissection. Temporary relief may occur with swallowing ice water or topical anesthetic solutions. Epigastric pain may develop in combination with the chest pain or as an isolated initial symptom. Severe abdominal pain, when associated with involuntary rebound and guarding, may simulate an acute abdominal process. Varying degrees of dyspnea occur in 50% of patients. Hematemesis may accompany rupture of the esophagus but rarely progresses to persistent or massive bleeding.

Vital signs may initially remain normal or rapidly progress to profound hemodynamic collapse. The chest examination may appear unremarkable or demonstrate rales and decreased breath sounds if a pleural effusion or pneumothorax occurs. The presence of cervical subcutaneous emphysema is the major clinical finding that separates esophageal rupture from the alternative cardiopulmonary diagnoses—other than spontaneous pneumomediastinum—that have similar presenting manifestations. Unfortunately, palpable crepitance may take several hours to develop and remain absent in up to 50% of patients. Mediastinal air may be detectable in up to 20% of patients with esophageal rupture by the presence of Hamman's sign, which is a "crunching"

or "clicking" sound that occurs synchronously with heart beats and changes in intensity with respiration and patient position.

The chest radiograph provides important diagnostic information in patients with esophageal rupture. Typical features of a pneumomediastinum include lucencies along the left cardiac border and posteriorly and inferiorly along the lateral edge of the aorta. Streaks of air commonly track along the trachea and major vessels in the superior mediastinum. A "V"-shaped linear density (Naclerio's V-sign) appears in the retrocardiac region, representing dissection of air through the fascial planes of the mediastinal and diaphragmatic pleurae.

Because the site of rupture is usually longitudinal in the left posteriolateral aspect of the esophagus a few centimeters proximal to the cardia, a left-sided pleural effusion with or without a left lower lobe infiltrate commonly develops hours after onset of symptoms. Pleuropulmonary findings, however, may be right-sided or bilateral in distribution. Pneumothorax may develop with extension of mediastinal air into the pleural space, and the presence of a hydropneumothorax in the setting of a pneumomediastinum is highly suggestive of esophageal rupture. Widening of the mediastinum after establishment of mediastinitis may also occur.

The diagnosis may be confirmed in patients with pleural effusions when thoracentesis demonstrates food particles and squamous epithelial cells in pleural fluid, which usually has a low pH and an elevated salivary amylase content once the mediastinal pleura tears. In most patients, however, an esophageal contrast study is required to demonstrate the presence and location of the esophageal rupture. The initial examination is performed with water-soluble Gastrografin, which undergoes rapid absorption in the mediastinum without causing intense tissue reaction. Aspiration should be avoided because of the risks of pulmonary edema from the hypertonic contrast media. Because Gastrografin may fail to detect up to 25–50% of esophageal ruptures, negative studies should be pursued with esophageal swallows using barium sulfate compounds, which have better radiographic density and adherence to mucosal surfaces but may induce fibrosis in the mediastinum in the presence of frank esophageal leakage. Negative contrast studies in clinically suspicious instances should be followed with thoracic CT scanning, which can demonstrate air and fluid tracking into the region of the lower esophagus. The safety and sensitivity of esophagoscopy have not been adequately demonstrated in Boerhaave's syndrome.

Management requires prompt diagnosis, rapid fluid resuscitation, initiation of broad-spectrum antibiotics, and surgical intervention to drain the mediastinum and pleural space and seal the esophageal perforation. Most studies identify an increasing mortality with surgical delay. Rarely, patients with an esophageal rupture confined to the periesophageal tissue without frank leakage into the mediastinum accompanied by minimal symptoms may respond to conservative therapy consisting of nasogastric drainage, broad-spectrum antibiotics, and total parenteral nutrition for several weeks.

The present patient underwent a Gastrografin swallow study because of the pain relief noted with drinking iced water and the severity of pain beyond that anticipated with an uncomplicated spontaneous pneumomediastinum. Constrast material migrated into the mediastinum from the distal esophagus. The patient underwent a thoracotomy with closure of the esophageal perforation and drainage of the mediastinum, and experienced an uncomplicated recovery.

Clinical Pearls

1. Boerhaave's syndrome may occur in the setting of severe thoracoabdominal straining despite the absence of a history of emesis.

2. A hydropneumothorax associated with mediastinal emphysema is highly suggestive of Boerhaave's syndrome.

3. Relief of substernal pain with drinking iced water in a patient with pneumomediastinum suggests esophageal rupture.

REFERENCES

1. Ward WG. Cold water polydipsia: unheralded marker of spontaneous esophageal rupture. South Med J 1986;79:1161–1162.
2. Jaworski A, Fischer R, Lippmann M. Boerhaave's syndrome. Computed tomographic findings and diagnostic considerations. Arch Intern Med 1988;148:223–224.
3. Pate JW, Walker WA, Cole FH Jr, et al. Spontaneous rupture of the esophagus: a 30-year experience. Ann Thorac Surg 1989;47:689–692.
4. Attar S, Hankins JR, Suter CM, et al. Esophageal perforation: a therapeutic challenge. Ann Thorac Surg 1990;50:45–51.

PATIENT 70

A 50-year-old man with cirrhosis and dyspnea on exertion

A 50-year-old man was referred for evaluation of a 2-year history of dyspnea on exertion without wheezing, hemoptysis, chest pain, fever, or night sweats. The patient had known gastric varices secondary to alcoholic cirrhosis, and a 20-pack-year history of cigarette smoking, but had quit smoking 1 year earlier. He had no history of exposure to asbestos or tuberculosis.

Physical Examination: Temperature 97.6°; pulse 100; respirations 24; blood pressure 120/80. Skin: multiple truncal spider angiomata. Chest: clear. Cardiac: regular rhythm; normal S1 and S2 with an S3. Abdomen: mildly protuberant with shifting dullness. Extremities: cyanotic nail beds; clubbing; pedal edema.

Laboratory Findings: Hct 45%; WBC 6,300/μl; prothrombin time 13.5 sec. ABG (RA): pH 7.47; PCO_2 28 mmHg; PO_2 58 mmHg. ABG (100% O_2 face mask): pH 7.47; PCO_2 28 mmHg; PO_2 107 mmHg. Pulmonary function studies: FVC 4.31 L (80% predicted); FEV_1 3.13 L (81% predicted); FEV_1/FVC 73%; DL/VA 85% of predicted. Chest radiograph: shown below.

Question: Which specialized tests would assist in establishing the diagnosis?

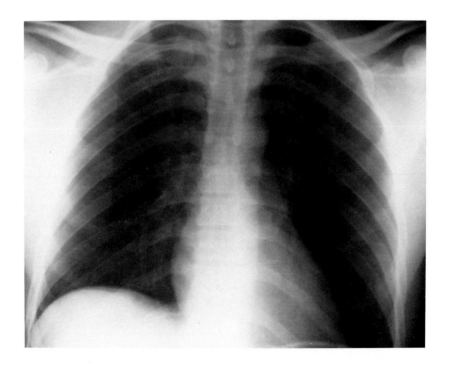

Diagnosis: Hepatopulmonary syndrome secondary to cirrhosis.

Discussion: Patients with liver disease frequently experience concomitant respiratory abnormalities. For instance, ascites with or without transduction of peritoneal fluid into the pleural space may elevate the diaphragms and restrict pulmonary function. The presence of severe liver dysfunction with accompanying immunosuppression increases the risk for respiratory infections, such as bronchitis and pneumonia. Some underlying systemic conditions may be associated with both liver and pulmonary dysfunction as occurs in alpha-1-antitrypsin deficiency and primary biliary cirrhosis.

One of the most common pulmonary disorders in patients with liver disease is mild to moderate hypoxemia, which may occur in up to one-third of patients with cirrhosis. This condition, termed "hepatopulmonary syndrome," has been attributed to several functional and anatomic abnormalities that may share some pathophysiologic features with the hepatorenal syndrome. Classically, patients present with dyspnea on exertion and platypnea (dyspnea in the erect position, relieved with recumbency). Clubbing, cyanosis, and cutaneous spider telangiectasia are common physical findings. Hepatosplenomegaly and ascites are usually present, although some patients may have already progressed to a small, cirrhotic liver by the time hypoxemia is noted.

Several pathophysiologic explanations exist for hepatopulmonary syndrome, including the presence of "pleuropulmonary telangiectasis," previously suspected as a cause of right-to-left intrapulmonary shunting. The most plausible mechanism, however, invokes the presence of abnormally dilated precapillary vessels that promotes a "diffusion-perfusion defect," resulting in incomplete oxygenation of pulmonary artery blood. These precapillary dilatations cause a rapid transit of erythrocytes through the alveolar capillary with insufficient time for loading of oxygen onto hemoglobin. As cardiac output increases and transit time is further shortened, the severity of hypoxemia worsens.

The functional nature of hepatopulmonary syndrome is supported by its reversibility. Improvement in liver function has resulted in resolution of the hypoxemia, clubbing, and cyanosis. Likewise, liver transplantation has produced similar results, altering the previously held belief that patients with hypoxemia should be excluded from consideration for liver transplantation.

Routine laboratory studies in patients suspected of having hepatopulmonary syndrome may demonstrate elevated transaminases and bilirubin and various visceral protein abnormalities associated with liver dysfunction. Patients also may have erythrocytosis if the arterial hypoxemia has been long-standing. Arterial blood gases usually show hypocapnia and respiratory alkalosis. The hypoxemia, caused by *combined* shunting and diffusion defects, may respond to supplemental oxygen to a greater degree than observed in patients with conditions that cause a pure cardiopulmonary shunt. Orthodeoxia (decrease in oxygenation in the supine position) is a classic manifestation of the disease thought to occur because of the primarily basilar location of the vascular abnormalities. The lung examination is often normal, but low-grade systolic cardiac flow murmurs are commonplace.

Several imaging studies assist in establishing the diagnosis of hepatopulmonary syndrome. Scanning with technetium-99-labeled macroaggregated albumin (used in the perfusion portion of ventilation-perfusion lung scans) can demonstrate the presence of the abnormally dilated precapillary vessels. The cross-sectional diameter of normal pulmonary capillaries is 8–15 μm, and the diameter of labeled albumin is 20 μm. In the absence of an intracardiac or intrapulmonary shunt, venous injections of the macroaggregated albumin should not pass through the cardiopulmonary circulation to the visceral organs. Demonstration of measurable radioactivity over the kidneys and brain suggests intracardiac or intrapulmonary shunt. Cardiopulmonary angiography may be useful in some patients to exclude an intracardiac shunt or intrapulmonary arteriovenous malformation. Although the intrapulmonary, precapillary dilatation of hepatopulmonary syndrome may be demonstrable by pulmonary angiography, this study is generally not needed to definitively establish the diagnosis. Contrast echocardiography is probably the most useful diagnostic test. In hepatopulmonary syndrome, the study shows microbubble contrast material in the left heart approximately 3–6 cycles after appearance of contrast in the right ventricle. Intracardiac shunt may be differentiated by the appearance of microbubbles in the left heart concurrently or within 1 or 2 cardiac cycles of their appearance in the right heart.

At present there is no specific medical treatment for hepatopulmonary syndrome. Any measures that can reverse or improve liver function should be initiated. If the hypoxemia is sufficiently severe and inadequately responsive to supplemental oxygen, liver transplantation should be considered.

The present patient underwent a ventilation-perfusion lung scan that showed a single subsegmental mismatch considered unlikely to represent pulmonary thromboemboli. Unfortunately, visceral organs were not scanned after injection of the macroaggregated albumin because the diagnosis of hepatopulmonary syndrome had not yet been considered. Cardiopulmonary angiography showed no evidence of pulmonary embolism, intracardiac shunt, or pulmonary arteriovenous malformation. A contrast echocardiogram demonstrated an intrapulmonary shunt compatible with hepatopulmonary syndrome. The patient's presentation with cirrhosis, clubbing, hypoxemia that had a moderate response to supplemental oxygen, and a normal chest radiograph was suggestive of the diagnosis. The patient discontinued all alcohol consumption, and his dyspnea and hypoxemia improved.

Clinical Pearls

1. Hepatopulmonary syndrome should be considered in patients with liver disease, hypoxemia, clubbing, and cyanosis.

2. The condition most likely results from abnormally dilated precapillary vessels that produce a diffusion-perfusion defect.

3. Contrast echocardiography is a sensitive test for demonstrating intrapulmonary shunting in hepatopulmonary syndrome.

4. Hypoxemia from hepatopulmonary syndrome should not be considered a contraindication to liver transplantation if the patient is otherwise an appropriate candidate.

REFERENCES

1. Agusti AGN, Roca J, Rodriguez-Roisin R. The lung in patients with cirrhosis. J Hepatol 1990;10:251–257.
2. Eriksson LS, Soderman C, Ericzon BG, et al. Normalization of ventilation/perfusion relationships after liver transplantation in patients with decompensated cirrhosis: evidence for a hepatopulmonary syndrome. Hepatology 1990;12:1350–1357.
3. Thorens JB, Junod AF. Hypoxaemia and liver cirrhosis: a new argument in favour of a "diffusion-perfusion defect." Eur Respir J 1992;5:754–756.
4. Krowka MJ, Cortese DA. Hepatopulmonary syndrome: current concepts in diagnostic and therapeutic considerations. Chest 1994;105:1528–1537.

PATIENT 71

An 18-year-old woman with hypertension, dyspnea, and an abdominal bruit

An 18-year-old white woman was admitted because of hypertension and progressive dyspnea over a 7-day period. Her ankles had begun to swell 3 days earlier and a severe headache on the day of admission prompted her to seek medical attention. The patient had received medical care at the age of 12 for an unknown childhood condition but had discontinued follow-up. She took no medications and denied drug usage.

Physical Examination: Temperature 38.2°C; pulse 92; respirations 14; blood pressure 220/120 (right arm) and 180/98 (left arm). General: uncomfortable because of a severe headache. Fundi: narrowing of retinal arteries with scattered hemorrhages. Chest: normal. Cardiac: active precordium with a grade II/VI systolic ejection murmur over the aortic region that radiated into the carotids; diminished left brachial pulse. Abdomen: soft bruit in the epigastrium. Extremities: mild edema without hyperreflexia.

Laboratory Findings: Hct 31%; WBC 10,900/μl; platelets normal; electrolytes normal; BUN 20 mg/dl; creatinine 1.3 mg/dl; calcium 10.1 mg/dl. Urinalysis: no proteinuria or cells. ECG: voltage criteria for left ventricular hypertrophy. Chest radiograph: shown below left. Chest CT: shown below right.

Question: What childhood condition underlies this patient's medical problems?

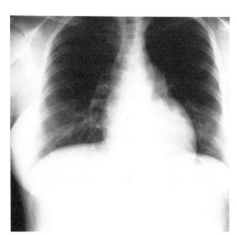 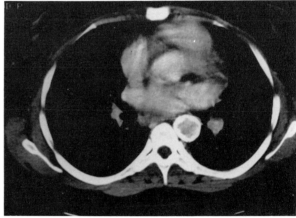

Answer: Takayasu's arteritis with secondary hypertension.

Discussion: Takayasu's arteritis is a chronic segmental inflammatory process that involves the aorta, the aorta's major branches, and occasionally the pulmonary vasculature, and eventually leads to vascular occlusion, aneurysmal dilatation, and ischemic tissue damage. First described as an ophthalmologic condition with ocular ischemia and retinal microaneurysmal formation, subsequent observations characterized Takayasu's arteritis as a large-vessel vasculitis mainly affecting Asian or Central American women in their second to third decades of life. More recently, its worldwide distribution in young women from all nationalities and races has been recognized. In the United States, Takayasu's arteritis occurs in 2.6 patients per million population, which is similar to the incidence of polyarteritis nodosa.

Takayasu's arteritis classically progresses through three pathophysiologic stages. Initially, a systemic inflammatory phase causes nonspecific constitutional manifestations such as fever, myalgias, arthralgias, weight loss, night sweats, anorexia, and pleuritic pain. Various skin findings may be present and include erythema nodosum, pyoderma gangrenosum, erythema induratum, tuberculoid eruption, and cutaneous polyarteritis nodosa. Subsequently, a vascular inflammatory phase presents as pain over palpable large arteries or nonspecific chest pain. Spontaneous resolution of symptoms may occur or patients may continue within a period of months or years to the final "burned out" or "pulseless" phase of the disease, which is characterized by arterial stenosis, vascular occlusion, aneurysmal formation, and end organ ischemia. Conversely, ischemic events may develop at any stage of the disease or patients may present with well-established pulseless symptoms without a preexisting systemic inflammatory course.

Although of unknown etiology, the histopathologic manifestations of Takayasu's arteritis confirm its inflammatory nature and correspond to the clinical stages of the disease. Initially, lymphocytes, plasma cells, and histiocytes invade the adventitia and media, producing granulomas with or without giant cell formation. A fibrosing process then ensues with scar formation that replaces the adventitia and media. Medial degeneration disrupts the elastic lamellae, causing aneurysmal dilatation, intravascular thrombosis, and vascular calcifications. Invasion of the intima by connective tissue cells leads to the arterial stenosis and vascular occlusion with organ ischemia characteristic of the third stage of the disease.

Vaso-occlusive complications in various organ systems are the clinical hallmarks of Takayasu's arteritis. Patients may present with upper extremity or masseter muscle claudication (pain with chewing), vascular bruits, or absent pulses. Secondary hypertension, as occurred in the present patient, results from renovascular involvement. Visual disturbances develop as a consequence of hypotensive ischemic retinopathy.

The cerebrovascular complications are the most profound cause of morbidity in patients with Takayasu's arteritis. The carotid and subclavian arteries are the most commonly involved aortic branches. Resultant occlusion of both the internal carotid and external carotid arteries along with the vertebral branches of the subclavian arteries severely restricts central nervous system perfusion. Episodes of aphasia, hemiplegia, or lethal cerebrovascular events subsequently ensue.

Congestive heart failure is another major manifestation of Takayasu's arteritis. Aortic regurgitation followed by mitral insufficiency results from aneurysmal dilatation of the aortic root. Left ventricular failure also may occur after prolonged poor control of secondary hypertension. Occasionally patients may develop an inflammatory or granulomatous cardiomyopathy—up to 80% of patients with Takayasu's arteritis have histologic evidence on endomyocardial biopsies of inflammatory myocardial abnormalities. Also, ischemic cardiomyopathy from stenosis, kinking, fistula formation, or aneurysmal dilatation of the coronary arteries may occur. Fifty percent of patients with Takayasu's arteritis will have pulmonary artery involvement, although only rare patients manifest signs or symptoms of dyspnea, pleuritic chest pain, or pulmonary hypertension.

The diagnosis of Takayasu's arteritis in the early stages of the disease requires a high clinical suspicion when patients present with nonspecific constitutional symptoms. Although a high erythrocyte sedimentation rate is characteristic of the disease, no pathognomonic clinical or laboratory features exist to confirm the diagnosis. Pathologic confirmation based on artery biopsy specimens at this clinical stage is rare.

Most patients undergo diagnostic studies when vaso-occlusive symptoms develop. Angiographic evidence of vascular ectasia or occlusion with saccular or fusiform aneurysms in a young woman with organ ischemia supports the diagnosis. Chest radiographs or CT scan imaging may demonstrate vascular calcifications or dilatation, as in the present patient. Ultasonography can assist by excluding intravascular thrombosis of the major aortic branches as the primary cause of ischemic symptoms. Although extensive clinical experience with magnetic resonance imaging and angiography in patients with Takayasu's arteritis is lacking, these imaging techniques may be valuable in diagnosing and monitoring the disorder.

No definitive therapy exists for patients with Takayasu's arteritis. The clinical efficacy of corticosteroids during the inflammatory stage of the disease is not universally acknowledged. Administered in doses of 1 mg/kg/day, prednisone may alleviate constitutional symptoms and vascular pain as well as improve survival by preventing progression to vascular occlusive complications. A trial of cytotoxic agents such as cyclophosphamide or methotrexate may be of value in patients not responding to 4 weeks of corticosteroids. Patients with established vaso-occlusive symptoms do not dramatically improve with medical management, although antihypertensive therapy remains critically important.

Patients with clinical manifestations of vascular occlusion who do not improve after 3–6 months of corticosteroid therapy with or without cytotoxic agents or who demonstrate early deterioration are candidates for vascular reconstructive surgery. Right ventricular hypertrophy, ocular ischemia, aortic insufficiency, and aneurysmal dilatation are associated with an especially poor prognosis unless surgically managed. Emphasis for timing of surgery is placed on interceding before ischemic events occur. This approach is especially important for stroke prevention in patients with innominate or carotid arteries that exhibit hemodynamically significant stenoses. The presence of congestive heart failure does not obviate surgical repair because cardiac decompensation usually improves with control of hypertension.

Reconstructive surgery is complex and technically demanding, with early series complicated by graft occlusion. Acceptance of the importance of graft placement with anastomoses at uninvolved vascular segments has improved patency—balloon angioplasty, patch angioplasty, and endarterectomy have been associated with disappointing long-term results. Coronary artery bypass surgery may be necessary in patients with aortic disease at the coronary ostia or direct involvement of the coronary vasculature with arteritis.

The present patient had an ectatic descending aorta with linear calcifications apparent on the routine chest radiograph. The chest CT confirmed the presence of dense aortic calcification. An aortogram revealed segmental aortic disease with aneurysmal dilatation and stenosis along with stenotic narrowing or occlusion of the aorta's major branches. The patient refused further evaluation for surgical repair but improved after initiation of antihypertensive therapy.

Clinical Pearls

1. Takayasu's arteritis segmentally affects the aorta, the major aortic branches, and the pulmonary arteries, with mononuclear inflammation that progresses to transmural fibrosis, vascular stenosis, and aneurysmal dilatation.

2. Takayasu's arteritis classically proceeds through three clinical stages: a nonspecific inflammatory stage with nonspecific constitutional symptoms, a localized vascular phase with vascular tenderness, and a "pulseless" stage with vaso-occlusive manifestations.

3. Congestive heart failure may result from secondary hypertension, valvular insufficiency from aortic aneurysmal dilatation, inflammatory cardiomyopathy, or ischemic cardiomyopathy from stenosis, kinking, fistula formation, or aneurysmal dilatation of the coronary arteries.

4. Corticosteroid therapy may improve inflammatory symptoms but usually does not reverse established vaso-occlusive manifestations. Although not universally accepted, early corticosteroid therapy may prevent progression to the "pulseless" stage of the disease.

REFERENCES

1. Leavitt RY, Fauci AS. Pulmonary vasculitis. Am Rev Respir Dis 1986;134:149–166.
2. Weaver FA, Yellin AE, Campen DH, et al. Surgical procedures in the management of Takayasu's arteritis. J Vasc Surg 1990;12:429–439.
3. Amano J, Suzuki A. Coronary artery involvement in Takayasu's arteritis. J Thorac Cardiovasc Surg 1991;102:554–560.
4. Giordano JM, Leavitt RY, Hoffman G, et al. Experience with surgical treatment of Takayasu's disease. Surgery 1991;109:252–258.
5. Jorens PG, Williame LM, Tombeur JP, et al. Takayasu's disease and artherosclerosis. J Cardiovasc Surg 1991;32;373–375.
6. Krachman JE, Cunniff DJ, Kramer N, Rosenstein ED. Takayasu's arteritis. N J Med 1991;88:341–344.
7. Talwar KK, Kumar K, Chopra P, et al. Cardiac involvement in nonspecific aortoarteritis (Takayasu's arteritis). Am Heart J 1991;122:1666–1670.

PATIENT 72

A 42-year-old man with acute myelogenous leukemia, dyspnea, and bilateral pleural effusions

A 42-year-old retired Navy radar worker was transferred for evaluation and treatment of acute leukemia. He had presented to his local hospital with sudden onset of dyspnea and left anterior chest pain that was not relieved by over-the-counter analgesics. The patient reported epistaxis on the day of admission but denied fevers, chills, or cough.

Physical Examination: Temperature 100.4°; pulse 96; respirations 24; blood pressure 140/75. General: dyspneic with ambulation but otherwise in no acute distress. Chest: dullness to percussion with decreased fremitus over the left posterior chest. Cardiac: normal. Abdomen: no organomegaly. Skin: nonpalpable purpura on both upper and lower extremities.

Laboratory Findings: Hct 21%; WBC 47,000/μl with 10% blasts; platelets 15,000/μl. PT 13 sec; PTT 25 sec. Chest radiograph (below left): bilateral pleural effusions; mild cardiomegaly; apical bullous changes; and increased interstitial markings. Chest CT (below right): bilateral effusions with atelectasis and several soft tissue extrapleural densities. Pleural fluid: serosanguinous. Nucleated cells 3162/μl with 35% neutrophils, 15% lymphocytes, 7% eosinophils, 21% macrophages, 20% others. Erythrocytes 16,000/μl; total protein 4.0 g/dl; LDH 293 IU/L; glucose 109 mg/dl. Gram stain: negative.

Question: What is the likely cause of the bilateral pleural effusions?

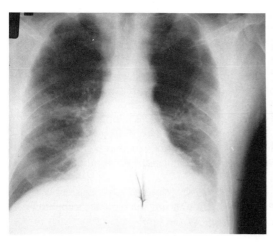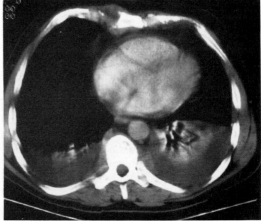

Diagnosis: Leukemic involvement of the pleura.

Discussion: The presence of pleural effusions in patients with acute and chronic leukemia presents a differential diagnosis that includes tuberculosis, pulmonary infarction, pneumonia, heart failure, and subphrenic processes such as splenic infarction due to leukemic infiltration of the spleen. In some patients, however, pleural effusions may develop as a direct result of pleuropulmonary infiltration by leukemia cells.

The exact incidence of pleuropulmonary involvement in leukemia is not well-defined because many patients experience no respiratory symptoms. Autopsy studies indicate that up to 24–64% of patients with acute and chronic leukemias have postmortem evidence of microscopic infiltration of the lungs by leukemia cells. This tissue infiltration contributes to the premorbid clinical course in only 7% of patients. Only 8–22% of patients with autopsy evidence of leukemic infiltration have abnormal chest radiographs. Frequently, the respiratory symptoms noted in patients shown later to have leukemic infiltration can be attributed to coexisting pulmonary edema, alveolar hemorrhage, or pneumonia. Patients with symptoms clearly resulting from pulmonary leukemic infiltration invariably have diffuse bilateral interstitial or reticulonodular infiltrates and frequently rapidly progress to respiratory failure.

From 4–15% of patients with leukemia have autopsy evidence of leukemic infiltration of the pleura, and approximately one-half of these patients have no accompanying pulmonary parenchymal involvement. Some autopsy series, however, indicate that up to 20% of patients with leukemia have postmortem pleural effusions, most of which do not have corresponding histologic evidence of direct pleural invasion. Subpleural infarction with surrounding zones of parenchymal leukemic infiltration is frequently noted in these patients. Only 50% of patients with leukemia with autopsy detection of pleural effusions have premorbid radiographic evidence of pleural fluid, which is usually accompanied by mediastinal adenopathy. In contrast to pulmonary parenchymal involvement, which is usually asymptomatic, visceral pleural infiltration is commonly associated with respiratory symptoms related to the presence of pleural effusions. Pulmonary ischemia or infarction from leukemic infiltration of the pleura, impaired lymphatic drainage of the pleural space, and increased capillary permeability may underlie the pathogenesis of leukemic pleural effusions.

Autopsy series indicate that the incidence of leukemic infiltration of the lungs in patients with acute leukemia is unaffected by a history of chemotherapy treatment. Visceral pleural involvement likewise occurs with a similar frequency in patients with or without a history of chemotherapy treatment. In the largest autopsy series to date, the incidence of pleural metastasis in acute lymphocytic leukemia was 37%, 3% in chronic myelogenous leukemia, and 19% in acute myelogenous leukemia.

Evaluation of patients by chest CT has not demonstrated a high incidence of pleural involvement in acute or chronic leukemia. Only one example of pleural involvement was identified in a retrospective review of 43 chest CT scans from 29 patients with leukemia. The pleural involvement appeared as plaquelike pleural thickening, with areas of interstitial subpleural thickening extending from the pleura. The latter finding probably represents subpleural leukemic infiltration in perivascular and peribronchial tissues.

The clinical evaluation of patients with leukemia and pleural effusions requires thoracentesis and careful exclusion of infectious etiologies. Morphologic, cytochemical, and immunochemical methods for evaluating blood and pleural fluid leukocytes in conjunction with the clinical findings assist in establishing the cytodiagnosis of leukemic effusions. In some patients, percutaneous pleural biopsy with specialized staining techniques may be required to confirm the diagnosis. Patients with pulmonary infiltrates compatible with leukemic infiltration similarly require exclusion of infectious etiologies, which often depends on a transbronchial or open lung biopsy. Histologic examination of biopsy specimens must differentiate leukemic infiltration from simple aggregation of circulating leukemic blast cells within the pulmonary vasculature. Leukemic infiltration is characterized by an interstitial location of blast cells typically around smaller bronchi, alveolar septi, and blood vessels often in a nodular distribution. Several patients with pulmonary leukemic infiltration have been reported to be diagnosed by bronchoalveolar lavage with the detection of leukemic cells in the lavage specimen. Contamination of the specimen by blood that contains circulating blasts must be excluded.

Examination of the present patient's bone marrow biopsy specimen made the diagnosis of acute myelogenous leukemia. Results of a thoracentesis excluded pleural infection. The pleural fluid contained 20% blasts, supporting the diagnosis of a leukemic pleural effusion; specialized stains confirmed the diagnosis. The patient was treated with daunorubicin and cytosine arabinoside and, after 3 weeks of therapy, demonstrated resolution of the pleural effusions and extrapleural masses that had been noted on the chest CT scan (previous page).

Clinical Pearls

1. Leukemic infiltration of the lung is a common autopsy finding, occurring in 24–64% of patients, but usually does not cause premorbid symptoms.

2. Leukemic involvement of the visceral pleura is usually associated with respiratory symptoms referable to the presence of a pleural effusion.

3. Leukemic pleural effusions probably result from increased capillary permeability induced by malignant cells, pulmonary ischemia or infarction, and impaired lymphatic drainage of the pleural space.

4. The diagnosis leukemia-related pleural effusions is established by morphologic, cytochemical, and immunochemical analysis of pleural fluid leukocytes in conjunction with the clinical findings after exclusion of intrapleural infection.

REFERENCES

1. Green RA, Nichols NJ. Pulmonary involvement in leukemia. Am Rev Respir Dis 1959;86:833–844.
2. Klatte EC, Yardley J, Smith EB, et al. The pulmonary manifestations and complications of leukemia. Am J Roentgenol Radium Ther Nucl Med 1963;89:598–609.
3. Ross JS, Ellman L. Leukemic infiltration of the lungs in the chemotherapeutic era. Am J Clin Pathol 1974;61:235–241.
4. Viadana E, Bross IDH, Pickren JW. An autopsy study of the metastatic patterns of human leukemias. Oncology 1978;35:87–96.
5. Janckila AJ, Yam LT, Li C-Y. Immunocytochemical diagnosis of acute leukemia with pleural involvement. Acta Cytologica 1985;29:67–72.
6. Kovalski R, Hansen-Flaschen J, Lodato RF. Localized leukemic pulmonary infiltrates: diagnosis by bronchoscopy and resolution with therapy. Chest 1990;97:674–678.
7. Kim FM, Fennessy. Pleural thickening caused by leukemic infiltration: CT findings. AJR 1994;162:293–294.

PATIENT 73

A 21-year-old woman with a tracheostomy and progressive dyspnea

A 21-year-old woman presented with a 3-month history of progressive dyspnea on exertion and purulent sputum. At 3 years of age, she had undergone multiple laryngeal polyp resections and an eventual tracheostomy for a diagnosis of recurrent respiratory papillomatosis (juvenile laryngeal papillomatosis). She received close follow-up monitoring until 1 year previously when she went to college. Her laryngeal disorder had stabilized during the past several years and her chest radiograph had always been normal.

Physical Examination: Vital signs normal. Skin: normal. Mouth: normal. Neck: tracheostomy tube in place with healthy appearing stoma. Chest: diffuse basilar crackles, no rubs or wheezes. Cardiac: normal. Abdomen: no hepatosplenomegaly. Extremities: clubbing.

Laboratory Findings: Hct 32%; WBC 11,000/μl. Electrolytes and renal indices: normal. ABG (RA): pH 7.45; PCO_2 34 mmHg; PO_2 61 mmHg. Sputum Gram stain: > 25 PMNs/hpf, mixed bacteria. Chest radiograph: shown below.

Question: What is the likely cause of the patient's dyspnea and chest radiographic abnormalities?

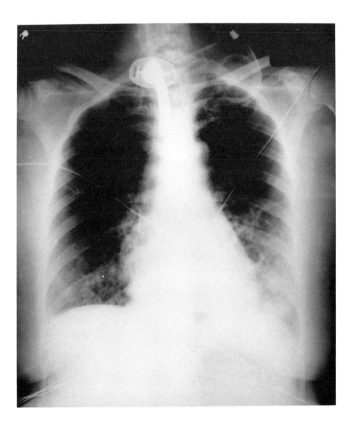

Answer: Broncholoalveolar papillomatosis.

Discussion: Benign papillomas of the larynx are the most common respiratory tract tumors of infancy and childhood. Originally termed "juvenile laryngeal papillomatosis," the potential for occurrence at any age and the inclination for recurrence after excisional therapy favor the designation "recurrent respiratory papillomatosis."

The laryngeal papillomas have the histologic appearance of benign epithelial neoplasms with a central fibrous connective tissue core covered by squamous epithelium. If epithelial atypia occurs, it tends to be mild without any evidence of invasion of normal adjacent tissue. The occurrence of multiple or solitary laryngeal papillomas in a range of age groups has prompted classification of the disorder into four clinical groups called juvenile or adult multiple and juvenile or adult single papillomatosis.

Infection with human papillomaviruses appears to be the cause of multiple recurrent respiratory papillomatosis. Of the 50 different papillomaviruses, types 6 and 11 are most strongly associated with the disorder. The role of papillomavirus infection in patients with solitary laryngeal papillomas is less well defined. An equal female-male ratio in juvenile patients supports the impression that papillomavirus is spread from mother to child before or during birth. The predominance of men in the adult group indicates an alternative route of infection other than activation of a latent infection originating from maternal transmission.

Laryngeal papillomas develop most commonly in children under 4 years of age. Initial symptoms include an abnormal cry or hoarseness that progresses to cough, dyspnea, and stridor. Papillomata may spread into the trachea and involve the entire respiratory tract from the nasal cavities to the lungs. Multiple resections of polyps with resulting airway scarring and recurrence of disease may require a tracheostomy for relief of airway obstruction. Although several medical reviews indicate that childhood laryngeal papillomas may regress at puberty, few data exist to support this impression.

Laryngeal papillomas have malignant potential, with a respiratory tract carcinoma developing in 2–14% of patients. The incidence of malignant transformation is greatest in patients who smoke and those who undergo laryngeal irradiation to control the laryngeal papillomatosis. Single laryngeal papilloma of the adult has a very high rate of malignant transformation and may actually represent a well-differentiated squamous cell carcinoma at its inception rather than a virally induced papilloma.

The mean time to diagnosis of laryngeal carcinoma after onset of recurrent respiratory papillomatosis is 32 years with a range of 20–37 years.

Typically local invasion occurs with little involvement of regional lymph nodes or distant metastases. Cytologic criteria for malignancy may or may not exist.

Pulmonary spread of papillomata rarely occurs (1% of patients) but is a particularly lethal form of the disease. Lung involvement tends to be in dependent regions and occurs on average 13 years after diagnosis of the laryngeal disease. Foci of proliferating squamous epithelium grow within the lung, using alveolar walls as a supporting framework. As further circumferential growth occurs, obliteration of the blood supply and central necrosis transforms multicentric nodules to cavitary disease. The mechanism of spread to the lungs is poorly defined but may result from contiguous extension or aerosolization of the virus into peripheral airways. The latter route of spread is supported by the peripheral, subpleural location of pulmonary lesions in patients with normal-appearing bronchi beyond the carina and the high incidence of pulmonary disease in patients managed with tracheostomies or other airway manipulations.

Patients with broncholoalveolar papillomatosis are often diagnosed incidentally on follow-up chest radiographs. Symptoms of cough and dyspnea may be incorrectly attributed to the laryngeal disease. Clubbing occurs only with extensive pulmonary involvement. Repeated parenchymal infections and aggressive formation of multiple papillomata may result in progressive respiratory failure. Focal malignant transformation is difficult to diagnose in patients with extensive background lung involvement with destructive papillomatosis.

The initial chest radiograph in broncholoalveolar papillomatosis may demonstrate multiple or solitary nodules that progress to thick or thin-walled cavities with a predilection for the lower lobes. Less common radiographic signs include consolidation, a large solitary mass, and bronchiectasis. CT findings include solid round nodules in the posterior lung segments, cavitating nodules, dilated and irregular bronchi, and consolidation of atelectatic peripheral lung segments.

Multiple therapies have been tried for recurrent respiratory papillomatosis that include mechanical surgical excision, cryosurgery, cauterization, ultrasound, laser surgery, topical chemotherapy as an adjunct to surgical laser excision, photodynamic therapy with photosensitive dyes, podophyllum, antibiotics, autogenous vaccine, and interferon. Now carbon dioxide laser has superseded other forms of treatment because excessive scarring of the normal underlying laryngeal tissue can be avoided. Treatment is symptomatic because new lesions appear de novo in areas adjacent to removed papillomata. Therapeutic approaches to arrest progression of broncholoalveolar papillomatosis are limited; parenchymal disease may spontaneously arrest but rarely if ever regresses.

The present patient had radiographic evidence for cavitary infiltrates suggestive of the diagnosis of broncholoalveolar papillomatosis. The preceding laryngeal polyps and a characteristic chest CT scan further supported the diagnosis. The patient improved with antibiotic therapy for a presumed bacterial superinfection and remains in long-term follow-up.

Clinical Pearls

1. Respiratory infection with papillomavirus types 6 and 11 is the etiology of multiple recurrent respiratory papillomatosis.

2. Pulmonary involvement occurs in 1% of patients with recurrent respiratory papillomatosis and may result from inhalational spread of viral particles after manipulation of laryngotracheal polyps.

3. In patients with broncholoalveolar papillomatosis, foci of pulmonary squamous epithelium present as lung nodules that progressively outstrip their vascular supply, becoming multiple thin or thick-walled pulmonary cavities.

4. Broncholoalveolar papillomatosis has malignant potential. Radiographic detection of focal malignant transformation is complicated by the background of diffuse pulmonary destruction from underlying nodular and cavitary papillomatosis.

REFERENCES

1. Glazer G, Webb R. Laryngeal papillomatosis with pulmonary spread in a 69-year-old man. AJR 1979;132:820–822.
2. Kawanami T, Bowen A. Juvenile laryngeal papillomatosis with pulmonary parenchymal spread. Pediatr Radiol 1985;15:102–104.
3. Kramer SS, Wehunt WD, Stocker JT, Kashima H. Pulmonary manifestations of juvenile laryngotracheal papillomatosis. AJR 1985;144:687–694.
4. Lindeberg H, Elbrond O. Laryngeal papillomas: clinical aspects in a series of 231 patients. Clin Otolaryngol 1989;14:333–342.
5. Quiney RE, Hall D, Croft CB. Laryngeal papillomatosis: analysis of 113 patients. Clin Otolaryngol 1989;14:217–225.

PATIENT 74

**A 38-year-old man with cough, pleuritic chest pain, hemoptysis,
and progressive dyspnea following a rash**

A 38-year-old man presented with a 1-week history of worsening dyspnea, a nonproductive cough with pleuritic chest pain, fever, and chills preceded several days earlier by blood-streaked sputum. He denied headache, nausea, vomiting, or diarrhea but had experienced the onset of a pruritic rash 5 days before his respiratory symptoms.

Physical Examination: Temperature 100.2°; pulse 100; respirations 30. General: moderate respiratory distress. Chest: bilateral diffuse end-expiratory wheezes. Abdomen: right upper quadrant tenderness to deep palpation. Skin: diffuse papulovesicular eruptions.

Laboratory Findings: Hct 37%; WBC 10,000/μl; ABG (RA): pH 7.50; PCO_2 30 mmHg; PO_2 48 mmHg. Chest radiograph: shown below.

Question: What is the most likely cause of the patient's clinical presentation?

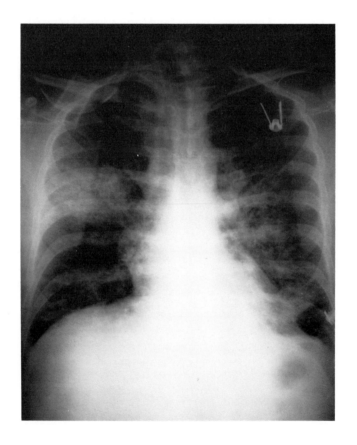

Diagnosis: Varicella-zoster pneumonia.

Discussion: Varicella is a highly communicable disease that primarily affects children and has a 90% attack rate among household contacts. Primary infection results in chickenpox and can occur by direct skin-to-skin contact or by inhalation of respiratory secretions. Most children with the disease experience a mild, self-limited illness. Although only 2% of the total cases of chickenpox are attributable to patients over 20 years of age, nearly 25% of the fatalities occur in this adult age group.

The incubation period for chickenpox ranges from 3–21 days, with the onset of disease heralded by a rash. Pneumonia, the major complication in the previously normal adult, is noted radiographically in 16–50% of adults with chickenpox but causes symptoms in only 10–20%. Symptoms of fever, cough, dyspnea, pleuritic chest pain, and minimal hemoptysis when present typically occur 1–6 days after the onset of the rash. The chest physical findings of wheezes and crackles may be minimal and correlate poorly with the severity of the disease. Pneumonia most often develops in adults who have the severe cutaneous manifestations of chickenpox. The course of the pneumonia is most severe during the period of maximum skin involvement. Chickenpox pneumonia without any accompanying rash has not been reported.

The chest radiograph demonstrates an interstitial pneumonia, diffuse nodular infiltrates (1–10 mm), hilar adenopathy, peribronchial infiltrates, and infrequently pleural effusions. Occasionally, varicella pneumonia may present with a miliary pattern.

Pneumonia occurs more frequently in immunologically compromised adults and during pregnancy. Gestational age at onset of the infection is a significant risk factor, with the greatest risk for pneumonia occurring in the third trimester. Patients receiving immunosuppressive drugs, including corticosteroids, are also at increased risk. A history of smoking, advanced age, and the presence of a solid malignancy or chronic obstructive pulmonary disease have been suggested to be additional risk factors for varicella pneumonia. Varicella pneumonia in the normal adult is usually a self-limited illness. Mortality approaches 10–30% in immunocompromised and pregnant patients.

Microscopic examination of lung tissue in patients with varicella pneumonia demonstrates interstitial pneumonitis with mononuclear infiltration of the alveolar walls. Fibrinous exudates with macrophages are found within the alveoli. Endothelial damage in the small blood vessels results in focal hemorrhagic necrosis. Vesicles may occur on the pleural surfaces and within the tracheobronchial tree.

A presumptive diagnosis of varicella pneumonia may rest on the presence of the characteristic papulovesicular skin eruption, typical radiographic findings, and a history of exposure. Scrapings from cutaneous lesions may assist the diagnosis by demonstrating multinucleated giant cells and intranuclear inclusion bodies with a Tzank smear. The virus can be isolated from vesicular fluid inoculated into human embryonic lung fibroblasts. Complement fixation studies can confirm the diagnosis by demonstrating an antibody titer rise by 2–4 weeks.

Adult patients with varicella pneumonia require prompt initiation of antiviral therapy. Acyclovir, which is the most thoroughly studied agent for this infection, is used with an intravenous dose of 10–15 mg/kg every 8 hours or an oral dose in mild cases of 800 mg five times daily. Immunocompromised patients should receive intravenous therapy. Recent studies suggest that oral acyclovir given during the incubation period may prevent clinical manifestations of varicella infections. Vidarabine and foscarnet have been less successful as therapeutic options.

In considering the pregnant patient with varicella pneumonia, acyclovir is listed as a category C drug with fetal risk unknown. However, no fetal abnormalities attributed to acyclovir therapy have been reported to the Burroughs Wellcome Acyclovir Registry as of the publication of this text. Zoster immunoglobulin will modify the severity of the illness, particularly in the immunocompromised patient. The incidence of clinical varicella may be reduced by 50% if immunoglobulin is given within 72–96 hours of exposure. Active immunization with a vaccine appears to be relatively safe in normal and immunocompromised patients and may be of benefit up to 3 days after exposure. Vaccine efficacy appears to be greater in children. The role of corticosteroids in the treatment of varicella pneumonia remains controversial.

Secondary bacterial infections, sepsis, pulmonary hemorrhage, and pulmonary emboli can complicate the recovery of patients with varicella pneumonia. Patient recovery occurs at a variable rate. The chest radiograph may clear as soon as 9 days or as long as several months after the onset of respiratory symptoms. After resolution of the pneumonia, the radiographic infiltrates rarely may calcify in a nodular pattern predominantly at the lung bases and simulate old, healed histoplasmosis. Spirometry typically returns to normal, although decreased diffusion capacity may persist long after recovery. Isolated case reports exist of persistent restrictive ventilatory impairment.

Long-term alterations in the FEF 25–75 suggest the presence of small airways disease.

The present patient required short-term mechanical ventilation secondary to hypoxic respiratory failure. He eventually recovered and his pulmonary symptoms resolved, although spirometric studies demonstrated a persistent mild restrictive ventilatory defect.

Clinical Pearls

1. The presence of a typical papulovesicular skin eruption, a history of chickenpox exposure, and a compatible chest radiograph are adequate to make a presumptive diagnosis of varicella pneumonia and warrant the initiation of acyclovir therapy.

2. Varicella pneumonia, which has not been reported to develop in the absence of an accompanying skin rash, occurs 1–6 days after onset of the skin eruptions.

3. Varicella pneumonia should be considered as a possible cause of interstitial pneumonia in any immunocompromised or pregnant patient.

4. After resolution of varicella pneumonia, the radiographic infiltrates may rarely calcify in a nodular pattern predominantly at the lung bases and simulate old, healed histoplasmosis.

REFERENCES

1. Bocles JS, Ehrenkranz NJ, Marks A. Abnormalities of respiratory function in varicella pneumonia. Ann Intern Med 1964;60:183–195.
2. Hockberger RS, Rothstein RJ. Varicella pneumonia in adults: a spectrum of disease. Ann Emerg Med 1986;15:931–934.
3. Schlossberg D, Littman M. Varicella pneumonia. Arch Intern Med 1988;148:1630–1632.
4. Smego RA, Asperilla MO. Use of acyclovir for varicella pneumonia during pregnancy. Obstet Gynecol 1991;78:1112–1115.
5. Rodrigues J, Niederman MS. Pneumonia complicating pregnancy. Clin Chest Med 1992;13:679–691.
6. Feldman S. Varicella-zoster virus pneumonitis. Chest 1994;106:22S–27S.

PATIENT 75

A 54-year-old obese man with cough, fever, and pulmonary infiltrates

A 54-year-old man presented with fever, chills, cough, purulent sputum, and progressive dyspnea. He had been in good health until 6 months earlier when he developed severe headaches. Hypertension was diagnosed at that time and therapy was initiated with hydrochlorothiazide and metoprolol. Since then, he has experienced marked weight gain and generalized weakness.

Physical Examination: Temperature 100°; pulse 110; respirations 28; blood pressure 180/100. General: truncal obesity; moderate respiratory distress. Head: round face. Chest: bilateral crackles with dullness at the right posterior base. Cardiac: grade II/VI systolic murmur. Abdomen: markedly obese; no organomegaly. Extremities: no clubbing. Neurologic: generalized weakness without focal deficits.

Laboratory Findings: Hct 36%; WBC 9,000/μl with 85% polymorphonuclear cells and 8% band forms. Na$^+$ 145 mEq/L; K$^+$ 2.5 mEq/L; HCO$_3^-$ 34 mEq/L; Cl$^-$ 100 mEq/L; glucose 195 mg/dl; BUN 25 mg/dl; Cr 1.9 mg/dl. ABG (RA): pH 7.50; PCO$_2$ 37 mmHg; PO$_2$ 52 mmHg. Sputum Gram stain: gram positive coccobacilli with an irregularly stained, beaded appearance. Chest radiograph: shown below.

Questions: What is the etiology of the patient's pulmonary disorder? What underlying condition might exist?

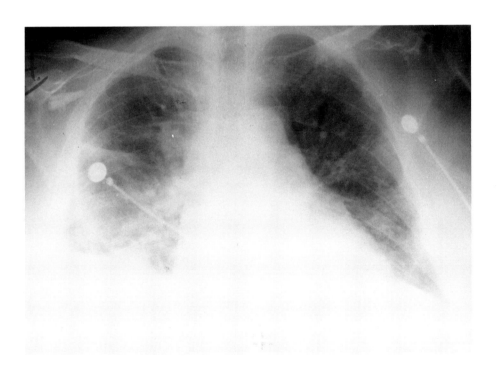

Diagnosis: Nocardial pneumonia due to immunosuppression from an adrenocorticotropin (ACTH)-secreting tumor.

Discussion: It is well known that glucocorticoid therapy depresses normal immunity and lowers resistance to infection by a host of viral, bacterial, fungal, and parasitic agents. Although emphasized by Cushing in the 1930s, it is less well recognized that patients with endogenous hypercortisolism related to Cushing's syndrome are also immunosuppressed and at risk for opportunistic infections. This infectious risk occurs predominantly in patients with ectopic-adrenocorticotropin (ACTH)-secreting tumors and adrenal tumors but also develops to a lesser extent in patients with pituitary causes of Cushing's syndrome.

The specific mechanisms by which corticosteroids alter immunocompetence remain unclear partly because these compounds can affect nearly every limb of the immune system to some degree. Although humoral immunity is relatively preserved, circulating B-lymphocytes may be depressed and plasma concentrations of IgA and IgG lowered after prolonged, high-dose corticosteroid treatment. Corticosteroids appear not to have major effects on the neutrophilic functions of chemotaxis, phagocytosis, and phagocytic killing. Other neutrophilic activities such as leukocyte adhesion, diapedesis, and migration through tissue, however, may be suppressed. Corticosteroids have a major effect on inhibiting the bactericidal and fungicidal functions of monocytic and macrophage cell lines.

T-lymphocytes are the most susceptible cells to the effects of increased plasma concentrations of corticosteroids. The mechanism of T-cell depression is uncertain but may result from a redistribution of circulating T-cell populations to other body compartments or inhibition of T-cell–effector cell interactions. Functional reactivity of T-lymphocytes as measured by blastogenic response to antigens has been shown to be depressed in patients with exogenous hypercortisolism and those with Cushing's syndrome.

The corticosteroid-induced alterations of host defenses in patients with Cushing's syndrome translate to an increased risk of infection from a variety of pathogens. Mucocutaneous fungal infections, postoperative wound infections, localized and systemic bacterial infections, and reactivation tuberculosis are commonly associated conditions. The more serious infections that involve the lungs in patients with Cushing's syndrome reflect the primary effect of corticosteroids on altering macrophage and T-cell function. The four most common of these pulmonary infections include cryptococcosis, aspergillosis, nocardiosis, and pneumocystosis. These infections may exist confined to the lung or rapidly disseminate in patients with Cushing's syndrome.

It appears that a dose-response effect exists in Cushing's syndrome between the severity of hypercortisolism and the degree of immunocompromise, as has been observed in patients undergoing corticosteroid therapy. This relationship is shown by the high incidence of opportunistic infections in patients with Cushing's syndrome due to adrenal tumors or ectopic ACTH-secreting tumors, which have higher levels of corticosteroid production compared to pituitary causes of Cushing's disease. Furthermore, the etiology of the Cushing's syndrome affects the type of opportunistic infection that may occur. Patients with ectopic ACTH-secreting tumors have massive elevations of plasma cortisol and a high risk for *Pneumocystis* pneumonia. Patients with lesser degrees of hypercortisolism more commonly develop cryptococcosis.

The association of Cushing's syndrome with opportunistic infections has profound diagnostic and therapeutic implications. Patients who present with an infection as the initial manifestation of Cushing's syndrome may not have timely recognition of their underlying immunocompromised condition. Delays in initiating aggressive diagnostic techniques in favor of empirical therapy for common infections and failure to control the hypercortisolism may subsequently ensue. Conversely, patients presenting with newly diagnosed Cushing's syndrome may have an underlying infection masked or obscured in severity by the antiinflammatory effects of hypercortisolism. Patients with Cushing's syndrome may manifest *Pneumocystis* pneumonia only after control of plasma cortisol levels, as occurs in patients with lymphoma or leukemia undergoing tapering of corticosteroid therapy.

Because opportunistic infections in patients with uncontrolled endogenous hypercortisolism are usually fatal, urgent lowering of plasma cortisol levels combined with appropriate antimicrobial therapy is the cornerstone of therapy. Detection of elevated morning cortisol levels in a patient with a deep-seated infection should be treated immediately with aminoglutethimide (an agent that inhibits conversion of cholesterol to pregnenolone) and metyrapone (an 11, beta-hydroxylase inhibitor) that can correct hypercortisolism and restore immunocompetence to normal within several days. More urgent needs to lower plasma cortisol levels require surgical interventions to control steroidogenesis.

The present patient presented with clinical and roentgenographic features of a bacterial pneumonia with a parapneumonic effusion. The generalized weakness, hypertension, truncal obesity, and moon facies indicated the possibility of Cushing's syndrome complicated by an opportunistic infection. The severity of the patient's hypokalemic metabolic alkalosis, lymphopenia, and hyperglycemia strongly suggested an adrenal tumor or an ACTH-secreting neoplasm rather than pituitary Cushing's disease. He was started on trimethoprim-sulfamethoxasole because of sputum Gram-stain evidence of a *Nocardia* species, which subsequently grew from the patient's sputum and pleural fluid. Despite prompt initiation of aminoglutethimide and metyrapone after a morning plasma cortisol level returned markedly elevated ($220\mu g/dl$, normal 5–22 $\mu g/dl$) followed by emergency bilateral adrenalectomies, the patient expired. At autopsy, a thymic tumor was found and presumed to be the source of ectopic ACTH; disseminated nocardiosis was also present.

Clinical Pearls

1. Patients who have Cushing's syndrome and uncontrolled hypercortisolism are at increased risk for opportunistic infections.

2. The four most common pulmonary infections in Cushing's syndrome are cryptococcosis, aspergillosis, nocardiosis, and pneumocystosis.

3. Patients with adrenal tumors or ectopic-ACTH secreting tumors have higher levels of plasma cortisol and a greater risk of opportunistic infections compared to patients with pituitary Cushing's disease.

4. Infected patients with Cushing's syndrome and uncontrolled hypercortisolism require urgent medical or surgical interventions to lower the plasma cortisol level. Deep-seated infections in patients with Cushing's syndrome are medical emergencies that commonly have a fatal outcome.

5. The clinical manifestations of *Pneumocystis* pneumonia may first appear after control of plasma cortisol levels, as occurs in patients with lymphoma undergoing a taper of corticosteroid therapy.

REFERENCES

1. Higgins TL, Calabrese LH, Sheeler LR. Opportunistic infections in patients with ectopic ACTH-secreting tumors. Cleve Clin Q 1982;49:43–49.
2. Fulkerson WJ, Newman JH. Endogenous Cushing's syndrome complicated by *Pneumocystis carinii* pneumonia. Am Rev Respir Dis 1984;129:188–189.
3. Graham BS, Tucker WS Jr. Opportunistic infections in endogenous Cushing's syndrome. Ann Intern Med 1984;101:334–338.
4. Dunlap NE, Grizzle WE, Heck LW Jr. Unsuspected Cushing's disease in a patient with fatal staphylococcal bacteremia and multiple pituitary adenomas. Am J Med 1989;86:217–221.

PATIENT 76

A 47-year-old woman with a 6-week history of dyspnea on exertion and a nonproductive cough

A 47-year-old woman was seen in a local emergency department with a 6-week history of progressive dyspnea on exertion and a nonproductive cough. She denied fever, chills, or hemoptysis. Three months earlier, the patient had stopped smoking cigarettes when she was told she had chronic obstructive pulmonary disease (COPD). She had a history of chronic atrial fibrillation and pulmonary embolism managed with warfarin.

Physical Examination: Temperature 98.8°; pulse 100; respirations 30. General: moderate respiratory distress. Chest: bilateral diffuse rhonchi with rare end-expiratory wheezes. Extremities: no clubbing or edema.

Laboratory Findings: Hct 36%; WBC 8,500/μl. ABG (RA): pH 7.38; PCO_2 30 mmHg; PO_2 50 mmHg. PT 17.8 sec; PTT 40.7 sec. Spirometry (3 months earlier): FEV_1 = 1.44 L (65% predicted); FVC = 2.04 L (68% predicted); FEV_1/FVC = 71%. Spirometry (at presentation): FEV_1 = 0.70 L (32% of predicted); FVC = 1.39 L (47% of predicted); FEV_1/FVC = 51%. Chest radiograph (shown below): hyperinflation with bilateral peribronchial interstitial infiltrates.

Question: What clinical condition could explain the patient's clinical presentation?

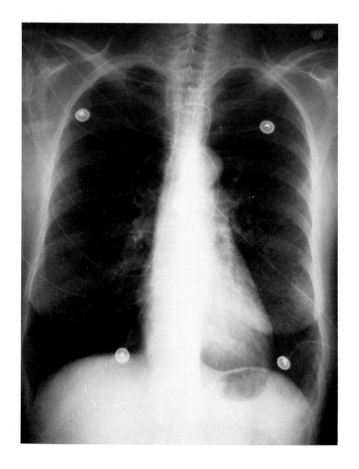

Diagnosis: Constrictive bronchiolitis obliterans.

Discussion: Bronchiolitis and bronchiolitis obliterans (BO) are general terms used to describe an inflammatory disease that primarily affects the small conducting airways, often spares a considerable portion of the interstitium, and occasionally extends into the alveolar ducts. Characteristically, there is partial or total obliteration of the affected airways by an organizing exudate and granulation tissue that projects into the lumen in a polypoid fashion. In some cases, there is complete destruction of the small airways. The lesion results from damage to the bronchiolar epithelium, and the repair process leads to excessive proliferation of granulation tissue.

Acute bronchiolitis, seen in infants and young children, usually is associated with viral infection, most commonly the respiratory syncytial virus. In the adult, BO was previously considered rare, although recently it has been found to represent as many as 4% of patients previously diagnosed with COPD. Approximately 10–54% of long-term survivors with heart-lung transplants and 3–10% of long-term bone marrow transplant patients have developed BO. Bronchiolitis obliterans has been associated with connective tissue diseases (rheumatoid arthritis, lupus, and systemic sclerosis), penicillamine therapy, toxic fume exposure (NO_2, SO_2, cocaine), and infection (adenovirus, legionella, mycoplasma, nocardia); an idiopathic form of the disease has also been recognized. The idiopathic cases and those associated with connective tissue disease are often confused with COPD or idiopathic pulmonary fibrosis.

The clinical presentation varies according to the etiology. Those cases classified as idiopathic BO may represent a subset of patients with unrecognized viral syndrome or toxic fume exposure. Patients usually are in the fifth to sixth decade of life, with men and women equally affected. A persistent, nonproductive cough is the most common presenting symptom, which is closely followed by dyspnea on exertion; fever, chest pain, rales, and wheezes are rare. The onset of symptoms is over months to years. Spirometry demonstrates severe airflow obstruction but restriction or a mixed pattern may be present. Diffusion capacity is decreased or normal. Variable degrees of hypoxemia and hypercapnia may be present.

The most common radiographic finding is hyperinflation with or without interstitial infiltrates. Nodular densities, a miliary pattern, and alveolar infiltrates are uncommon and pleural involvement is rare. The chest radiograph may be normal. CT scan shows widespread areas of increased attenuation of a patchy nature, even in patients with normal radiographs.

A definitive diagnosis requires an open lung biopsy. The clinical diagnosis requires a high index of suspicion with the characteristic findings of rapid progression of symptoms, severe airflow obstruction not attributable to other causes of COPD, no improvement with bronchodilators, and > 25% neutrophils on bronchoalveolar lavage (BAL). Additional diagnostic clues include age < 40 years, a modest or absent smoking history, severity of obstruction out of proportion to tobacco use, and rapid progression of symptoms after discontinuation of smoking. Neutrophil products, including collagenase and myeloperoxidase, have been recovered in increased amounts, suggesting a role in the pathogenesis of the airway lesions.

Treatment is corticosteroids (prednisone 1 mg/kg) for 8–16 weeks or until maximal improvement occurs with gradual tapering over months to 20 mg/day. Treatment should be continued for 2 years at the lowest alternate-day dose, with the goal of stable lung function. There is a significant improvement in FEV_1 and reduction in BAL neutrophils in responders.

The present patient had a BAL that demonstrated 35% neutrophil with negative stains and cultures. She was treated with corticosteroids with marked improvement at 2 months.

Clinical Pearls

1. BO is an inflammatory disease of the small airways that produces a rapidly progressive (few months to years) form of obstructive lung disease.

2. The most common radiographic finding is hyperinflation with or without interstitial infiltrates.

3. Rapid progression of symptoms, severe airflow obstruction not attributable to other causes of COPD, absence of physiologic improvement with bronchodilators, and > 25% neutrophils on BAL without evidence of infection provide a clinical diagnosis.

4. A rapid progression of symptoms after discontinuation of smoking is an additional diagnostic clue to BO.

REFERENCES

1. Kindt GC, Weiland JE, Davis BW, et al. Bronchiolitis in adults. Am Rev Respir Dis 1989;140:483–492.
2. King TE. Bronchiolitis obliterans. Lung 1989;167:69–93.
3. Lentz D, Bergin CJ, Berry GJ, et al. Diagnosis of bronchiolitis obliterans in heart lung transplantation patients. Am J Roentgenol 1992;159:463–467.
4. Kraft M, Mortenson RL, Colby TV, et al. Cryptogenic constrictive bronchiolitis. Am Rev Respir Dis 1993;148:1093–1101.
5. St. John RC, Dorinsky PM. Cryptogenic bronchiolitis. Clin Chest Med 1993;14:667–675.

PATIENT 77

A 46-year-old man with HIV infection and nosocomial pneumonia

A 46-year-old man with known HIV infection presented with cough, shortness of breath, fever, and bilateral alveolar infiltrates (chest radiograph, below left). Bronchoalveolar lavage specimens were positive for *Pneumocystis carinii* on direct fluorescent antibody staining. After initiation of pentamidine and corticosteroids, the patient improved until the third hospital day when a left-sided spontaneous pneumothorax required chest tube placement. On the sixth hospital day, dyspnea rapidly worsened and was associated with delirium, cough with watery sputum, diarrhea, and profound hypoxemia. The patient was intubated and transferred to the ICU.

Physical Examination: Temperature 103°; pulse 80; respirations 22 on assist-control ventilation; blood pressure 110/70. General: moderate respiratory distress. Neck: shoddy supraclavicular adenopathy. Chest: diffuse rales with consolidative findingss over the left upper lobe. Cardiac: no murmurs or rubs. Abdomen: no organomegaly. Neurologic: delerious.

Laboratory Findings: Hct 30%; WBC 11,200/μl with 95% PMNs, 3% bands. Na$^+$ 129 mEq/L; K$^+$ 3.5 mEq/L; Cl$^-$ 95 mEq/L; HCO$_3^-$ 25 mEq/L; BUN 32 mg/dl; creatinine 1.9 mg/dl, LDH 450 IU/l. ABG (100% FiO$_2$): pH 7.50; PCO$_2$ 32 mmHg; PO$_2$ 58 mmHg. Sputum Gram stain: many PMNs without bacteria. Chest radiograph: below right.

Question: What is the possible cause of the patient's respiratory deterioration?

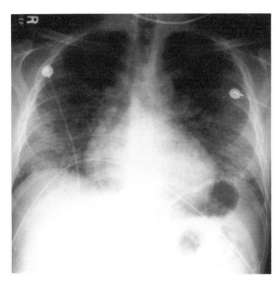 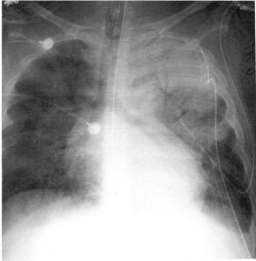

Diagnosis: Nosocomial pneumonia with *Legionella pneumophila.*

Discussion: More than 90% of patients with HIV infection experience a complicating pulmonary infection at some time during the course of their disease. Although *Pneumocystis carinii* is the most common cause of opportunistic pneumonia in this patient population, HIV disease also promotes an increase risk of pulmonary infections from a variety of common and unusual bacterial pathogens. Pyogenic bacteria, such as *Streptococcus pneumoniae* and *Haemophilus influenzae,* cause pneumonia with increased frequency because of an AIDS-related abnormality in B-cell and neutrophil function. Pulmonary infections with intracellular facultative pathogens such as *Legionella pneumophila* occur as a result of the profound abnormalities in T-cell function and cellular immunity associated with HIV infection.

Legionella pneumonia may occur in patients with HIV infection both as a nosocomial and community-acquired disease. In the hospital setting, small numbers of *Legionella* bacteria in the incoming water supply can survive at 40–60°C and multiply, reaching extremely high concentrations in inadequately chlorinated systems. Although human-to-human transmission does not occur, *Legionella* species can survive in aerosolized droplets of 1–5 microns in diameter generated from potable water sources that can enter the lower respiratory tract by inhalation. Direct inoculation of the tracheobronchial tree in intubated patients is an additional cause of *Legionella* pneumonia.

Once established in the airway, *Legionella* species may cause a mild flu-like illness or a severe pneumonia with or without extrapulmonary manifestations such as pericarditis, endocarditis, and cutaneous abscesses. Most patients with HIV infection are at risk for the latter course of the disease. Fever is the most constant clinical feature of *Legionella* pneumonia. Other described classic findings, such as diarrhea, hypophosphatemia, hyponatremia, relative bradycardia, altered mental status, and rhabdomyolysis, are insufficiently sensitive or specific features when considered independently to assist in the diagnosis of individual patients. The combination of several of these findings, however, in a patient with severe pneumonia and compromised immune defenses may suggest the diagnosis. The absence of bacteria in leukocyte-laden, watery sputum in a patient with an untreated pneumonia is further suggestive evidence of *Legionella* pneumonia.

Patients with HIV infection complicated by *Legionella* pneumonia have unilateral and unilobular pulmonary infiltrates that cavitate more commonly than other forms of nosocomial pneumonia. Pleural effusions frequently occur, although frank empyema is an uncommon finding. Differentiation from *Pneumocystis* pneumonia is aided by the localized distribution of the consolidative infiltrates in *Legionella* infection, although diffuse, patchy infiltrates may also occur.

Culture techniques remain the only absolute method for confirming the diagnosis of *Legionella* pneumonia. Sputum cultures take several days to grow *Legionella* species; positive blood cultures are associated with a high mortality. Bronchoalveolar lavage specimens should be acquired using water rather than saline, which interferes with growth of *Legionella* species. A serologic diagnosis depends on demonstration of a single high titer of specific antibody greater than 1:128 or a four-fold rise in acute and convalescent antibody titers. Patients with HIV infection commonly fail to produce an antibody response. Direct fluorescent antibody test of bronchial or tracheal aspirates can aid the rapid diagnosis of *Legionella* pneumonia. This test, however, is less sensitive than culture techniques. Urinary antigen detection appears to be a valuable test with reported sensitivities of 70–86%. Only *L. pneumophila* serogroup 1 are detected, but this is the most common serotype to cause disease.

Erythromycin remains the drug of choice for *Legionella* pneumonia supplemented with rifampin in severe infections. Doxycycline, trimethoprim-sulfamethoxazole, and the azalide antibiotics (azithromycin and clarithromycin) are alternative agents. The quinolones have in vitro activity against *Legionella* species, but demonstration of efficacy awaits clinical trials. Prompt initiation of antibiotic therapy can decrease the 25–70% mortality of *Legionella* pneumonia to less than 15%.

The present patient presented with the acquired immunodeficiency syndrome complicated by *Pneumocystis* pneumonia. His subsequent nosocomial pneumonia appeared to be bacterial in etiology. The absence of bacteria despite leukocytes on Gram stain of his sputum suggested the possibility of *Legionella* pneumonia. He was started on intravenous erythromycin and a third-generation cephalosporin and recovered after undergoing extensive pulmonary cavitation and prolonged hypoxic respiratory failure. Subsequent cultures of a tracheal aspirate were positive for *Legionella pneumophila.* In retrospect, the infection control team observed that a portable water-based cooling unit had been placed without their knowledge near the patient's room during a power failure several days before the onset of his nosocomial pulmonary infection.

Clinical Pearls

1. Patients with HIV infection are at increased risk for infection from *Legionella* species because of defects in cell-mediated immunity.

2. Legionella pneumonia may occur by inhalation of contaminated water droplets less than 5 μ in diameter or by direct inoculation of the lower airway by aspiration or airway instrumentation.

3. Patients with HIV infection develop pulmonary cavitation more commonly with *Legionella* pneumonia than from other causes of nosocomial pneumonia.

4. Bronchoalveolar lavage specimens should be acquired with sterile water rather than saline since the latter interferes with growth in culture of *Legionella* species.

REFERENCES

1. Kirby BD, Snyder KM, Meyer RD, Finegold SM. Legionaires' disease: report of sixty-five nosocomially acquired cases and review of the literature. Medicine 1980;59:188–205.
2. Murray JF, Garay SM, Hopewell PC, et al. Pulmonary complications of the acquired immunodeficiency syndrome: an update. Am Rev Respir Dis 1987;135:504–509.
3. Amorosa JK, Nahass RG, Nosher JL, Gocke DJ. Radiologic distinction of pyogenic pulmonary infection from *Pneumocystis carinii* pneumonia in AIDS patients. Radiology 1990;175:721–724.
4. Ruf B, Schürmann D, Horbach I, et al. Prevalence and diagnosis of *Legionella* pneumonia: a 3-year prospective study with emphasis on application of urinary antigen detection. J Infect Dis 1990;162:1341–1348.
5. Roig J, Aguilar X, Ruiz J, et al. Comparative study of *Legionella pneumophila* and other nosocomial-acquired pneumonia. Chest 1991;99:344–350.

PATIENT 78

A 42-year-old man with chronic renal failure and progressive dyspnea

A 42-year-old man with diabetes mellitus since age 16 was referred for evaluation of progressive dyspnea and recurrent pleural effusions. Two thoracenteses during the preceding 6 months showed a hemorrhagic, mononuclear-predominant exudate that was culture negative for tuberculosis. The patient had diabetic neuropathy, retinopathy, and nephropathy managed by peritoneal dialysis for 5 years. A pericardial window had been done 3 years earlier for uremic pericarditis.

Physical Examination: Temperature 97.5°; pulse 100 and regular; respiratory rate 36; blood pressure 160/95. General: chronically ill appearing. Chest: decreased-to-absent breath sounds at bases without adventitious sounds. Cardiac: regular tachycardia; S4. Extremities: trace edema.

Laboratory Findings: Hct 25%; WBC 7,000/μl; BUN 75 mg/dl, creatinine 8 mg/dl. FVC 0.92 L (27% of predicted), FEV_1 0.92 (23% of predicted), TLC 2.73 (36% of predicted), D_L/VA 4.12 (85% of predicted), ABG (RA): pH 7.36; PCO_2 35 mmHg; PO_2 79 mmHg. Chest radiograph: below left. Chest CT: below right.

Questions: What is the cause of the patient's dyspnea? What therapeutic options are available?

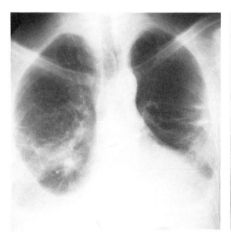
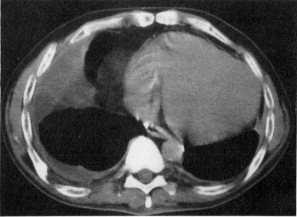

Diagnosis: Fibrosing uremic pleuritis.

Discussion: Pleural disease is a common problem in patients with chronic renal insufficiency. At autopsy, pleural effusions, acute fibrinous pleuritis, or pleural adhesions are noted in up to 20–70% of uremic patients. Furthermore, many patients with uremia develop pleural friction rubs and pleural effusions that are otherwise unexplained. Pleural effusions also have been reported as a companion finding in patients with uremic pericarditis. The consistency of reports of pleural disease in patients with chronic renal insufficiency supports the concept that uremic pleurisy is a distinct clinical entity, albeit with an as-of-yet undefined pathogenesis.

It is estimated that uremic pleural effusions develop in 3–10% of patients with chronic insufficiency. The incidence actually may be higher, however, considering that many of the effusions are asymptomatic. The typical patient with uremic pleural effusions has been undergoing hemodialysis or peritoneal dialysis for 1–2 years, with a range of a few months to greater than 4 years. Patients usually but not always have symptoms at the onset of the effusion, with fever, cough, or chest pain predominating. Dyspnea is an unusual presenting manifestation. Pericardial and pleural rubs are heard in 30–50% of patients. The pleural rub usually persists for 2 or 3 days.

The chest radiograph typically shows a unilateral, moderate to large pleural effusion without accompanying pulmonary infiltrates. Some patients may have coexisting uremic pneumonitis. Massive and bilateral pleural effusions also have been described. The cardiac silhouette is usually enlarged.

Thoracentesis most often reveals a serosanguinous to bloody exudate, although the fluid may be serous. The nucleated cell count ranges from 80–3,700/μl with a lymphocyte predominance averaging 70% of the cells. A neutrophil predominance has not been described and only rare cases of pleural fluid eosinophilia have been reported. Pleural fluid glucose approximates serum glucose, and pleural fluid acidosis has not been observed. The creatinine concentration is high, reflecting the blood creatinine, but the ratio of pleural fluid to serum fluid creatinine is less than 1.0.

Uremic pleurisy remains a diagnosis of exclusion, as no pathognomonic test is available. More common causes of pleural effusions in patients with chronic dialysis must be considered and include congestive heart failure, parapneumonic effusion, and atelectasis. A less frequent but important cause of effusions in this setting is tuberculous pleurisy.

Pleural effusions generally resolve with continued dialysis over several weeks, although the effusions may later recur. Some patients have been reported to progress to a fibrothorax, resulting in severe pulmonary restriction. Despite the abnormal bleeding tendency that exists in patients with renal insufficiency, the reported experience with decortication for uremia-induced fibrothorax has been favorable. Maximum return of pulmonary function has generally occurred 6–8 months after surgery. Decortication has even been performed in patients with an FVC as low as 30% of predicted.

The present patient's chest radiograph showed bilateral pleural opacities that were not free-flowing on decubitus radiographs. The CT scan confirmed that the opacities represented marked pleural fibrosis. He underwent a right decortication with improvement of symptoms.

Clinical Pearls

1. A uremic pleural effusion should be considered the presumptive diagnosis in the chronic dialysis patient when a hemorrhagic, lymphocyte-predominant exudate is found, and alternative diagnoses, particularly tuberculous pleurisy, have been excluded.

2. Patients with uremic pleurisy typically present with fever, cough, chest pain, and a transient pleural rub, although many patients may be asymptomatic.

3. Most uremic pleural effusions resolve with continued dialysis, although severe fibrosing pleuritis with pulmonary restriction that requires decortication develops in some patients.

REFERENCES
1. Berger HW, Rammohan G, Neff MS, et al. Uremic pleural effusion. Ann Intern Med 1975;82:362–364.
2. Galen MA, Steinberg SM, Lowrie EG, et al. Hemorrhagic pleural effusions in patients undergoing chronic hemodialysis. Ann Intern Med 1975;82:359–361.
3. Rodelas R, Rakowski TA, Argy WP, et al. Fibrosing uremic pleuritis during hemodialysis. JAMA 1980;243:2424–2425.
4. Maher JF. Uremic pleuritis. Am J Kidney Dis 1987;10:19–22.

PATIENT 79

A 48-year-old woman with atrial fibrillation and an intrathoracic mass

A 48-year-old woman presented with a 2-week history of left-sided chest pain, weight loss, and shortness of breath. Her past medical history was negative except for a chronic cough and a heavy smoking habit.

Physical Examination: Temperature 36.7°C; pulse 120 and irregular; respirations 25; blood pressure 120/60. General: thin-appearing woman with mild respiratory distress. Eyes: equal pupils. Neck: flat neck veins; no lymphadenopathy. Chest: left basilar dullness with crackles and decreased breath sounds. Cardiac: no murmurs or rubs.

Laboratory Findings: Hct 33%; WBC 10,500/μl; electrolytes and renal indices: normal; albumin 3.1 g/dl. ECG: atrial fibrillation with rapid ventricular response. Chest radiograph: below top. CT scan at the level of the hilum: below bottom.

Question: What etiology of atrial fibrillation is suggested by the CT scan?

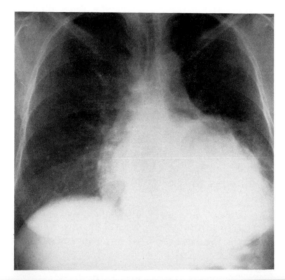

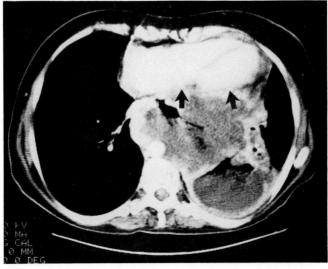

Diagnosis: Cardiac metastases with atrial fibrillation.

Discussion: Metastatic cancer to the heart represents the most common form of cardiac neoplasia, and occurs 10–40 times more often than primary cardiac tumors. Autopsy studies indicate that up to 1.5–20% of patients with underlying cancer have cardiac metastases at the time of death. Recent observations suggest that the incidence of cardiac metastatic disease is increasing with the use of aggressive multimodality cancer therapy that prolongs patient survival and extends the opportunity for cardiac metastases to occur.

Nearly every tumor cell type has been associated with cardiac metastases. Lung cancer, however, is the most commonly found underlying neoplasm followed in frequency by leukemias, lymphomas, and malignant melanomas. Patients with malignant melanoma or leukemias have the highest risk, compared to other cell types, of developing cardiac metastases at some time during the course of their disease, with reported incidences of 50% and 35%, respectively.

Cardiac metastases are classified on the basis of their anatomic location. Commonly involved cardiac sites include the pericardium, cardiac valves, and endocardial surfaces, including intracavitary tumor extension, coronary arteries, and myocardium. Pericardial involvement most commonly causes pericardial effusions with cardiac tamponade but also may produce clinical manifestations of pericardial constriction. Endocardial or valvular metastases rarely occur but when present may cause ventricular outflow obstruction or valvular insufficiency. Intracavitary tumor extension is most often associated with renal cell carcinomas or hepatomas, which may simulate the cardiac manifestations of a right atrial myxoma. Embolization of tumor fragments into coronary arteries may produce myocardial infarction.

Direct metastatic invasion of the myocardium may develop as focal nodular tumors, as occurs with malignant melanomas, or as diffuse infiltrating disease, as observed in patients with leukemia. Access routes to the myocardium include embolization of the coronary arteries, seeding through the vena cavae or lymphatics, and direct extension of pulmonary or mediastinal tumor into adjacent myocardium. Tumors that extend directly into the myocardium also may protrude through the endocardium into the cardiac chambers as polypoid masses.

The antemortem diagnosis of direct myocardial metastases is complicated in that 90% of patients do not have signs or symptoms of cardiac disease. The remainder of patients may have clinical manifestations that are insufficiently unique to suggest the diagnosis. Therefore any patient with an underlying malignancy who presents with a new cardiac disorder should be evaluated for the possibility of myocardial metastases. Common manifestations include arrhythmias, conduction blocks, congestive heart failure, chest pain, and myocardial rupture. Atrial fibrillation and atrial flutter are the most commonly observed arrhythmias, and occur as a result of atrial invasion. The electrocardiogram may show prolonged and pronounced ST-segment elevation in the absence of Q waves over the region of myocardial replacement by tumor infiltration. The chest radiograph may reveal cardiomegaly with or without evidence of primary or metastatic pulmonary or mediastinal tumors.

The echocardiogram in patients with myocardial metastases may detect ventricular hypokinesis, increased thickness of the myocardial septum or free walls, or an intracavitary extension of tumor. MRI or CT may also reveal myocardial tumor invasion. The role of transesophageal echocardiography in patients with myocardial metastases is not yet clearly defined.

Therapy for patients with myocardial tumor invasion is directed at supportive care for hemodynamic stabilization and measures to arrest tumor growth. Radiotherapy and chemotherapy are employed for patients with sensitive tumor cell types. Surgical intervention is more commonly employed for patients with intracavitary tumors who present with ventricular outlet obstruction than for patients with myocardial invasion. Occasional patients with myocardial invasion who have intracavitary extensions and radioresistant tumors, however, may benefit from palliative surgical resection. Regardless of therapy, the prognosis is poor in the presence of myocardial metastases.

The present patient had radiographic evidence of an intrathoracic tumor that appeared on CT scan to compress the posterior aspect of the heart (solid arrows on CT scan, previous page). An echocardiogram demonstrated an intra-atrial tumor mass that extended through the myocardial wall. Bronchoscopic biopsy of left lower lobe endobronchial lesions demonstrated large-cell cancer. After control of the patient's ventricular rate, she began therapy with radiation therapy.

Clinical Pearls

1. Metastatic tumors to the heart are the most common form of cardiac malignancies.

2. Malignant melanomas and leukemias are the tumor cell types most commonly associated with cardiac metastases.

3. Although 1.5–20% of patients with metastatic malignancies have autopsy evidence of cardiac involvement, antemortem diagnosis is complicated by the absence of cardiac symptoms in 90% of patients.

4. Electrocardiographic evidence of pronounced and prolonged ST-segment elevation in patients with an underlying malignancy is highly suggestive of myocardial tumor invasion.

REFERENCES

1. Stark RM, Perloff JK, Glick JH, et al. Clinical recognition and management of cardiac metastatic disease: observations in a unique case of alveolar soft-part sarcoma. Am J Med 1977;63:653–659.
2. Weinberg BA, Conces DJ Jr, Waller BF. Cardiac manifestations of noncardiac tumors. Part II: Direct effects. Clin Cardiol 1989;12:347–354.
3. Tallon JM, Montoya DR. Acute cor pulmonale secondary to metastatic tumor to the heart: a case report and literature review. J Emerg Med 1990;8:721–726.
4. Labib SB, Schick EC Jr, Isner JM. Obstruction of right ventricular outflow tract caused by intracavitary metastatic disease: analysis of 14 cases. J Am Coll Cardiol 1992;19:1664–1668.

PATIENT 80

A 43-year-old woman with dyspnea, cough, and blurred vision

A 43-year-old woman was referred for evaluation of a nonproductive cough and progressive shortness of breath. Three weeks earlier, an urgent-care physician diagnosed "asthmatic bronchitis" and treated her with erythromycin and inhaled albuterol without success. The patient then noted the rapid onset of blurred vision. There was no history of hemoptysis, fever, night sweats, or exposure to tuberculosis.

Physical Examination: Temperature 99.4°; pulse 110; respirations 22; blood pressure 138/62. General: mildly obese; frequent coughing. Lymph nodes: normal. Chest: bibasilar crackles. Abdomen: no hepatosplenomegaly. Rectal: Hemoccult-positive stool. Extremities: no clubbing, cyanosis, or skin lesions. Neurologic: dysconjugate gaze with loss of lateral gaze in the right eye.

Laboratory Findings: Hct 34%; WBC 14,00/μl; erythrocyte sedimentation rate 38 mm/hr. ANA: negative. HIV test: negative. Calcium 9.3 mg/dl; glucose 96 mg/dl; albumin 3.1 g/dl; alkaline phosphatase 430 IU/L; LDH, 535 IU/L; SGOT 63 IU/L. PPD: negative with positive controls. ABG (RA): pH 7.46; PCO_2 33 mmHg; PO_2 65 mmHg. Lumbar puncture: WBC 0 cells; glucose 67 mg/dl; protein 26 mg/dl; India ink negative; cryptococcal antigen negative. Chest radiograph (below left): right unilateral reticular interstitial infiltrates and pleural effusion. Head CT: normal. Chest CT: shown below right.

Question: Consider the differential diagnosis and the next diagnostic test.

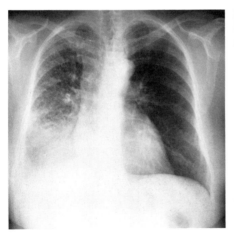 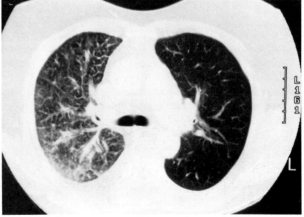

Diagnosis: Lymphangitic carcinomatosis (gastric primary).

Discussion: The combination of a cranial nerve palsy and infiltrative lung disease presents a unique differential diagnosis that includes infectious, malignant, and vasculitic disorders in addition to sarcoidosis. The list of infectious diagnoses is extensive, but the more common disorders that affect the cranial nerves and lung include nocardiosis, tuberculosis, histoplasmosis, cryptococcosis, brucellosis, mucormycosis, rat bite fever, and the meningitides. Vasculitides that should be considered are scleroderma, Sjögren's disease, systemic lupus erythematosus, and Wegener granulomatosis. The malignancies include metastatic carcinoma, lymphoma, and leukemia.

In considering metastatic malignancy, lymphangitic carcinomatosis is the most likely form of the disease to present with diffuse infiltrative lung disease. A relatively unusual pattern of metastasis, lymphangitic carcinomatosis is characterized by malignant infiltration of pulmonary and pleural lymphatics. The most common sites of primary cancer are the stomach, breast, bronchus, pancreas, and prostate. The disorder appears to be more commonly associated with adenocarcinoma than other cell types.

Various mechanisms for tumor spread exist in patients with lymphangitic carcinomatosis. Some pathologic studies suggest that the route of metastasis is primarily hematogenous with secondary involvement of the lymphatic channels. Other investigations support a primarily lymphatic mode of spread with subsequent involvement of the bronchovascular bundle. It also appears that tumor cells can spread through the lymphatics in an antegrade direction toward the hilum or retrograde along obstructed lymphatic channels.

It is often difficult to diagnose lymphangitic carcinomatosis because symptoms referable to the primary neoplasm are often absent. Recognition of the suggestive history and chest radiographic findings can accomplish an early diagnosis, especially when the patient has a known underlying malignancy. The most common symptoms are breathlessness and cough; however, patients may be relatively asymptomatic or develop severe manifestations of subacute, progressive cor pulmonale. Factors contributing to pulmonary hypertension include vascular occlusion by tumor, interstitial fibrosis secondary to a desmoplastic reaction, and interstitial edema due to lymphatic obstruction.

Typical radiographic manifestations of lymphangitic carcinomatosis include reticular densities, Kerley B lines, and subpleural edema. Hilar and mediastinal adenopathy and pleural effusions are frequent additional findings. Notably, the degree of dyspnea may be out of proportion to the radiographic findings in some patients. High-resolution CT shows highly characteristic findings of thickened and beaded interlobular septal lines associated with polygonal structures and prominent peripheral arcades, as seen in the present patient (figure, previous page). Pulmonary function tests usually demonstrate a restrictive defect and a diffusion abnormality. Ventilation-perfusion lung scans have been found, in retrospective analyses, to reveal multiple peripheral defects with normal ventilation.

Although a presumptive diagnosis can be made by the history and radiographic evaluation, cytologic or pathologic specimens are required for confirmation. Cytologic evaluation of bronchial washings, bronchoalveolar lavage samples, transthoracic needle aspirates, and blood aspirated from a pulmonary artery catheter during balloon inflation may establish the diagnosis in some instances. Although the least invasive and most sensitive procedure for diagnosis appears to be transbronchial biopsy, the small sample size and heterogeneity of study groups make it difficult to determine the best diagnostic procedure for patients with lymphangitic carcinomatosis.

Lymphangitic carcinomatosis portends a poor prognosis in most patients. In one study of patients with breast cancer and lymphangitic carcinomatosis, responders to chemotherapy and/or radiation therapy lived 7 months, whereas nonresponders and those not treated lived only 1 month.

The present patient underwent transbronchial biopsies that showed "clusters of cohesive epithelioid cells within the air spaces" thought to be "reactive type II pneumocytes or carcinoma cells." Before a thoracoscopic lung biopsy could be scheduled, the patient's respiratory status worsened, and she expired. An autopsy established the diagnosis of metastatic adenocarcinoma of gastric origin with lymphagitic spread throughout the lung.

Clinical Pearls

1. Malignancy, infectious disease, sarcoidosis, and vasculitis should be considered when a patient presents with infiltrative pulmonary parenchymal disease and cranial nerve palsy.

2. Lymphangitic carcinomatosis is most commonly found with gastric, breast, lung, pancreas, and prostate primaries.

3. Patients with lymphangitic carcinomatosis may present with dyspnea out of proportion to the chest radiographic abnormalities of reticular densities, Kerley B lines, and subpleural edema.

4. The combination of thickened and beaded interlobular septal lines associated with polygonal structures and prominent peripheral arcades on high-resolution CT scan is highly characteristic of lymphangitic carcinomatosis.

5. Lymphangitic carcinomatosis should be considered in the differential diagnosis of illnesses that cause subacute cor pulmonale.

REFERENCES

1. Goldsmith HS, Bailey HD, Callahan EL, Beattie EJ. Pulmonary lymphangitic metastasis from breast carcinoma. Arch Surg 1967;94:483–488.
2. Green N, Kern W, Levis R, et al. Lymphangitic carcinomatosis of the lung: pathologic, diagnostic, and therapeutic considerations. Int J Radiat Oncol Biol Phys 1977;2:149–153.
3. Munk PL, Muller NL, Ostrow DN. Pulmonary lymphatic carcinomatosis: CT and pathologic findings. Radiology 1988;166:705–709.

PATIENT 81

A 30-year-old woman with a portacaval anastomosis and dyspnea, syncope, and hemoptysis

A 30-year-old woman was admitted for evaluation of a history of 2 years of progressive dyspnea on exertion recently complicated by syncope, chest pain, and hemoptysis. Her past history included neonatal omphalitis and portal vein thrombosis, which required portacaval anastomosis at the age of 9 to manage bleeding esophageal varices.

Physical Examination: Pulse 120; respirations 25; blood pressure 102/90. Neck: jugular venous distention with hepatojugular reflux. Chest: clear. Cardiac: right ventricular lift, loud pulmonic second sound, grade 3/6 systolic murmur over the left second intercostal space. Abdomen: no organomegaly. Extremities: mild ankle edema without cyanosis.

Laboratory Findings: Hct 45%. ABG (RA): pH 7.41; $PaCO_2$ 35 mmHg; PaO_2 90 mmHg. ECG: right ventricular hypertrophy. Pulmonary function test results: normal. Radionuclide lung scan: normal. Echocardiogram: dilated right ventricle and atrium. Cardiac catheterization: pulmonary artery pressure 70/30 mmHg; pulmonary capillary wedge pressure 7 mmHg; cardiac output 4.5 L/min. Chest radiograph: shown below.

Questions: What diagnosis is most probable? How would you proceed?

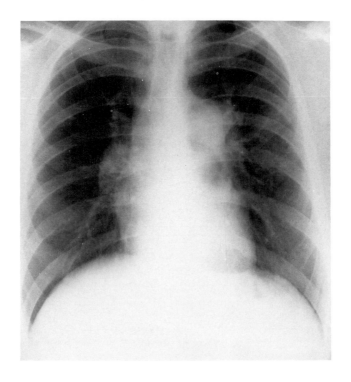

Diagnosis: Primary pulmonary hypertension associated with portal hypertension and portacaval anastomosis.

Discussion: Progressive symptoms of dyspnea on exertion, easy fatigability, substernal chest pain, syncope, and hemoptysis with signs of right-sided cardiac failure are characteristic features of pulmonary hypertension. In the absence of left ventricular dysfunction, congenital heart disease, valvular heart disease, pulmonary parenchymal disorders, and systemic diseases that increase pulmonary vascular resistance, primary pulmonary hypertension becomes a likely clinical diagnosis.

For nearly four decades, there have been numerous reports of an apparent association between primary pulmonary hypertension and increased portal vein pressure. First described in patients with liver cirrhosis, an increased incidence of pulmonary hypertension has also been noted in patients with extrahepatic portal vein obstruction without underlying liver disease. A common feature shared by these patients is the presence of a surgically placed or spontaneous portalsystemic shunt.

The cause of pulmonary hypertension in this setting can only be speculated. Early theories suggested that portal vein thrombosis developed in patients with portal hypertension, becoming a source of thromboembolic disease. In patients with portosystemic anastomoses, clinically occult, recurrent emboli enter the pulmonary circulation, eventually causing extensive vascular occlusion and progressive pulmonary hypertension.

Although reports of pulmonary hypertension in patients with portal vein thrombosis exist, most patients with pulmonary hypertension have not demonstrated clear-cut evidence of intravascular thrombosis in the splanchnic circulation. Furthermore, radionuclide lung scans and pulmonary angiograms have typically failed to identify pulmonary emboli in these patients.

These observations, combined with the absence of major pulmonary thromboemboli in autopsy studies, indicate that portal vein thrombosis with resultant pulmonary emboli is not a major cause of pulmonary hypertension.

Several necropsy series supply useful insight into pathogenetic mechanisms. In the small pulmonary arteries, researchers have found microscopic evidence of medial hypertrophy, concentric intimal proliferation, and plexiform lesions, which are characteristic features of primary pulmonary hypertension. The presence of these vascular abnormalities suggests that the pulmonary circulation is responding to circulating toxic or vasoconstrictive agents from the splanchnic bed that would normally be detoxified by the liver. In the presence of raised portal pressures and portosystemic shunts, these agents bypass the liver and directly contact pulmonary endothelial surfaces, causing cellular injury and deranged vascular anatomy.

At present, there are no experimental data to support this hypothesis. However, the occurrence of cardiac abnormalities in patients with hepatic metastases of serotonin-secreting carcinoid tumors supports the concept that the liver is important in preventing systemic vascular injury from splanchnic toxins. Furthermore, the pulmonary vascular abnormalities that have been observed in patients who ingested toxins, such as the appetite suppressants aminorex and fenfluramine, which were previously available in Europe, indicate that certain dietary substances can damage the pulmonary circulation.

The symptoms of pulmonary hypertension may occur from 2–15 years after the diagnosis of portal hypertension is clearly established, although the two conditions have developed simultaneously in rare instances. The onset of respiratory symptoms may be insidious or surprisingly abrupt.

Mean pulmonary artery pressures range from 25–100 mmHg, and no clinical features separate patients with pulmonary hypertension and portal hypertension from those with pulmonary hypertension and normal portal venous pressures.

The course of this disease varies considerably; death occurs from two months to five years after the diagnosis of pulmonary hypertension has been made. No medical regimen has been noted to significantly improve outcome.

The present patient underwent careful diagnostic evaluation to exclude the presence of any correctable causes of pulmonary hypertension, such as intracardiac left-to-right shunts and pulmonary thromboemboli. In the absence of these disorders, primary pulmonary hypertension was diagnosed and the patient was treated symptomatically.

Clinical Pearls

1. Primary pulmonary hypertension occurs with an increased incidence in patients with portal hypertension and surgical or spontaneous portosystemic shunts.

2. Pulmonary thromboemboli are not a necessary feature of the disorder.

3. Although pathogenetic mechanisms can only be speculated, portosystemic shunts may allow splanchnic toxins to bypass liver metabolism, causing pulmonary vasoconstriction and vascular injury.

REFERENCES

1. Mantz FA, Craige E. Portal axis thrombosis with spontaneous portacaval shunt and resultant cor pulmonale. Arch Pathol 1951;52:92–97.
2. Cohen MD, Rubin W, Taylor WE, et al. Primary pulmonary hypertension: an unusual case associated with extrahepatic portal hypertension. Hepatology 1983;3:588–592.
3. McDonnell PJ, Toye PA, Hutchins GM. Primary pulmonary hypertension and cirrhosis: are they related? Am Rev Respir Dis 1983;127:437–441.
4. Goenka MK, Mehta SK, Malik AK, et al. Fatal pulmonary arterial hypertension complicating noncirrhotic portal fibrosis. Am J Gastroenterol 1992;87:1203–1205.
5. Case records of the Massachusetts General Hospital. Case 25—1992. A 33-year-old woman with cirrhosis and right ventricular failure. N Engl J Med 1992;326:1682–1692.

PATIENT 82

A 26-year-old woman with multiple skin lesions, mediastinal adenopathy, and a right upper lobe infiltrate

A 26-year-old woman presented for evaluation of multiple skin lesions that primarily affected her torso and lower extremities. She had been well until 7 months earlier when she had sustained a splinter in her right palm. Over the next 4 months, multiple skin lesions developed that were biopsied and found to be histologically consistent with vegetative pyoderma gangrenosum. A systemic workup was negative and the patient was begun on prednisone 60 mg daily and intermittent antibiotics with only moderate improvement. The patient denied fevers, chills, productive cough, dyspnea, changes in mental status, and risk factors for HIV infection.

Physical Examination: Vital signs: normal. General: cushingoid. HEENT: normal. Lymph nodes: small left axillary lymph nodes with bilateral inguinal adenopathy. Chest: normal. Skin (shown below left): multiple, vegetative oval plaques with a friable verrucous surface and blackened punctate collections on both thighs, right palm, right shoulder, posterior torso and buttocks; rolled borders at the periphery of the plaques; several plaques with draining gelatinous purulent material.

Laboratory Findings: Hct 43%; WBC 14,300 /μl; platelet count 285,000/μl. Liver function tests: normal. Pregnancy test: negative. Chest radiograph: shown below right.

Questions: What diagnosis could explain the entire clinical presentation? What is the appropriate therapy?

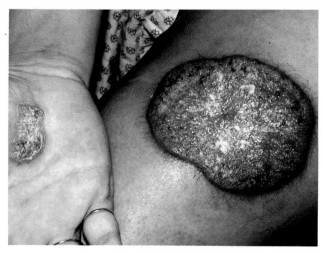
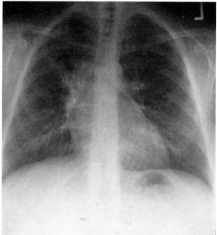

Diagnosis: Disseminated blastomycosis.

Discussion: Blastomycosis is an uncommon but potentially serious infection caused by the thermal dimorphic fungus *Blastomyces dermatitidis*. The spectrum of illness ranges from an asymptomatic self-limited pulmonary disease to rapid fatal dissemination.

Although it is likely that the soil is the source of the fungus, it has been extremely difficult to culture the organism from the environment. The growth of blastomyces may depend on specific conditions of temperature, humidity, and nutrition that have not yet been defined.

B. dermatitidis is co-endemic with histoplasmosis over much of the central United States; however, coastal South Carolina, North Carolina, Virginia, Wisconsin, and northern Minnesota are endemic areas for blastomycosis alone. Direct exposure to an infected site is probably necessary for an infection with *B. dermatitidis* to occur. Therefore, blastomycosis is seen most commonly in rural areas among individuals with outdoor jobs or interests.

There is a male predominance of clinical cases, and half of the reported patients are between the ages of 20 and 50. The portal of entry is always the lung. Microconidia of fungus can be inhaled when a person is exposed to a contaminated site. The initial response to infection is an intense neutrophilia in the lung. A specific cell-mediated immunologic response resulting in a mixed pyogenic and granulomatous reaction occurs within 1–2 weeks.

Acute pulmonary blastomycosis may develop with or without symptoms but symptomatic patients usually experience a self-limited course. Some patients, however, fail to manage the primary infection and progress to a chronic pulmonary form of the disease. Because seeding of distant sites may occur during primary infections, patients with primary infections may present with associated evidence of dissemination to varied tissue sites. Reactivation blastomycosis also may occur. Some patients with reactivated disease present with isolated skin lesions and a normal chest radiograph without recollecting symptoms of a preceding primary pulmonary infection. Such patients further attest to the observation that the initial infection often is asymptomatic or associated with minimal, nonspecific complaints.

When symptomatic, patients with primary blastomycosis may follow a course typical of an acute bacterial pneumonia with fever, pleuritic chest pain, myalgias, and a productive cough. Symptoms usually last less than 2 weeks but radiographic abnormalities may persist for several months. The chest radiographic findings are variable, ranging from a single nodule or unilobar consolidation to diffuse alveolar infiltrates. The chance of reactivation appears highest during the 1–2 years immediately following the primary infection.

Most patients with blastomycosis who seek medical care have already progressed to the more chronic form of the disease. They usually do not recount a history of the preceding acute pneumonia but may report an insidious progression of symptoms. Chronic cough, low-grade fever, night sweats, and weight loss are the primary manifestations. The chest radiograph may show a fibronodular infiltrate with areas of cavitation or a single large perihilar mass suggestive of lung cancer. Dissemination is common in chronic pulmonary blastomycosis, with skin (50%), bone (30%), and the genitourinary tract (20%) being the most common sites. The clinician should consider blastomycosis in any patient who presents with a chronic pulmonary infiltrate and associated disorders in these tissue sites.

Skin disease is common with chronic pulmonary blastomycosis but may occur without evidence of infection elsewhere. Characteristic lesions are raised and crusted with irregular borders. They commonly occur on the face or extremities and have the distinguishing feature of small microabscesses at the periphery of the lesions. Blastomycosis is very uncommon in patients with AIDS, probably because of a lower likelihood of exposure to an infected site while immunocompromised and a small reservoir of patients with remote blastomycosis that could reactivate.

The diagnosis is established by demonstrating the characteristic broad-necked, single-budding yeast in the sputum. The organisms also may be demonstrated in aspirates of skin lesions or prostatic secretions. Gomori methenamine silver and periodic acid–Schiff stains are best for diagnosis in biopsy specimens. Growth of *B. dermatitidis* on primary isolation can take 1–3 weeks or more.

There is no reliable skin test for blastomycosis. The complement-fixation test is not sensitive or specific. An agar gel double-diffusion test has been found to be more helpful in chronic and extrapulmonary infections. A new enzyme immunoassay is more sensitive but less specific than immunodiffusion.

Acute pulmonary blastomycosis does not require specific treatment if the disease is mild and is resolving at the time of diagnosis. Follow-up is indicated because patients may present later with disease at distant sites despite an apparently self-limited primary infection. All patients with moderate or severe primary infection, chronic pulmonary infection, or disseminated disease require treatment. If the patient is not seriously ill and the disease does not involve the meninges, itraconazole may be used for initial treatment. Itraconazole appears to be more potent and less toxic than ketoconazole. Patients with meningeal or other life-threatening disease should be treated with intravenous amphotericin B to a total dose of 2 gm.

The present patient was diagnosed by isolation of fungal elements from the skin lesions. The chest radiograph with a right perihilar mass was typical of the disease. The patient was treated with itraconazole and experienced a full clinical recovery.

Clinical Pearls

1. Direct exposure to an infected site is probably necessary for blastomycosis to occur; therefore, the disease most commonly occurs in rural areas in individuals with outdoor jobs or interests.

2. Many patients with isolated cutaneous blastomycosis have a normal chest radiograph and no recollection of a previous pneumonia. Because the portal of entry is always the lung, the primary infection is often asymptomatic.

3. Dissemination is common in chronic pulmonary blastomycosis, with skin, bone, and the genitourinary tract being the most common sites.

4. Acute pulmonary blastomycosis does not require treatment if the disease is mild or resolving at diagnosis. All patients with moderate or severe primary infection, chronic pulmonary infection, or disseminated disease require treatment.

REFERENCES

1. Laskey WL, Sarosi GA. Endogenous reactivation of blastomycosis. Ann Intern Med 1978;88:50–52.
2. Sarosi GA, Davies SF. Blastomycosis. Eur J Clin Microbiol Infect Dis 1989;8:474–479.
3. Brown LR, Swensen SJ, Van Scoy RE, et al. Roentgenologic features of pulmonary blastomycosis. Mayo Clin Proc 1991;66:29–38.
4. Dismukes WE, Bradsher RW Jr, Cloud GC, et al. Itraconazole therapy for blastomycosis and histoplasmosis. Am J Med 1992;93:489–497.
5. Winer-Muram HT, Beals DH, Cole FH Jr. Blastomycosis of the lung: CT features. Radiology 1992;182:829–832.

PATIENT 83

A 57-year-old man with a sore throat, difficulty swallowing, and stridor

A 57-year-old man was admitted to an Arizona hospital for evaluation of a 10-day history of sore throat, hoarseness, difficulty swallowing, and a cough productive of greenish sputum. He also noted a 20-pound weight loss over the previous several months. His past medical history included a non–Q-wave myocardial infarction and coronary artery bypass graft surgery 2 years earlier. He was a heavy smoker and carried the diagnosis of emphysema.

Physical Examination: Temperature 98.6°; pulse 95; respirations 20; blood pressure 128/75. General: chronically ill appearing; obvious difficulty swallowing. Mouth: drooling; no oral lesions; edentulous. Neck: mild inspiratory stridor; no lymphadenopathy. Chest: hyperresonant to percussion; scattered rales over the posterior upper lung fields. Cardiac: normal heart tones without murmur. Abdomen: scaphoid without organomegaly.

Laboratory Findings: Hct 32.6%; WBC 5,900 with 81% granulocytes, 5% bands, 9% lymphocytes. Electrolytes and renal indices: normal. Serum albumin: 2.3 gm/dl. Sputum examination: greater than 25 granulocytes/hpf with mixed flora on Gram stain; acid-fast smear negative. Chest radiograph: below left. Soft tissue roentgenographic view of the neck: below right.

Question: What diagnosis might explain this patient's symptoms and roentgenographic abnormalities?

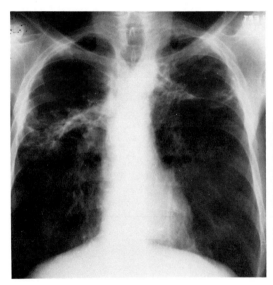
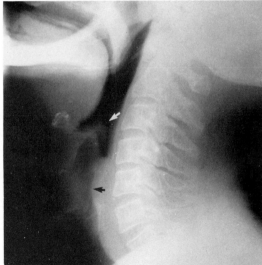

Diagnosis: Disseminated histoplasmosis with laryngeal and chronic cavitary pulmonary infection.

Discussion: Histoplasmosis is a common infection caused by the dimorphic fungus *Histoplasma capsulatum*. In hyperendemic regions along the Mississippi and Ohio river valleys, up to 90% of the population will have skin test reactivity to histoplasmin that documents previous infection. Fortunately, less than 1% of those infected develop serious conditions that require medical management.

H. capsulatum is a thermal dimorphic fungus found in highest concentrations in soil enriched by bird or bat guano. It grows in nature at 24°C as mycelia with microconidia and distinctive tuberculate macroconidia. Disturbance of heavily contaminated soil around starling roosts and within chicken coops and caves promotes aerosolization and inhalation of these conidiospores, which are sufficiently small to penetrate through distal airways to alveolar structures. Once established in tissue at 37°C, the fungus assumes the characteristics of a small (2–4 μm) budding yeast.

The three important clinical forms of histoplasmosis are primary pulmonary infection, chronic cavitary infection, and disseminated disease. Primary pulmonary histoplasmosis develops after inhalation of spores that convert to the yeast phase in the distal alveoli. Establishing an acute pneumonitis characterized by the influx of polymorphonuclear leukocytes followed by monocytes and macrophages, *H. capsulatum* spreads via the lymphatics to the hilar lymph nodes and into the bloodstream. The organisms are phagocytized in the reticuloendothelial system but retain viability, multiplying intracellularly within tissue phagocytes. In most instances, this transient fungemia does not lead to true dissemination but underlies the calcified granulomas frequently detected in livers and spleens of patients from endemic regions.

Although more than 50% of patients with primary pulmonary histoplasmosis remain asymptomatic, symptoms when present usually develop 2 weeks after spore inhalation. Influenza-like manifestations with fever, myalgias, and nonproductive, brassy cough are common clinical features. Patients less commonly develop erythema nodosum, arthralgias, and acute arthritis. Heavy spore exposure or underlying immunocompromise may promote diffuse infiltrates and varying degrees of dyspnea. The typical roentgenographic appearance, however, is that of patchy nonsegmental pulmonary infiltrates with mediastinal adenopathy. Most patients recover spontaneously, although rare long-term complications may develop, such as fibrosing mediastinitis, pericarditis, and broncholithiasis. Patients with severe symptoms or respiratory compromise during the acute pneumonitis may require therapy with amphotericin B.

Chronic cavitary histoplasmosis typically resembles pulmonary tuberculosis with bilateral upper lobe fibronodular infiltrates and cavitation. In contrast to tuberculosis, however, chronic histoplasmosis does not represent reactivation of latent infection but rather progression of primary disease in abnormal lungs. The most common lung abnormality is centrolobular emphysema. Approximately one-third of patients with chronic pulmonary infections progress to widespread fibrosis and lung destruction. Clinical manifestations include night sweats, fever, and weight loss. Patients with chronic cavitary histoplasmosis require therapy with amphotericin B or ketoconazole, with the latter drug reserved for patients with mild to moderate and slowly advancing disease.

Disseminated histoplasmosis can follow a rapidly fatal course in the "infantile" form of the disease characterized by fever, hepatosplenomegaly, and pancytopenia; a more indolent pattern in older adults presents with weight loss, low-grade fevers, and oropharyngeal ulcers. Adults may present with either a nonspecific illness or a localized infection of the meninges, skin, head and neck, or gastrointestinal tract. Tissue biopsies usually demonstrate well-formed granulomas and phagocytized yeast in the adult form of the disease. Diagnosis can be assisted in patients with nonspecific presentations by serologic studies, which are positive in 50% of patients. Rapidly progressive disease, however, requires aggressive evaluative efforts with pathologic examination of multiple tissue biopsy samples.

Patients with HIV infection are at increased risk for disseminated histoplasmosis and have an especially poor prognosis. A granulomatous inflammatory response may not occur, which lowers the probability of an adequate response to antifungal therapy.

Pharyngeal and laryngeal mucosal lesions develop in 40–75% of patients with disseminated histoplasmosis and represent the initial manifestation of disease in 30% of patients who experience a fatal outcome. Lesions appear as painful ulcers with firm, heaped-up margins and typically occur on the tongue, laryngeal structures, and buccal mucosa. In the early stages of infection, verrucous and plaque-like lesions occur that may simulate pharyngeal and laryngeal cancer or tuberculosis. Patients usually present with varying combinations of sore throat, hoarseness, dysphagia, and painful gums.

Diagnosis of mucosal histoplasmosis is promoted by a high clinical suspicion. A swab specimen taken from the center of ulcerative lesions may be submitted for culture and smear. Gomori's methenamine-silver (GMS) and periodic acid–Schiff stains may demonstrate the yeast within macrophages, obviating the need for excisional biopsy. Tissue biopsy specimens typically demonstrate granulomatous inflammation composed of lymphocytes, plasma cells, and multinucleated giant cells. The yeast may be detected by hematoxylin-eosin stains appearing as a stippled background. Tissue fixation may cause retraction of the organism from its cell wall, giving the false appearance of a capsule. Multiple buds with narrow bases are frequently observed and require differentiation from *Candida albicans, Cryptococcus,* and *Torulopsis.*

Once diagnosed, disseminated histoplasmosis requires initiation of antifungal therapy. Immunocompetent hosts with subacute or indolent disease can be treated with ketoconazole for 6–12 months. Immunocompromised patients with AIDS may respond to a total dose of 40 mg/kg of amphotericin B if eventual return of T-cell function occurs. Patients with disseminated histoplasmosis due to AIDS represent a special clinical situation.

Complete eradication of infection with amphotericin B rarely occurs and patients require chronic suppressive therapy. Current guidelines recommend intravenous amphotericin B to a total dose of 1–2 gm followed by life-long suppressive therapy with 50–100 mg of amphotericin B given 2–4 times a month, which is associated with relapse in 20% of patients. Recent studies suggest that maintenance therapy with itraconazole (200 mg bid) has similar and possibly superior efficacy compared to amphotericin B in patient with AIDS.

The present patient presented with fibrocavitary pulmonary infiltrates compatible with histoplasmosis. Soft tissue roentgenographic views of the neck (previous page) showed swelling of the epiglottis (white arrow) and narrowing of the endolarynx below the arytenoid cartilages (black arrow). Biopsy of ulcerative laryngeal lesions demonstrated multinucleated giant cells, granulomas, and tissue necrosis. GMS stains detected numerous yeast-like organisms that subsequently were identified in culture as *Histoplasma capsulatum.* Because the patient tested positive for HIV, he underwent aggressive antifungal therapy with amphotericin B, and gradually improved symptomatically.

Clinical Pearls

1. Unlike pulmonary tuberculosis, chronic cavitary histoplasmosis does not represent reactivation of latent infection but rather progression of primary disease in patients with underlying lung abnormalities.

2. Patients with HIV infection and disseminated histoplasmosis have an especially poor prognosis. Outcome is more favorable if the patient can mount a granulomatous response in infected tissue.

3. Pharyngeal and laryngeal mucosal lesions develop in 40–75% of patients with disseminated histoplasmosis and represent the initial manifestation of disease in 30% of patients who experience a fatal outcome.

4. Mucosal lesions in disseminated histoplasmosis are characteristically painful and appear as ulcerative lesions with firm, heaped-up margins. Although the otolaryngologic examination may suggest laryngeal cancer, the presence of fibronodular pulmonary infiltrates should indicate the possibility of disseminated histoplasmosis.

REFERENCES
1. Pillsbury HC, Sasaki CT. Granulomatous diseases of the larynx. Otolaryngol Clin North Am 1982;15:539–551.
2. Schlech WF, Carden GA. Fungal and parasitic granulomas of the head and neck. Otolaryngol Clin North Am 1982;15:493–513.
3. O'Hara M. Histopathologic diagnosis of fungal diseases. Top Clin Microbiol 1986;7:78–84.
4. Johnson PC, Sarosi GA. Community-acquired fungal pneumonias. Semin Respir Infect 1989;4:56–63.
5. Johnson P, Sarosi G. Current therapy of major fungal diseases of the lung. Infect Dis Clin North Am 1991;5:635–645.
6. Wheat J, Hafner R, Wulfsohn M, et al. Prevention of relapse of histoplasmosis with itraconazole in patients with the acquired immunodeficiency syndrome. Ann Intern Med 1993;18:610–616.

PATIENT 84

A 66-year-old man with fatigue, weakness, and bilateral pleural effusions following laryngectomy

A 66-year-old man with a history of heavy alcohol abuse presented with a 2-month history of increasing weakness, fatigue, and bilateral pleural effusions. Eighteen months earlier, he had undergone total laryngectomy with a left thyroid lobectomy, left modified radical neck dissection, and radiation therapy for squamous cell carcinoma of the left true vocal cord. He denied fever, chills, nausea, vomiting, or diarrhea but did note cold intolerance and pruritus.

Physical Examination: Temperature 97°; pulse 68 and regular; respirations 20; blood pressure 110/70. General: thin; no acute distress. Skin: dry. Lymph nodes: no adenopathy. Chest: decreased breath sounds in the bases bilaterally; scattered rhonchi. Cardiac: distant heart sounds; no gallops or murmurs. Extremities: mild ankle edema.

Laboratory Findings: Hct 35%; WBC 4,800/μl. Electrolytes, renal indices: normal. Albumin: 2.4 g/dl; total protein 5.1 g/dl; LDH 90 IU/L. Thyroid function tests: T4 3.3 μg/dl; T3 45 ng/dl; TSH 211 μU/ml. ABG (RA): pH 7.43; PCO_2 41 mmHg; PO_2 68 mmHg. Chest radiograph (shown below): small bilateral pleural effusions with hyperinflation. Pleural fluid: shown below right.

Question: What is the most likely cause of the patient's bilateral pleural effusions?

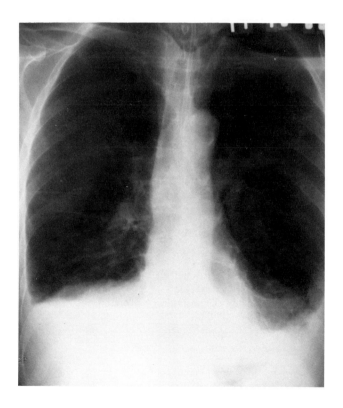

Pleural Fluid Analysis

Appearance: serous

Nucleated cells:
150/μl
14% neutrophils
28% lymphocytes
58% macrophages

Erythrocytes: 1,266/μl

Total protein: 1.5 g/dl

LDH: 34 IU/L

Glucose: 96 mg/dl

Amylase: 14 IU/L

pH: 7.41

Gram stain: negative

Cytology: negative

Diagnosis: Hypothyroid pleural effusion.

Discussion: Hypothyroidism may lead to varied functional derangements in multiple organs. One manifestation that may be particularly preplexing to the clinician is the onset of hypothyroid-related effusions in different body cavities. These effusions may result in ascites, pericardial effusions, middle ear effusions, joint effusions, uveal effusions, and hydrocele in addition to pleural effusions. The presence of the effusions may present a diagnostic challenge because they may precede the onset of more obvious manifestations of hypothyroidism considered more suggestive of the disease.

Pleural effusions were previously considered rare in the setting of hypothyroidism and have not been mentioned often in reports of large patients series with thyroid disease. Recently, however, pleural effusions have been reported with greater frequency associated with hypothyroidism. In one autopsy study of 10 patients with an antemortem diagnosis of myxedema, four had hydrothoraces, all in association with ascites. A recent study of 28 hospitalized patients with hypothyroidism indicated that most pleural effusions were due to other diseases, such as pneumonia or congestive heart failure. Only 1 of the 28 patients had a pleural effusion that was associated with a pericardial effusion; 5 of the 28 patients had pleural effusions attibutable solely to hypothyroidism. The frequency of hypothyroid-related pleural effusions has been underestimated previously because the effusions are usually small and of minor clinical importance. When present, the effusions may be the only serous cavity fluid collection or associated with other effusions such as ascites or pericardial fluid.

Although the pathogenesis of hypothyroid pleural effusions remains poorly defined, several potential explanations have been suggested. The high protein content in hypothyroid-related pleural effusions and the presence of pleural fluid cells that stain positive with periodic acid–Schiff support the possibility that extravasation of hydroscopic mucopolysaccharides into the pleural space occurs. Documentation of increased capillary permeability of the skin in hypothyroidism that resolves with thyroid replacement therapy suggests the possibility of a pleural membrane permeability defect. Additional potential explanations include impaired lymphatic drainage and inappropriate secretion of antidiuretic hormone.

Hypothyroid pleural effusions are typically small, unilateral or bilateral, serous or serosanguinous fluid collections that may be either exudates or transudates. They have low nucleated cell counts with a mononuclear predominance. Reports exist, however, of early neutrophil predominance with subsequent conversion to a lymphocyte predominance. A low pleural fluid glucose and pleural fluid acidosis have not been reported. Patients with hypothyroid pleural effusions are usually asymptomatic from their effusions and require no therapeutic intervention other than thyroid hormone replacement. The presence of these effusions does not appear to be predictable based on the degree of chemical hypothyroidism or clinical signs or symptoms.

The present patient was treated with thyroid replacement with resolution of his pleural effusions over several weeks.

Clinical Pearls

1. Peritoneal, pericardial, middle ear, joint, uveal, and pleural effusions have been described to occur in hypothyroidism. These effusions may precede the more typical manifestations of the disease.

2. Pleural fluid collections in patients with hypothyroidism commonly result from comorbid conditions or occur in association with pericardial effusions; however, pleural effusions may also occur independent of these other conditions.

3. Hypothyroid pleural effusions are typically small, unilateral or bilateral effusions that may be transudates or exudates and have a small number of mononuclear cells.

4. The presence of hypothyroid pleural effusions do not appear to be predictable based on the degree of chemical hypothyroidism or clinical signs or symptoms.

REFERENCES

1. Schneierson SJ, Katz M. Solitary pleural effusion due to myxedema. JAMA 1958;168:1003–1005.
2. Sachdev Y, Hall R. Effusions into body cavities in hypothyroidism. Lancet 1975;1:564–565.
3. Parving H-H, Hansen JM, Nielsen SL, et al. Mechanisms of edema formation in myxedema-increased protein extravasation and relatively slow lymphatic drainage. N Engl J Med 1979;301:460–465.
4. Gottehrer A, Roa J, Stanford GG, et al. Hypothyroidism in pleural effusions. Chest 1990;98:1130–1132.

PATIENT 85

A 73-year-old woman with diffuse infiltrates, anemia, and renal insufficiency

A 73-year-old woman experienced a flu-like illness that progressed to weakness, fatigue, and a nonproductive cough. She was admitted 2 weeks later with severe shortness of breath. She denied cigarette abuse, fevers, hemoptysis, or purulent sputum. Her only medication was hydrochlorothiazide.

Physical Examination: Temperature 100°; pulse 110; respirations 32; blood pressure 125/90. Skin: no lesions. Chest: diffuse crackles with decreased breath sounds throughout. Cardiac: normal heart sounds. Abdomen: normal.

Laboratory Findings: Hct 22%; WBC 15,600/μl with 90% neutrophils, 2% bands. Na^+ 129 mEq/L; Cl^- 92 mEq/L; K^+ 6.7 mEq/L; HCO_3^- 22 mEq/L; BUN 63 mg/dl; creatinine 3.5 mg/dl. ABG (nonrebreather oxygen mask): pH 7.48; PO_2 52 mmHg; PCO_2 32 mmHg. Urinalysis: red cell casts. Chest radiograph (after intubation): shown below.

Hospital Course: The patient required intubation, mechanical ventilation, and hemodialysis for oliguric renal failure. A transbronchial fiberoptic lung biopsy demonstrated alveolar hemorrhage without antibasement membrane fluorescent staining. Two days after admission, the following blood tests results were available: ANA negative; anti-glomerular basement membrane antibody negative; cANCA negative; pANCA positive.

Question: What diagnosis is most likely on the basis of the clinical and laboratory presentation?

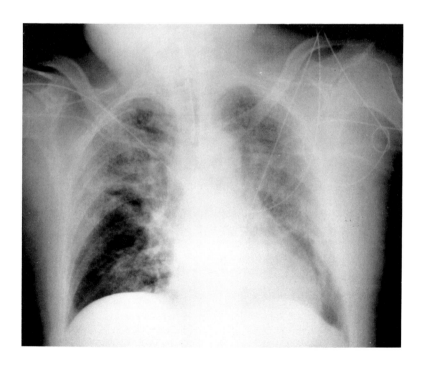

Diagnosis: Pulmonary hemorrhage due to rapidly progressive glomerulonephritis.

Discussion: Patients with primary vasculitides commonly present with diagnostic dilemmas to their physicians because the nonspecific nature of their clinical manifestations often fail to suggest the underlying disorder. Consequently, the time from first presentation to a specific diagnosis may amount to as long as 13 months in some vasculitis-associated disorders, such as Wegener's granulomatosis. Vasculitis classification systems that have relied heavily on the histologic features of vascular inflammation can seem to further complicate diagnosis, in that many patients with normal tissue biopsies are found to have extensive vasculitis after death.

New serologic markers of vasculitis are emerging as a major aid in the diagnosis of patients with suspected vasculitis or patients with ill-defined clinical conditions. Antineutrophilic cytoplasmic antibodies (ANCA) represent a category of antibodies that were first noted in 1982 in a small number of patients with segmental necrotizing glomerulonephritis. Subsequently, some types of ANCA were defined as sensitive and specific markers for Wegener's granulomatosis. Detected by indirect immunofluorescence (IIF) on ethanol-fixed granulocytes, ANCA demonstrate characteristic staining patterns that vary on the basis of the underlying condition.

In patients with Wegener's granulomatosis, the occurrence of a cytoplasmic pattern of staining—termed cANCA—detects antibodies directed against the granular constituents of myeloid cells. The specific antigen determined by enzyme-linked immunoassay (ELISA) testing is proteinase-3 (Pr3), a third serine protease from the primary granules of myeloid cells, which is distinct from the other serine proteases elastase and cathepsin G. A positive IIF for cANCA followed by a positive ELISA for Pr3 is a sensitive and specific marker for Wegener's granulomatosis. Furthermore, some but not all clinical studies indicate that serial titration of cANCA by IIF correlates with disease activity and assists the management of patients with Wegener's granulomatosis. Increasing IIF titers may precede a flare of the underlying vasculitis by several weeks or months, allowing an increase of immunotherapy before clinical signs of an exacerbation occur.

Another pattern of fluorescence staining on ethanol-fixed granulocytes noted by IIF is perinuclear and detects the presence of pANCA. The perinuclear pattern is actually an artifact of the ethanol-fixed cells in that other fixation techniques result in cytoplasmic staining in the presence of pANCA. The specific antigen of importance in patients with pANCA is myeloperoxidase (MPO) in that the presence of anti-MPO antibodies is fairly specific for a necrotizing vasculitis, such as idiopathic necrotizing and crescentic glomerulonephritis with or without systemic vasculitis. Other conditions associated with pANCA due to anti-MPO include microscopic polyarthritis, Churg-Strauss syndrome, polyarteritis nodosa, and polyangiitis overlap syndrome. Anti-MPO has also been detected, however, in patients with antiglomerular basement membrane disease, systemic lupus erythematosus, during the acute or convalescent phase Kawasaki disease, and in 30% of children with recent acute illnesses.

The presence of pANCA that is not associated with anti-MPO is of limited diagnostic value. Associated conditions include ulcerative colitis, autoimmune liver diseases, and rheumatoid arthritis. The pANCA in these conditions appears to be directed against lactoferrin or other myeloid cytoplasmic antigens.

Several important observations can assist the initial interpretation of ANCA IIF tests. The sensitivity of cANCA depends on the extent and activity of Wegener's granulomatosis. In patients with clinical and pathologic manifestations of the disease limited to the respiratory tract, only 50% of patients may be cANCA positive. With increasingly active and widespread disease, 60–100% of patients will have a positive test for cANCA. A negative cANCA test does not exclude Wegener's granulomatosis, although the presence of cANCA in the correct clinical context essentially confirms the diagnosis. A positive pANCA is most often seen in patients without Wegener's granulomatosis but can occur in this disease. Only a small number of patients with Wegener's granulomatosis have anti-MPO, and existing series have not demonstrated the presence of both anti-Pr3 and anti-MPO in any one patient with this disease. The presence of cANCA by IIF is a fairly reliable indicator of anti-Pr3, but a positive pANCA is not specific for anti-MPO.

The present patient had renal failure with red cell casts and diffuse alveolar hemorrhage. Although the absence of fluorescent staining on the lung biopsy may have represented a sampling error, the patient's age, negative anti-GBM antibodies, and negative lung biopsy result made the diagnosis of antibasement membrane disease unlikely. An assay for anti-MPO was positive and the patient was considered to have idiopathic necrotizing glomerulonephritis with systemic vasculitis. She was treated with corticosteroids and cyclophosphamide, which resolved her pulmonary hemorrhage and permitted weaning from mechanical ventilation but failed to improve her renal function.

Clinical Pearls

1. The presence of cANCA due to anti-Pr3 essentially confirms the diagnosis of Wegener's granulomatosis in the correct clinical context.

2. Titers of cANCA correlate with disease activity, rising weeks to months before flares of Wegener's granulomatosis.

3. A positive pANCA by IIF can indicate antibodies against myeloperoxidase (MPO) or other cellular antigens. Anti-MPO is associated with necrotizing vasculitides.

4. The presence of cANCA by IIF is a fairly reliable indicator of anti-Pr3, but a positive pANCA is not specific for anti-MPO.

5. A positive pANCA without anti-MPO is of limited diagnostic value.

REFERENCES

1. Roberts DE. Antineutrophil cytoplasmic autoantibodies. Clin Lab Med 1992;12:85–98.
2. Batsakis JG, El-Naggar AK. Wegener's granulomatosis and antineutrophil cytoplasmic autoantibodies. Ann Otol Rhinol Laryngol 1993;102:906–908.
3. Hagen EC, Ballieux BE, van Es LA, et al. Antineutrophil cytoplasmic autoantibodies: a review of the antigens involved, the assays, and the clinical and possible pathogenetic consequences. Blood 1993;81:1996–2002.
4. Kallenber CGM. Autoantibodies in vasculitis: current perspectives. Clin Exp Rheumatol 1993;11:355–360.

PATIENT 86

A 47-year-old woman with a skin rash, arthralgias, and dyspnea

A 47-year-old woman was referred for the evaluation of dyspnea. One year earlier, she developed hand and shoulder arthralgias followed 6 months later by a skin rash involving her face, thighs, chest, back, and arms. Soon thereafter, she noted dyspnea on exertion. The patient denied Raynaud's phenomenon, dysphagia, skin tightness, or ingestion of tryptophan. She had undergone bilateral subcutaneous mastectomies for fibrocystic disease and implantation of silicone gel-filled breast implants 7 years earlier.

Physical Examination: Vital signs: normal. Skin: sharply demarcated hypopigmented and deep pigmented patches around nasolabial folds and right cheek; hyperpigmented areas on upper thighs, chest, and back. Breasts: firm scarred submuscular implants with nodularity on left. Lymph nodes: no adenopathy. Chest: decreased breath sounds at the bases bilaterally with end-inspiratory crackles.

Laboratory Findings: Hct 36%; WBC 8,100/μl with a normal differential; ESR 60 mm/hr. Rheumatoid factor: negative. ANA: positive at 1:80 (homogeneous). Anti-double-stranded DNA: positive at 1:80. Antibodies to Sm, Scl-70, RNP, SS-A, SS-B antigens: absent. Spirometry: FVC 1.85 L (64% of predicted), FEV$_1$ 1.70 L (77% of predicted), FEV$_1$/FVC 92%. TLC 62% of predicted, D$_L$/VA 95% of predicted. Chest radiographs (below): increased interstitial markings in the bases with pleural thickening.

Question: What possible cause of the patient's symptom complex should be considered?

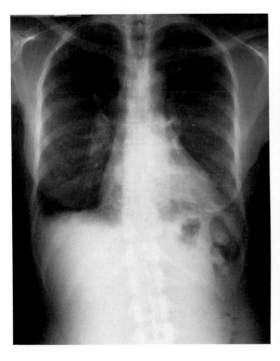
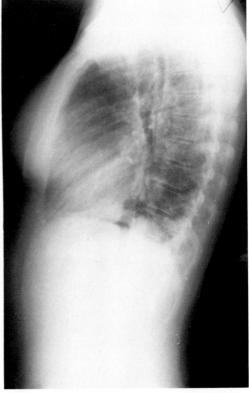

Diagnosis: Connective tissue disease (overlap syndrome of scleroderma and SLE) possibly secondary to silicone-gel breast implants.

Discussion: Since the silicone, gel-filled, elastomeric, envelope-type breast prosthesis was first introduced approximately 30 years ago, nearly 2 million women in the United States have undergone augmentation mammoplasty or breast reconstruction with this device. The Food and Drug Administration has become concerned about the long-term safety of these implants because of case reports of silicone-induced connective tissue diseases.

Emerging studies are beginning to formally investigate the risks of silicone breast implants relative to their potential induction of connective tissue diseases. A preliminary survey failed to reveal a significant increase in the incidence of connective tissue diseases in women with breast augmentation. The sample size of this study was small, however, severely limiting its ability to detect an increased risk. A recent population-based retrospective study examining the risk of a variety of connective tissue diseases and other disorders after breast implantation also found no association. Although 749 women with breast implants were followed for a mean of 7.8 years, the study did not have sufficient power to detect an association between silicone implants and the most rare connective tissue diseases, such as systemic sclerosis. The investigators estimated that a study would require 62,000 women with implants and 124,000 controls to adequately exclude such an association.

At present, therefore, it is reasonable on the basis of the numerous case reports to consider that an association may exist between connective tissue diseases (scleroderma, SLE, mixed connective tissue disease, rheumatoid arthritis, and Sjögren syndrome) and exposure to silicone. This relationship is supported by the demonstration that silicone-containing substances can spread from implants to connective tissue and regional lymph nodes where a foreign body reaction may be elicited. Reports exist of patients with connective tissue disease who have minute deposits of silicone in abnormal tissues affected by autoimmune disease. The silicone may leak through the Silastic envelope of an implant or escape by rupture of the prosthesis. It may also be true that silicone can cause disease by exposure to its various forms, such as silicon dust, Silastic arthroplasties, and silicon injections or implants. The factors that may potentially increase the risk of developing a connective tissue disease after silicone exposure include the host's immunogenetic background, the degree of leakage of silicone from the implant, and the extent of migration of the silicone to distant sites where an inflammatory response might occur.

It should be recognized, however, that detection of silicone within sites of inflammatory connective tissue diseases does not establish causation. The demonstration of silicone within sites of inflammation in association with improvement in symptoms following the removal of the implants and extravasated silicone, however, more strongly suggests a causal link.

In the present patient, a biopsy of the skin lesions was consistent with scleroderma. High-resolution CT of the lungs showed septal thickening with interstitial changes in the bases and minimal pleural thickening. At surgery, a ruptured left implant was found with free silicone in the chest wall. The implants were replaced with saline-filled prostheses. Two weeks after breast implant removal, the arthralgias, dyspnea, and skin manifestations were improved. She was treated with a several-month course of prednisone for continued lung restriction and dyspnea with moderate exertion. Three and a half years following presentation, the patient's overlap syndrome with features of systemic sclerosis and SLE resolved off corticosteroids.

Clinical Pearls

1. Silicone implants have been associated with the development of connective tissue disease in a number of case studies and small series.

2. Data suggest that the derivatives of silicon and silicone-gel can perturb the immune system and cause a human adjuvant disease.

3. The presence of silicone-containing material within sites of connective tissue disease supports a role for silicone in the pathogenesis of such conditions.

4. All patients with connective tissue disease should be questioned about exposure to various forms of silicone.

REFERENCES

1. Kumagai Y, Shiokaya Y, Medsger TA Jr. Clinical spectrum of connective tissue disease after cosmetic surgery: observations on 18 patients and a review of the Japanese literature. Arthritis Rheum 1984;27:1–12.
2. Varga J, Schumacher HR, Jimenes SA. Systemic sclerosis after augmentation mammoplasty with silicone implants. Ann Intern Med 1989;111:337–383.
3. Bridges AJ, Conley C, Wang G, et al. A clinical and immunologic evaluation of women with silicone breast implants in symptoms of rheumatic disease. Ann Intern Med 1993;118:929–936.
4. Silver RM, Sahn EE, Allen JA, et al. Demonstration of silicone in sites of connective-tissue disease in patients with silicon-gel breast implants. Arch Dermatol 1993;129:63–68.
5. Gabriel SE, O'Fallon M, Kurland LT, et al. Risk of connective-tissue diseases and other disorders after breast implantation. N Engl J Med 1994;330:1697–1702.

PATIENT 87

A 42-year-old woman with severe dyspnea, myalgias, and eosinophilia

A 42-year-old woman presented with severe respiratory distress that culminated a several-month illness. Previously well, she first noted a flu-like illness with body aches and fever 3 months earlier. The fever remitted but myalgias, fatigue, and weakness persisted. One week before admission she noticed a nonproductive cough and progressive shortness of breath. Her only medications were doxepin and diazepam; she had taken L-tryptophan for 1 month but had discontinued this agent 3 months earlier.

Physical Examination: Temperature 98.9°; pulse 128; respirations 30; blood pressure 160/98. General: marked respiratory distress. Skin: normal. Chest: bilateral crackles at bases. Cardiac: normal. Neurologic: normal.

Laboratory Findings: Hct 38%; WBC 18,000/μl with 55% neutrophils, 2% bands, 20% eosinophils, 23% mononuclear cells. Electrolytes and renal indices: normal. Urinalysis: normal. ABG (5 L O_2 nasal cannula): pH 7.40; PCO_2 45 mmHg; PO_2 46 mmHg. Chest radiograph (after intubation and Swan-Ganz catheter placement): shown below.

Question: What is the probable cause of the hypoxic, hypercapnic respiratory failure, and pulmonary infiltrates?

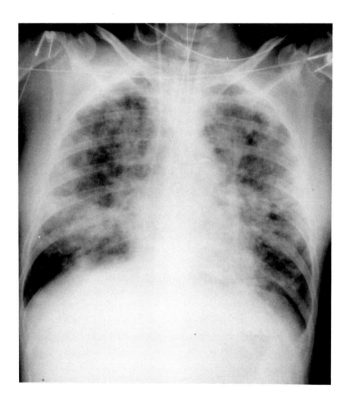

Diagnosis: Acute respiratory failure from L-tryptophan pulmonary toxicity.

Discussion: Pulmonary toxicity from ingestion of L-tryptophan-containing products was first described in 1988. The profound systemic manifestations of the disorder characterized most notably by severe myalgias and marked peripheral eosinophilia promoted the designation of this entity as eosinophilia-myalgia syndrome (EMS). It is presently estimated that more than 1,000 persons are affected by this condition in the United States despite removal of L-tryptophan-containing products from the market.

Although the Centers for Disease Control defines EMS by the occurrence of severe myalgias associated with a peripheral eosinophil count greater than $1000/\mu l$ in the absence of an infection or neoplasm that could explain these findings, the clinical manifestations of EMS are diverse. Either soon after initiation of therapy with L-tryptophan products or long after its discontinuation, patients experience a flu-like prodrome that progresses over several weeks to include variable combinations of symptoms. Myalgias are an important but inconsistent manifestation of the disease and may be intense and incapacitating. Respiratory complaints are common and patients also may experience rashes, weight gain, edema, fever, and encephalopathy.

Despite discontinuation of L-tryptophan, patients may progress to a chronic stage and experience weight loss, severe muscular weakness, muscle cramps, peripheral neuropathies, dry eyes, scleroderma-like skin changes, chronic fatigue, and hair loss. The physical examination is often relatively benign, although muscle tenderness, rashes and scleroderma-like skin changes, hepatomegaly without splenomegaly, extremity edema, and chest crackles may be found.

Nearly all patients with EMS will have some symptom related to the lungs ranging from mild dyspnea and cough to acute respiratory failure. Reports exist of pulmonary hypertension, interstitial lung disease, hypercapnic respiratory failure due to muscular weakness, and severe hypoxemia with ARDS occurring after ingestion of L-tryptophan. Pleuritic chest pain associated with pleural effusions has also been described.

All patients with EMS have striking peripheral eosinophilia ranging from $2000/\mu l$ to as high as $36,000/\mu l$, although eosinophil counts may normalize during the chronic stage of the disease. Bone marrow biopsies may also demonstrate proliferation of eosinophils and eosinophil precursors. Mild to moderate elevation of liver function tests (asparate aminotransferase, alanine aminotransferase, and γ-glutamyltransferase) commonly occurs. A distinctive pattern in a patient with EMS is an elevation of serum aldolase and a normal or minimally increased CPK. Muscle biopsies may show evidence of eosinophilic perimyositis or perivascular and interstitial inflammatory infiltrates with rare eosinophils.

Lung biopsies in patients with EMS and parenchymal lung disease demonstrate a unique form of nongranulomatous small-vessel vasculitis without alveolitis or evidence of tissue necrosis. Interstitial pneumonitis, interstitial fibrosis, and perivascular infiltrates of histiocytes, lymphocytes, eosinophils, and rare neutrophils may be found. One report indicated that proximal arteries may contain mural thrombi. Bronchiolitis obliterans with organizing pneumonia (BOOP) has also been described related to L-tryptophan ingestion.

The chest radiograph in EMS depends on the clinical presentation. Patients with minimal or no chest complaints may have a normal chest radiograph. Up to 16% of all patients, however, will have interstitial infiltrates and 15% will have pleural effusions. The radiographic appearance of ARDS may be apparent in patients with severe hypoxic respiratory failure.

Once the diagnosis is considered, therapy for EMS begins with discontinuance of L-tryptophan. The acute vasculitic phase of the condition may be responsive to corticosteroid therapy, as suggested by a sharp drop in eosinophil count, improvement in symptoms or radiographic infiltrates, and case reports of recurrence of respiratory symptoms after completion of corticosteroid therapy. The specific role of corticosteroid therapy, however, remains incompletely defined. Most patients in the chronic phase of the disease may not remit despite stopping L-tryptophan agents and initiating corticosteroids.

The present patient appeared to have EMS on the basis of her symptoms of myalgia, eosinophilia, and ingestion of L-tryptophan. Her respiratory failure was thought to be due to a combination of muscular weakness and ARDS caused by L-tryptophan toxicity. She underwent a thoracoscopic lung biopsy that demonstrated the characteristic pathologic features of EMS. She was treated with a course of corticosteroids that improved her pulmonary function and allowed extubation. The other symptoms of EMS, however, persisted and progressed.

Clinical Pearls

1. Although eosinophil-myalgia syndrome is defined by myalgias and peripheral eosinophilia greater than 1000/μl, the clinical manifestations are protean.

2. Respiratory failure may occur from muscular weakness or pulmonary parenchymal toxicity with a small vessel vasculitis.

3. A characteristic laboratory feature of EMS is a moderate elevation of serum aldolase with a normal or minimally increased CPK in a patient with disabling myalgias.

4. Because ARDS may occur with minimal accompanying symptoms of EMS, a history of L-tryptophan ingestion should be sought in any instance of acute respiratory failure of obscure etiology.

REFERENCES

1. Banner AS, Borochovitz D. Acute respiratory failure caused by pulmonary vasculitis after L-tryptophan ingestion. Am Rev Respir Dis 1991;143:661–664.
2. Philen RM, Eidson M, Kilbourne EM, et al. Eosinophilia-myalgia syndrome: a clinical case series of 21 patients. Arch Intern Med 1991;151:533–537.
3. Campagna AC, Blanc PD, Criswell LA, et al. Pulmonary manifestations of the eosinophilia-myalgia syndrome associated with tryptophan ingestion. Chest 1992;101:1274–1281.
4. Read CA, Clauw D, Weir C, et al. Dyspnea and pulmonary function in the L-tryptophan-associated eosinophilia-myalgia syndrome. Chest 1992;101:1282–1286.

PATIENT 88

A 78-year-old man with prostatic carcinoma and bilateral pleural effusions

A 78-year-old man presented with the insidious onset of dyspnea on exertion and a nonproductive cough. He denied hemoptysis, chest pain, decreased appetite, orthopnea, or nocturnal dyspnea. Eighteen months earlier, he had undergone a prostatectomy followed by a course of pelvic radiation for carcinoma of the prostate. The patient had a long smoking history but had discontinued this habit 3 years before admission.

Physical Examination: Temperature 98°; pulse 100 and regular; respirations 24; blood pressure 110/75. Chest: distant breath sounds; dullness to percussion and decreased fremitus at both bases. Cardiac: no jugular venous distention; no gallops; grade 2 systolic ejection murmur at the upper left sternal border. Abdomen: soft, nontender without evidence of ascites. Extremities: 2+ pretibial and ankle edema.

Laboratory Findings: Hct 28%; WBC 9,700/μl. Calcium 9.0 mg/dl; phosphorus 4.9 mg/dl; alkaline phosphatase 150 IU/L; LDH 180 IU/L; albumin 3.0 g/dl; total protein 6.8 g/dl; BUN 48 mg/dl; creatinine 2.7 mg/dl. ABG (RA): pH 7.41; PCO_2 37 mmHg; PO_2 66 mmHg. Chest radiograph (shown below left): small cardiac silhouette; enlarged central pulmonary arteries; evidence of emphysema, small bilateral effusions. High-resolution CT scan: no evidence of lymphangitic carcinomatosis or mediastinal adenopathy. Pleural fluid: shown below right.

Question: What is the most likely cause of the patient's bilateral transudative pleural effusions?

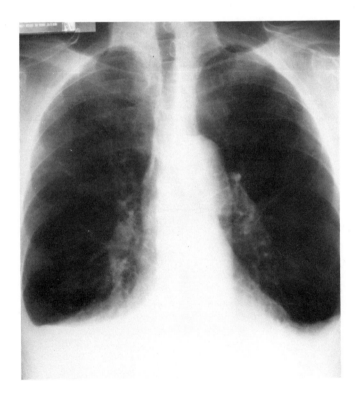

Pleural Fluid Analysis

Appearance: serous

Nucleated cells: 1050/μl

Differential:
  65% lymphocytes
  25% macrophages
  10% neutrophils

Erythrocytes: 850/μl

Total protein: 2.8 g/dl

LDH: 70 IU/L

Glucose: 90 mg/dl

Amylase: 40 IU/L

pH: 7.37

Cytology: positive

Diagnosis: Prostatic carcinoma metastatic to the pleura.

Discussion: Prostatic carcinoma follows lung and colon cancer as the third leading cause of cancer-related deaths in men. Between 12% and 46% of men over the age of 50 have evidence of prostatic carcinoma in postmortem studies. Furthermore, prostatic carcinoma frequently metastasizes, with the most common metastatic sites being lymph nodes and bone followed by the lungs and liver. Up to 5% of patients have pulmonary metastases on initial presentation. As the disease progresses to a more advanced stage, the incidence of pulmonary metastases increases to 25%. Pleuropulmonary metastases are found at autopsy in 25–50% of patients with prostatic carcinoma. Most of these lesions, however, appear as microscopic deposits and did not contribute to antemortem symptoms or radiographic findings. In a recent series of 603 patients with disseminated and treated prostate cancer, only 14 (2%) were found to have antemortem lung or pleural metastases.

An isolated pleural effusion without accompanying lymphangitic carcinomatosis or mediastinal lymph node metastases, as seen in the present patient, is an uncommon manifestation of prostatic carcinoma. The most common pattern of intrathoracic involvement in prostate metastases is pulmonary nodules followed by mediastinal lymphadenopathy, lymphangitic carcinomatosis, isolated pleural effusion, and microscopic tumor emboli.

The finding of a pleural effusion in a patient with a known malignancy is an ominous sign and predicts incurability in lung cancer and a worse prognosis compared to those without effusions in all types of malignancies. Patients with pleural effusions due to prostatic carcinoma, however, may be more likely to have resolution of effusions with chemotherapy than patients with other types of cancer.

The pathogenesis of pleural involvement appears to be pulmonary vascular invasion, embolization to the visceral pleural surface, exfoliation into the pleural space, and attachment to the dependent portion of the parietal pleura and the diaphragm.

Tumor cells may move across preformed or tumor-induced adhesions to attach to the parietal pleura. Although most patients with pleural metastasis from extrathoracic tumors have the liver as a secondary metastatic intermediary, this pattern of progression is not universally found.

The present patient had the unusual combination of a transudative malignant effusion with adenocarcinoma cells that stained positive for prostatic specific antigen (PSA), a glycoprotein produced only by normal and neoplastic prostate cells. Considered a sensitive and specific marker of prostatic carcinoma, a positive PSA stain in a metastatic site establishes the prostate as the primary site of cancer.

A malignant effusion is usually exudative with a protein concentration of about 4 g/dl with a reported range of 1.5–8 g/dl. The high range of protein concentrations occur almost solely in multiple myeloma or Waldenström macroglobulinemia. It is often overlooked that 2–19% of malignant pleural effusions are transudates. In a compilation of several series totaling 307 patients with malignant pleural effusions, 24 (7.8%) were transudates. Malignant transudates most commonly result from congestive heart failure, atelectasis from bronchial obstruction, or the early stages of mediastinal node metastases with lymphatic obstruction concomitant with exfoliation of malignant cells into the pleural space. Other causes of transudative effusions occurring coincident with an underlying malignancy, such as severe hypoalbuminemia, pulmonary embolism without infarction, and superior vena cava syndrome, also may account for a transudative pleural effusion in cancer patients. Exudative pleural effusions resulting from lymphatic obstruction require several weeks to develop.

The present patient received chemotherapy with partial resolution of pleural effusions and improvement in symptoms. He died 11 months after the diagnosis of malignant pleural effusions, and 17 months following the diagnosis of prostate cancer.

Clinical Pearls

1. At postmortem examination, microscopic pleuropulmonary metastases are found in 25% to 50% of patients with prostatic cancer. Most of these lesions did not cause antemortem symptoms.

2. Pleuropulmonary metastases may rarely be the initial manifestation of metastatic prostate carcinoma.

3. Transudative malignant pleural effusions account for $< 10\%$ of malignant effusions. They are most commonly associated with congestive heart failure, atelectasis from bronchial obstruction, and the early stages of mediastinal lymph node involvement.

4. A positive PSA stain of pleural fluid cells establishes the prostate as the primary site of cancer.

REFERENCES

1. Varkarakis MJ, Winterberger AR, Moore RH, et al. Lung metastases in prostatic carcinoma: clinical significance. Urology 1974;3:447–452.
2. Heffner JE, Duffey D, Schwarz MI. Massive pleural effusions from prostatic lymphangitic carcinomatosis: resolution with endocrine therapy. Arch Intern Med 1982;142:375–376.
3. Apple JS, Paulson DF, Baber C, et al. Advanced prostatic carcinoma: pulmonary manifestations. Radiology 1985;154:601–604.
4. Crawford ED, Eisenberger MA, McLeod DG, et al. A controlled trial of leuprolide with and without flutamide in prostatic carcinoma. N Engl J Med 1989;321:419–424.
5. Mestitz H, Pierce RJ, Holmes PW. Intrathoracic manifestations of disseminated prostatic adenocarcinoma. Respir Med 1989;83:161–166.
6. Carrascosa M, Perez-Castrillon JL, Mendez MA, et al. Malignant pleural effusion from prostatic adenocarcinoma resolved with hormonal therapy. Chest 1994;105:1577–1578.

PATIENT 89

A 52-year-old man with massive hemoptysis after coronary artery grafting

A 52-year-old man presented with chest pain diagnosed as an acute anterior myocardial infarction. Despite aggressive management, he experienced dyspnea and recurrent pain 2 days later. A Swan-Ganz catheter revealed a pulmonary artery occlusion pressure of 22 mmHg and a cardiac index of 2.2 L/min/m². Coronary arteriography demonstrated multiple high-grade obstructions. The patient underwent a three-vessel saphenous vein coronary artery bypass procedure successfully but developed massive bleeding through the endotracheal tube as he was being moved from the operating table to a gurney.

Physical Examination: Intubated patient with active bleeding through the endotracheal tube.

Laboratory Findings: Preoperative laboratory studies: normal. Preoperative chest radiograph with Swan-Ganz catheter in place: shown below.

Questions: What is a likely cause of the patient's airway hemorrhage? What immediate course of action is indicated?

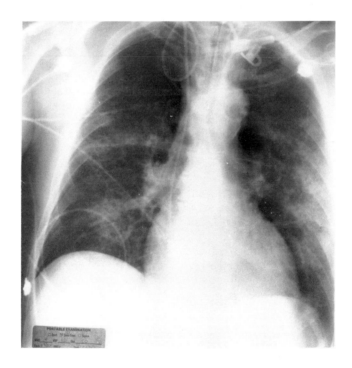

Diagnosis: Pulmonary artery perforation by a Swan-Ganz catheter.

Discussion: Perforation of a pulmonary artery is fortunately a rare complication of Swan-Ganz catheterization. In the ICU setting, risk factors for vascular perforation include advanced patient age (possibly due to fragile less elastic vessels), distal catheter migration, and balloon overinflation in an overly distal catheter tip position.

Catheter-induced pulmonary artery perforation is a distinct entity when it occurs in a patient undergoing cardiopulmonary bypass. It is estimated that vascular perforation occurs in 0.05–0.2% of bypass patients who have a pulmonary artery catheter in place. Several factors contribute to its pathogenesis. During decompression and manipulation of the heart, traction on the intra-cardiac portion of the catheter can cause a to-and-fro motion and perforate distal small pulmonary vessels. Furthermore, hypothermia during cardioplegia can stiffen the catheter, increasing the likelihood of vascular injury. Women are at increased risk for this injury apparently because of their relatively diminutive pulmonary vascular anatomy and lower tolerance for catheter motion.

Bypass-related pulmonary artery perforation may manifest as mild hemoptysis or major hemorrhage into the airway or pleural space. Bleeding is usually first evident during reinitiation of pulmonary artery flow as patients are being removed from cardiopulmonary bypass. Bleeding may be delayed, however, first developing after return to the ICU. Because catheter-induced injury also may create pulmonary artery dissections and false aneurysms, massive hemoptysis may also occur several days after surgery. The mortality of pulmonary artery perforation during cardiopulmonary bypass has been reported to be as high as 40% in some clinical series.

The immediate goals of managing a patient with catheter-induced pulmonary artery perforation is to maintain the airway and control the hemorrhage. If hemoptysis occurs before the patient leaves the operating room, cardiopulmonary bypass should be continued or reinstituted to allow surgical intervention. Patients who do not undergo surgical repair experience recurrence later, with life-threatening hemoptysis in 45% of instances. Reinitiation of cardiopulmonary bypass should control the hemorrhage as pulmonary artery pressures decrease. Possible interventions include vascular repair, which is commonly not possible because the perforation is usually intralobar. Lobectomy may be necessary but many patients may not be able to undergo this procedure because of diminished pulmonary reserve. Recent reports exist of placing a vascular loop that may be released later in the ICU after healing of the perforation occurs.

When hemoptysis first occurs in the ICU after return from the operating room, the severity of the bleeding and the patient's clinical stability are carefully assessed. Although patients with massive and unremitting hemoptysis may require emergency lobectomy, less severe degrees of hemorrhage may respond to angiography with vascular embolization therapy.

To prevent vascular injury, many surgeons avoid Swan-Ganz catheters in patients undergoing cardiopulmonary bypass surgery. If a catheter is thought to be necessary, it can be pulled back during surgery and refloated at the termination of the procedure.

The present patient continued to bleed through the endotracheal tube and required reinstitution of cardiopulmonary bypass. A right-sided proximal pulmonary artery perforation at a bifurcation of the vessel was located and repaired. Airway hemorrhage did not recur during the subsequent weaning from bypass, and the patient recovered without further complications.

Clinical Pearls

1. Pulmonary artery perforation by a Swan-Ganz catheter is a rare complication of cardiopulmonary bypass procedures, occurring in 0.05%–0.2% of patients.

2. Factors contributing to perforation include cardiac manipulation with resultant movement of the catheter tip and induced hypothermia, which decreases catheter pliability.

3. Airway hemorrhage related to vascular perforation usually occurs during weaning of cardiopulmonary bypass. Hemorrhage may be delayed in the presence of pulmonary artery dissection or false aneurysm formation.

4. Detection of pulmonary artery hemorrhage in the operating room requires reinitiation of cardiopulmonary bypass to allow surgical intervention. Patients with transient hemorrhage returned to the ICU without surgical intervention experience recurrence of life-threatening hemoptysis in 45% of instances.

REFERENCES

1. Connors JP, Sandza JG, Shaw RC, et al. Lobar pulmonary hemorrhage: an unusual complication of Swan-Ganz catheterization. Arch Surg 1980;115:883–885.
2. Barash PG, Nardi D, Hammond G, et al. Catheter-induced pulmonary artery perforation: mechanisms, management, and modifications. J Thorac Cardiovasc Surg 1981;82:5–12.
3. Fleischer AG, Tyers GFO, Manning GT, Nelems B. Management of massive hemoptysis secondary to catheter-induced perforation of the pulmonary artery during cardiopulmonary bypass. Chest 1989;95:1340–1341.
4. Urschel JD, Myerowitz PD. Catheter-induced pulmonary artery rupture in the setting of cardiopulmonary bypass. Ann Thorac Surg 1993;56:585–589.

PATIENT 90

A 77-year-old woman with a recurrent right-sided pleural effusion

A 77-year-old obese woman was referred because of a recurrent right-sided pleural effusion. Six months earlier, she noted the onset of dyspnea with exertion, fatigue, and a nonproductive cough. A local physician performed several diagnostic and therapeutic thoracenteses that revealed a serous transudate with negative cytology. Percutaneous pleural biopsy specimens showed no signs of malignancy or tuberculosis. An echocardiogram revealed an ejection fraction of 60% and no wall motion abnormalities.

Physical Examination: Temperature 99°; pulse 100; respirations 24; blood pressure 160/80. Chest: dullness to percussion and decreased fremitus at the right lung base. Cardiac: no jugular venous distention; heart sounds normal without gallops or murmurs. Abdomen: obese; no organomegaly or ascites. Extremities: bilateral pitting edema.

Laboratory Findings: Hct 33%; WBC 4,700/μl with a normal differential; ESR 24 mm/hr; PT 13.9 sec; PTT 31.2 sec; BUN 11 mg/dl; creatinine 0.9 mg/dl; AST 18 IU/L; alkaline phosphatase 222 IU/L; LDH 110 U/L; bilirubin 1.4 mg/dl; albumin 2.4 g/dl; amylase 14 IU/L; total protein 6.2 g/dl. Hepatitis B serology, ceruloplasmin, alpha-l-antitrypsin and antimitochondrial antibodies: normal or negative. Urinalysis negative. Chest radiograph: shown below left. Pleural fluid: results shown below right.

Questions: What is the most likely cause of the recurrent pleural effusion? What should be the next step to establish the diagnosis? What is the recommended therapy?

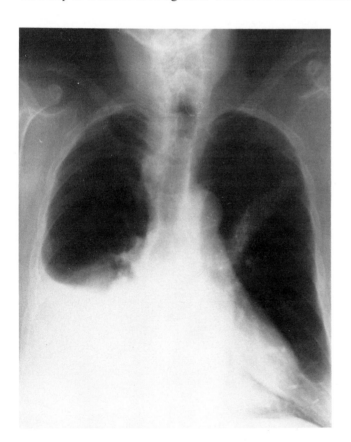

Pleural Fluid Analysis

Appearance: serous

Nucleated cell count: 149/μl
   87% macrophages

RBC: 30/μl

Total protein: 2.8 gm/dl

LDH: 63 IU/L

Amylase: 10 IU/L

pH: 7.48

Glucose: 120 mg/dl

Gram stain and culture: negative

Cytology: negative

Diagnosis: Hepatic hydrothorax without clinical ascites.

Discussion: Pleural effusions may accumulate in up to 10% of patients with cirrhosis of the liver and clinical ascites. Termed "hepatic hydrothorax," this condition appears to result from the movement of peritoneal fluid across the diaphragm through small diaphragmatic defects. These diaphragmatic defects, usually less than a centimeter in diameter, can easily be overlooked even at postmortem examination without the use of dyes or air bubble techniques. The higher pressure within the peritoneal space relative to the pleural cavity promotes a cephalad transfer of fluid. Occasionally, the diaphragmatic defect may be sufficiently large to allow a portion of the peritoneum to herniate into the chest, forming a peritoneal bleb. When the bleb ruptures, a rapid transfer of fluid occurs with the resulting sudden onset of respiratory symptoms.

The patient with hepatic hydrothorax usually has the physical stigmata of cirrhosis and clinically apparent ascites. Several reports have documented, however, that large to massive pleural effusions may occur due to liver disease in the absence of clinically demonstrable ascites, as was observed in the present patient. Many patients have only a small pleural effusion and experience dyspnea limited to exertion. Larger pleural effusions may cause more severe dyspnea, orthopnea, and nonproductive cough.

Asymptomatic pleural effusions may be commonly noted on routine chest radiographs in patients with ascites. The usual chest radiograph shows a normal cardiac silhouette and a right-sided effusion that may vary from small to massive. Effusions are isolated to the left pleural space in about 15% of patients and are bilateral in 15%. Thoracentesis typically shows a serous transudate with a low nucleated cell count and a predominance of mononuclear cells, pH > 7.40, a glucose similar to serum, and a low pleural fluid amylase. The fluid can be serosanguinous due to the underlying coagulopathy or the rupture of a pleural bleb but is never grossly bloody in the absence of another disease.

Pleural and ascitic fluids have similar characteristics so that a presumptive diagnosis can be established by a comparison of simultaneous thoracentesis and paracentesis results. The protein and LDH may be slightly higher in pleural fluid because increased portal pressure prevents the reabsorption of nonprotein-containing fluid by the peritoneum. Injection of a radiolabeled tracer into the ascitic fluid with detection on chest imaging within an hour supports a pleuroperitoneal communication through a diaphragmatic defect. Recently, the use of ultrafast gradient echo MR imaging and intraperitoneal contrast enhancement has confirmed hepatic hydrothorax and localized the diaphragmatic defect. In comparison with scintigraphy, MR offers a higher anatomic resolution of the diaphragm and adjacent peritoneal and pleural cavities with enhanced ability to localize the diaphragmatic defect.

Patients with hepatic hydrothorax without clinical ascites present with pulmonary symptoms and usually experience delayed diagnosis. A history of previous abdominal surgery often is obtained and radiographic imaging studies may or may not reveal minimal ascites.

Initial therapy should include a therapeutic thoracentesis, conservative management with fluid and sodium restriction, and diuretic therapy. Chest tube drainage is relatively contraindicated because it can lead to protein, fluid, and electrolyte depletion and iatrogenic empyema. Chemical pleurodesis is problematic because the pleural fluid rapidly recurs before pleural symphysis occurs. The use of a peritoneovenous shunt requires a substantial amount of ascites for success. The definitive procedure is thoracotomy with repair of the diaphragmatic defect and mechanical pleural abrasion; the substantial mortality of this procedure in this patient population limits its application.

The present patient had a CT scan that demonstrated a large right pleural effusion, a small liver with evidence of enlarged collateral veins, splenomegaly, and ascites principally on the right side of the abdomen. There was no evidence of mediastinal adenopathy or pulmonary lesions. She was treated with conservative methods with relief of symptoms and partial resolution of the pleural effusion.

Clinical Pearls

1. Hepatic hydrothorax may occur in the absence of clinical ascites.

2. Patients with hepatic hydrothorax in the absence of clinical ascites usually present with pulmonary symptoms and a large right pleural effusion. A history of previous abdominal surgery often is obtained.

3. Chest tube drainage is contraindicated because of the risks of iatrogenic empyema, and protein, electrolyte, and volume depletion.

4. Chemical pleurodesis is problematic due to the rapid reaccumulation of pleural fluid. Repair of the diaphragmatic defect with chemical abrasion may be successful but carries a high operative risk in these patients.

REFERENCES

1. Lieberman FL, Hidemura R, Peters RL, et al. Pathogenesis and treatment of hydrothorax complicating cirrhosis with ascites. Ann Intern Med 1966;64:341–351.
2. Singer JA, Kaplan M, Katz RL. Cirrhotic pleural effusion in the absence of ascites. Gastroenterology 1977;73:575–577.
3. Hartz RS, Bomalaski J, LoCicero J III, et al. Pleural ascites without abdominal fluid: surgical considerations. J Thorac Cardiovasc Surg 1984;87:141–143.
4. Runyon BA, Greenblatt M, Ming RHC. Hepatic hydrothorax as a relative contraindication to chest tube insertion. Am J Gastroenterol 1986;81:566–567.
5. Urhahn R, Gunther RW. Transdiaphragmatic leakage of ascites in cirrhotic patients: evaluation with ultrafast gradient echo MR imaging and intraperitoneal contrast enhancement. Magn Reson Imaging 1993;11:1067–1070.

PATIENT 91

A 54-year-old man with hyperpyrexia and respiratory failure

A 54-year-old man was admitted to the ICU after collapsing at a Fourth of July picnic. He had appeared in good health but began to talk strangely to friends during the late innings of a softball game. After improving in the dugout, he collapsed suddenly while chasing a fly ball in the outfield. Paramedics found him cyanotic and hypotensive with sinus tachycardia and transported him after intubation to the hospital.

Physical Examination: Temperature 41°; pulse 120; respirations 22; blood pressure 90/60. General: unconscious. Skin: warm and dry. Chest: diffuse rales. Cardiac: normal heart sounds. Neurologic: no focal findings.

Laboratory Findings: Hct 43%; WBC 14,000/μl with normal differential. Na^+148 mEq/L; K^+ 5.6 mEq/L; Cl^- 110 mEq/L; HCO_3^- 15 mEq/L; BUN 32 mg/dl; creatinine 1.2 mg/dl. SGOT 1,100 IU/L; CPK 8,700 IU/L. ABG (100% FiO_2, volume ventilator); PCO_2 31 mmHg; pH 7.31; PO_2 58 mmHg. ECG: sinus tachycardia, generalized ischemia. Chest radiograph: shown below.

Questions: What is the cause of the patient's collapse and respiratory failure? What measures should be initiated immediately?

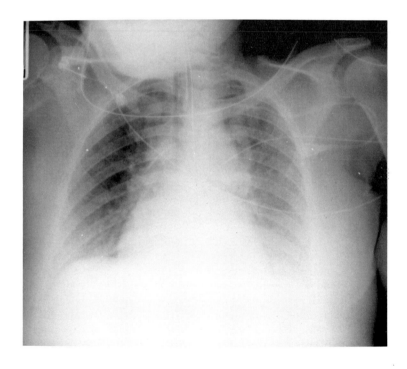

Diagnosis: Heatstroke with ARDS.

Discussion: Heatstroke is an environmental illness with a mortality greater than 25% that occurs when the homeostatic thermoregulatory mechanisms of the body are unable to meet the load of heat stress. Defined by a core temperature $> 41°C$ ($> 106°F$), unrelieved hyperpyrexia may progress to diffuse tissue destruction and eventual multiorgan failure.

Two general categories of heatstroke exist: classic heat stroke, which occurs in patients with failed thermoregulatory mechanisms passively exposed to high ambient temperatures, and exertional heatstroke, which occurs in previously healthy patients exercising vigorously in hot environments. The two forms differ in some ways in their clinical manifestations but share similar fundamental pathogenetic mechanisms.

To understand how heatstroke develops, one should consider that the body is constantly subject to sources of heat gain and dependent on physical methods of heat loss. Heat gain occurs through normal metabolism and exposure to high surrounding temperatures. Metabolic sources of heat are augmented by febrile conditions, physical exertion, and metabolic disorders, such as hyperthyroidism and pheochromocytoma. Heat dissipation occurs through radiation, convection, and evaporation. At moderate ambient temperatures, radiation of electromagnetic waves accounts for 65% of the body's heat loss with lesser contributions from the convective heat transfer by the air and water vapor molecules circulating around the body. As ambient temperatures increase above $35°C$ ($95°F$), cooling through evaporation of sweat becomes the major mechanism of heat dissipation, and radiation begins to become a source of net heat gain. As the ambient heat increases in settings of high humidity ($> 75%$), evaporative mechanisms of heat dissipation become less efficient.

Once body temperature begins to increase, additional regulatory mechanisms come into play. Cardiac output increases, cutaneous vasodilatation occurs, and circulating blood volume shunts away from visceral organs and toward the skin, promoting greater heat loss through evaporative cooling.

Multiple circumstances exist wherein thermoregulatory mechanisms may be impeded and heatstroke produced. Tight occlusive clothing or cutaneous disorders, such as scleroderma, interfere with heat loss through sweating. Furthermore, drugs such as anticholinergics (atropine, antiparkinsonian drugs, phenothiazines, tricyclic antidepressants, and antihistamines) impede sweating and salicylates uncouple oxidative phosphorylation and produce hyperthermia. Dehydration with hypernatremia increases the work of the cellular sodium-potassium ATPase pump, which can account for 20–45% of basal metabolic rate. Cardiac dysfunction can limit redistribution of an augmented cardiac output of blood volume toward the skin for enhanced body cooling. Sedatives and neuroleptic agents may interfere with thirst recognition, including dehydration that interferes with heat transfer to the skin. Finally, patients with obesity, fatigue, lack of sleep, or alcoholism are at increased risk.

Patients with heatstroke present with a rapid onset of disease in 80% of instances. Patients with classic heat stroke are usually elderly with comorbid disease and demonstrate the classic triad of hyperthermia, neurologic dysfunction, and anhidrosis with hot flushed skin. The absence of sweating may result from swelling of sweat gland ducts due to chronic exposure to salt and water. Patients with exertional heatstroke typically experience sudden collapse during or soon after vigorous exercise in a hot environment. A brief period of altered mental status or bizarre behavior may occur. Exertional heatstroke is most common in poorly conditioned adults or in those not acclimatized to hot suroundings.

Once established, heatstroke may progress rapidly (as fast as an egg can fry) to diffuse tissue injury and multiorgan failure. Manifestations of hepatic insufficiency occur in all patients with various abnormalities of liver function tests. An increased concentration of SGOT is such a uniform finding that an SGOT concentration less than 1,000 IU/L should suggest that clinically important hyperthermia is not present. Rhabdomyolysis is more likely to occur in patients with exertional heatstroke and is a major cause of renal insufficiency. Alterations in mental status rapidly progress to coma, and disseminated intravascular coagulation is a common and potentially life-threatening occurrence.

The adult respiratory distress syndrome (ARDS) has been a poorly recognized complication of heatstroke. Heatstroke does not appear on the list of causes of ARDS in most clinical reviews of respiratory failure and ARDS is not mentioned in most discussions of heatstroke. Episodes of hypoxemia in these patients have usually been ascribed to cardiogenic pulmonary edema, pulmonary hemorrhage, thromboembolic disease, or atelectasis. A recent series of patients with heatstroke undergoing Swan-Ganz catheterization, however, indicates that up to 25% of patients experience severe noncardiogenic pulmonary edema. As a historical note, Osler in 1896 describes the lungs of patients dying of heatstroke as "intensely congested."

Management of heatstroke requires an immediate response of measures to support hemodynamics, manage complications, and rapidly cool core temperatures. Survival does not appear to correlate with the severity of hyperthermia but does relate to the duration that hyperthermia persists. The goal of cooling is to decrease body temperature to less than 39°C (102°F) within 30 minutes of presentation. Cooling can begin in the field by dousing of the patient with water and fanning of the skin to promote evaporative cooling. Once in the emergency department, immersion in ice water is the preferred treatment because water has a 32-fold greater thermal conductivity compared to air. Adequate cooling may occur within 10–40 minutes as monitored with rectal or esophageal temperature probes. Recent studies suggest that equally rapid cooling may occur with immersion in water baths with temperatures of 15°–16°C (59°–61°F). Critically ill patients unable to be immersed in a bath may be unclothed, doused with water, fanned, and laterally packed with ice. Acetaminophen as an antipyretic is ineffective in this clinical setting and should be avoided because of the risks of compounding the hepatic injury.

The present patient presented with the clinical manifestations of exertional heatstroke complicated by hepatic injury, pulmonary edema, rhabdomyolysis, and coma. A Swan-Ganz catheter demonstrated a cardiac index of 5.5 L/min/m^2 and a pulmonary artery occlusion pressure of 10 mmHg. Despite rapid cooling from partial immersion in an iced bed-bath, he progressed to DIC and renal failure and died 10 days later, never regaining consciousness.

Clinical Pearls

1. Heatstroke occurs in a "classic" form in elderly debilitated patients and in an "exertional" form in vigorously exercising, previously healthy individuals.

2. Rhabdomyolysis is more common in patients with exertional compared to classic heatstroke; patients with rhabdomyolysis progress to myoglobinuric renal failure in 25% of instances.

3. ARDS appears to occur in up to 25% of patients with heatstroke.

4. A core temperature on admission less than 41°C does not exclude heatstroke because some cooling may have occurred during transport to the hospital.

REFERENCES

1. El-Kassimi FA, Al-Mashhadani S, Abdullah AK, Akhtar J. Adult respiratory distress syndrome and disseminated intravascular coagulation complicating heat stroke. Chest 1986;90:571–574.
2. Yarbrough BE, Hubbard RW. Heat-related illnesses. In Auerbach PS, Geeher EC (eds): Management of Wilderness and Environmental Emergencies, 2nd edition. St. Louis, Mosby, 1989, pp 119–143.
3. Hassanein T, Razack A, Gavaler JS, Van Thiel DH. Heatstroke: its clinical and pathological presentation, with particular attention to the liver. Am J Gastroenterol 1992;87:1382–1389.
4. Dahmash NS, Al Harthi SS, Akhtar J. Invasive evaluation of patients with heat stroke. Chest 1993;103:1210–1214.

PATIENT 92

A 68-year-old woman with 3 weeks of dyspnea

A 68-year-old previously healthy woman presented with a 3-week history of progressive dyspnea on exertion. Her tuberculin status was unknown, and she had a 30-pack-year history of cigarette smoking. There was no history of alcohol abuse.

Physical Examination: Temperature 99°; pulse 96; respirations 24; blood pressure 140/80. General: healthy appearing. Chest: dullness to percussion and decreased fremitus at both lung bases. Cardiac: no jugular venous distention, gallops or murmurs. Abdomen: soft without organomegaly. Extremities: no cyanosis, clubbing, or edema.

Laboratory Findings: Hct 42%; WBC 5,300/μl with a normal differential. Electrolytes and renal indices: normal. Total protein 6.6 g/dl; amylase 120 IU/L; LDH 120 IU/L. PPD: 10-mm induration. ABG (RA): pH 7.43; PCO_2 37 mmHg; PO_2 73 mmHg. Chest radiograph (shown below left): bilateral pleural effusion, right greater than left, normal cardiac silhouette, no parenchymal infiltrates. ECG: nonspecific ST and T wave changes. Pleural fluid (right thoracentesis): shown below right.

Questions: What is the most likely cause of the patient's bilateral pleural effusions? What chemical test would further support your clinical impression?

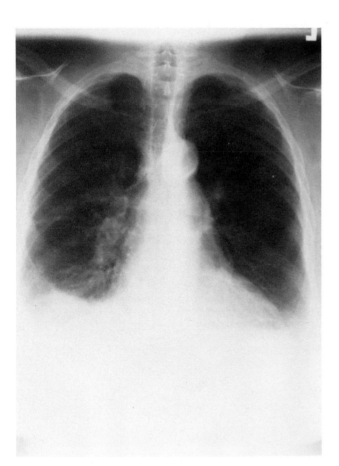

Pleural Fluid Analysis

Appearance: serous

Nucleated cells: 1,785/μl

Differential:
   43% macrophages
   49% lymphocytes
   8% neutrophils

RBC: 1,500/μl

Total protein: 3.8 gm/dl

LDH: 68 IU/L

Glucose: 114 mg/dl

pH: 7.32

Amylase: 150 IU/L

Gram stain and culture: negative

Diagnosis: Adenocarcinoma of the lung with pleural metastasis and an amylase-rich pleural effusion.

Discussion: Exudative pleural effusions present the clinician with an extensive differential diagnosis. Detecting an elevated amylase content in the pleural fluid substantially narrows the diagnostic possibilities. Defined as a pleural fluid amylase concentration that is above the upper limits of normal for serum or a pleural fluid/serum amylase ratio greater than 1, "amylase-rich" pleural effusions are primarily limited to patients with pancreatic disease, esophageal rupture, and malignancy. Less common causes of amylase-rich effusions include ruptured ectopic pregnancies, pneumonia, pulmonary tuberculosis, cirrhosis, and hydronephrosis. Considering all patients presenting with pleural effusions, up to 6–13% will be amylase-rich.

Considering the pancreatic disorders, both acute pancreatitis and pancreatic pseudocysts may produce amylase-rich pleural effusions. Effusions associated with pancreatic pseudocysts have a sustantially higher amylase level—often reaching levels above 100,000 IU/L—than those found in acute pancreatitis. Amylase-rich effusions associated with any type of pancreatic disorder have higher absolute amylase values and pleural fluid/serum amylase ratios than other causes of effusions associated with increased amylase concentrations. In a recent series, patients with pancreatic disease had a pleural fluid/serum amylase ratio approaching 20, whereas those with nonpancreatic diseases had a pleural fluid/serum amylase ratio of about 5. In patients with amylase-rich malignant effusions, the average pleural fluid to serum amylase ratio approximates 10, with the majority of patients having values less than 25.

Serum isoenzyme determination has proved useful in the differential diagnosis of hyperamylasemic states. In pancreatitis, the major isoenzyme isolated from the serum is the pancreatic type, which is almost solely produced by the pancreas. The specificity of this isoenzyme for the pancreas is attested by its observed rise in acute pancreatitis, fall in chronic pancreatic insufficiency, and disappearance after pancreatic ablation. A high concentration of pancreatic isoenzyme in the serum is virtually diagnostic of pancreatitis. A recent series has confirmed that an amylase-rich pleural effusion that contains predominantly pancreatic isoenzyme is specific for a pancreatic pleural effusion. In contrast, when amylase-rich pleural effusions contain predominantly a salivary isoenzyme, the most likely diagnosis is malignancy.

Amylase-rich pleural effusions are found in 10–15% of patients with malignancies, and the content of the salivary isoenzyme is usually greater than 90% of total amylase content. The most common malignancies associated with elevated amylase concentrations are adenocarcinomas of the lung and ovary, in that order. Other cancers metastatic to the pleura, however, have been associated with increased salivary isoamylase content, such as lymphomas and chronic lymphocytic leukemia.

The mechanism for increased amylase content in malignant pleural effusions is incompletely defined. It appears based on available data, however, that salivary amylase is secreted ectopically by tumors into the pleural space. Electron-dense granules suggestive of zymogen granules have been detected by electron microscopic study of malignant cells from pleural effusions. Pleural fluid amylase has been found to decrease following chemotherapy.

Amylase determination for exudative pleural effusions of uncertain etiology should be done routinely, as it can provide the first evidence of a malignant pleural process. When esophageal perforation is not a consideration, finding an amylase-rich effusion that is salivary in origin is highly suggestive of malignancy, most commonly lung cancer. Furthermore, a salivary isoamylase-rich effusion will help differentiate adenocarcinoma of the pleura from mesothelioma, as a mesothelioma that secretes amylase has not been reported.

The present patient had a pleural fluid amylase greater than the upper limit of normal for serum and a pleural fluid/serum amylase ratio of 1.25. Isoenzyme electrophoresis revealed 95% salivary amylase content. The pleural fluid cytology was positive for adenocarcinoma and chest CT showed a solitary peripheral lesion in the right lung compatible with an adenocarcinoma of the lung. A subsequent biopsy specimen confirmed the diagnosis of lung cancer.

Clinical Pearls

1. Finding an amylase-rich pleural effusion narrows the differential diagnosis toward pancreatic disease, esophageal rupture, and malignancy, although other less common causes of amylase-rich pleural effusions exist.

2. Pancreatic isoenzyme prominence in pleural fluid is specific for the diagnosis of pancreatic associated pleural effusion, while salivary isoenzyme suggests malignancy in the absence of esophageal rupture.

3. Up to 10–15% of patients with malignancies will have an amylase-rich pleural effusion.

4. Lung cancer is the most common cause of a nonpancreatic amylase-rich pleural effusion.

REFERENCES

1. Light RW, Ball WC Jr. Glucose and amylase in pleural effusions. JAMA 1973;225:257–260.
2. Buckler H, Honeybourne D. Raised pleural fluid amylase level as an aid in the diagnosis of the adenocarcinoma of the lung. Br J Clin Pract 1984;38:359–361 and 371.
3. Kramer MR, Saldana MJ, Cepero RJ, et al. High amylase levels in neoplasm-related pleural effusions. Ann Intern Med 1989;110:567–569.
4. Devuyst O, Lambert M, Scheiff JM, et al. High amylase activity in pleural fluid and primary bronchogenic carcinoma. Eur Respir J 1990;3:1217–1220.
5. Joseph J, Viney S, Beck P, et al. A prospective study of amylase-rich pleural effusions with special reference to amylase isoenzyme analysis. Chest 1992;102:1455–1459.

PATIENT 93

A 72-year-old woman with respiratory failure after extubation

A 72-year-old woman with multiple myeloma presented with acute left lower quadrant abdominal pain and positive peritoneal findings. An emergency laparotomy revealed uncomplicated diverticulitis that did not require colonic resection. The patient was transferred to the ICU where she was intubated, mechanically ventilated, and treated with intravenous fluids and antibiotics. Six hours later, she underwent extubation and immediately developed intense inspiratory stridor and severe dyspnea that required reintubation.

Physical Examination: Vital signs: normal. General: oral endotracheal tube in place; breathing with the mechanical ventilator. Neck: normal. Chest: clear. Cardiac: grade II/VI systolic murmur.

Laboratory Findings: Hct 38%; WBC 13,500/μl. Electrolytes: normal. Chest radiograph: shown below.

Question: What potential causes exist for the patient's postextubation respiratory failure?

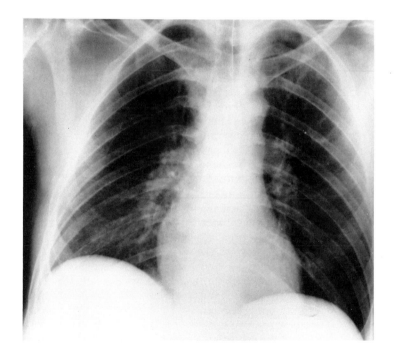

Diagnosis: Upper airway obstruction secondary to laryngeal edema.

Discussion: The sudden or progressive onset of respiratory failure within minutes or hours after tracheal extubation should prompt consideration of upper airway obstruction secondary to laryngeal injury. Damage to laryngeal structures may occur even after short periods of translaryngeal intubation in patients who undergo a seemingly uncomplicated airway placement procedure. The resultant narrowing of the laryngeal lumen remains clinically occult until after extubation when patients present with upper airway obstruction and varying degrees of respiratory compromise.

Although postextubation airway obstruction may result from throat packs, dentures, retained secretions, blood clots, or tissue swelling at surgical sites adjacent to the upper airway, patients should be evaluated for laryngeal causes of obstruction. These conditions include dislocation of arytenoid structures, laryngospasm, laryngeal edema, and bilateral vocal cord paralysis.

Dislocation of arytenoid structures can occur during complicated or uncomplicated intubations. After extubation, symptoms may be limited to painful swallowing or changes in voice quality. If both arytenoids are dislocated to a paramedian position, however, patients may experience glottic obstruction and respiratory failure. Patients with inspiratory stridor require early reintubation with subsequent examination of the upper airway. Early reduction may be possible by application of gentle pressure with a laryngeal spatula. Some patients may require prolonged intubation or a tracheotomy to enable healing of the dislocated joint.

Laryngospasm produces glottic occlusion with varying degrees of airway obstruction from sustained contraction of the intrinsic laryngeal muscles. The obstruction results variably from adduction of the true vocal cords, spasm of the arytenoepiglottic folds and false cords, or even spasm of the extrinsic laryngeal musculature. Probably emanating from a protective reflex mediated by the vagus nerves to prevent aspiration, laryngospasm is the most common cause of upper airway obstruction after tracheal extubation, occurring to some degree in 20% of children—and a smaller proportion of adults—undergoing tonsillectomy. The occurrence of laryngospasm may relate to local irritation of glottis secretions, vomitus, or blood, repeated intubation attempts, or the depth of anesthesia at the time of extubation.

Patients with laryngospasm awakening from anesthesia may benefit from positive-pressure face-mask breathing in the "sniff" position and an increased depth of anesthesia until spasm of the laryngeal musculature abates. The laryngeal structures should be visualized immediately to exclude other causes of airway obstruction. Some patients may require reintubation with the assistance of neuromuscular blocking agents with delayed extubation. Intravenous atropine has not been found to be of value, and intravenous lidocaine has provided variable benefit. Patients may improve with spraying 4% lidocaine directly on the laryngeal structures.

Laryngeal edema presents the greatest risk for airway obstruction in children and neonates undergoing extubation because of the small intrinsic caliber of their airways. The edema is localized either to the supraglottic, retroarytenoid, or subglottic regions. Patients with mild instances of laryngeal edema may be approached with a warmed and humidified inhaled gas mixture. Nebulized epinephrine may provide transient relief. Patients with respiratory compromise may require reintubation with a smaller caliber endotracheal tube. Corticosteroids to accelerate resolution of the edema are not of proven value.

Vocal cord paralysis is an interesting and rare complication of translaryngeal intubation. The anterior branches of the recurrent laryngeal nerves lie beneath the endolaryngeal mucosa in a location medial to the lamina of the thyroid cartilage where they are susceptible to compression by the endotracheal tube. Bilateral nerve injury results in bilateral vocal cord paralysis, which leaves the cords in an adducted position, thereby obstructing inspiration. Patients with complete paralysis require reintubation with subsequent tracheostomy until recovery of delayed cord function occurs, which is usually complete without residual defects.

The present patient underwent fiberoptic laryngoscopy, which demonstrated severe laryngeal edema possibly aggravated by her low serum oncotic pressure. Her chest radiograph showed no other cause of respiratory compromise. She failed a second extubation attempt several days later and required a tracheotomy. The tracheotomy was removed 2 weeks later and the patient fully recovered.

Clinical Pearls

1. Postextubation respiratory failure should prompt evaluation of the larynx for intubation-related damage.

2. Laryngospasm is the most common cause of postextubation airway obstruction and occurs most frequently in children undergoing tonsillectomy.

3. An endotracheal tube may injure the recurrent laryngeal nerves in the endolarynx, causing bilateral vocal cord paralysis and upper airway obstruction.

4. Dislocation of the arytenoids may occur even during uncomplicated intubations. Reduction is often successful with gentle pressure on the arytenoids using a laryngeal spatula.

REFERENCES

1. Rex MAE. A review of the structural and functional basis of laryngospasm and a discussion of the nerve pathways involved in the reflex and its clinical significance in man and animals. Br J Anaesth 1970;42:891–898.
2. Blanc VF, Tremblay NAG. The complications of tracheal intubation: a new classification with a review of the literature. Anesth Analg 1974;53:202–213.
3. Gibbin KP, Egginton MJ. Bilateral vocal cord paralysis following endotracheal intubation. Br J Anaesth 1981;53:1091–1092.
4. Hartley M, Vaughan RS. Problems associated with tracheal extubation. Br J Anaesth 1993;71:561–568.

PATIENT 94

A 44-year-old white woman with positive sputum cultures
for *Mycobacterium abscessus*

A 44-year-old white woman without a smoking history presented with a 5-year history of fever, cough, hemoptysis, and chest pain. At the outset of her symptoms, a chest radiograph showed a lingular infiltrate and sputum smears, and cultures were positive for *Mycobacterium avium-intracellulare* (MAC). She was treated with isoniazid, rifampin, and ethambutol. After 12 months of therapy, her symptoms improved, the infiltrate resolved, her sputum smear became negative for acid-fast bacilli, and sputum cultures were negative for MAC but positive for *Mycobacterium abscessus*. She completed 2 years of antituberculous therapy, becoming completely asymptomatic, but *M. abscessus* continued to be cultured from her sputum. The patient denied esophageal disease, alcohol consumption, or known risk factors for HIV infection.

Physical Examination: Vital signs: normal. General: healthy appearing. Chest: normal breath sounds without adventitious sounds. Cardiac: normal. Abdomen: normal. Extremities: normal.

Laboratory Findings: Hct 38%; WBC 5,700/μl; ESR 15 mm/hr. FVC 3.38 L (97% of predicted), FEV_1 2.73 L (101% of predicted), FEV_1/FVC ratio 81%. Chest radiographs (below): linear densities in the lingula (arrow); no pleural disease or adenopathy.

Question: How should this patient be managed?

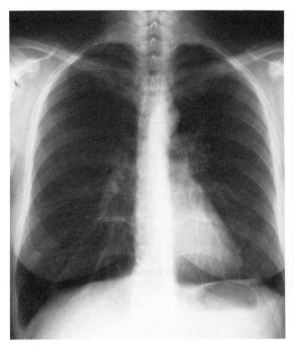
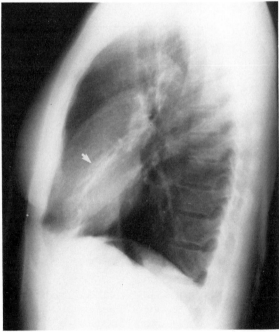

Diagnosis: Lung infection with *Mycobacteria abscessus.*

Discussion: The major pathogens in group IV of the Runyon classification of acid-fast bacilli (AFB) are the rapidly growing bacteria *Mycobacterium fortuitum* and *M. abscessus* (previously classified as *M. chelonei*, subspecies *M. abscessus*). Only in the last few decades have these organisms been recognized as human pathogens. Their pathogenicity had previously gone unnoticed because of the low incidence and insidious nature of lung infections caused by these organisms. Furthermore, group IV AFB present a radiographic appearance distinct from *M. tuberculosis* and often escape microbiologic isolation because of their greater susceptibility to sputum AFB concentration and decontamination procedures. Also, a lack of standard criteria for diagnosing the disease and the belief that single or multiple positive sputum cultures for these pathogens may be present in the absence of disease have further delayed the recognition of these pathogens as causing clinically important pulmonary infections. It is now understood, however, that rapidly growing mycobacteria cause lung disease that shares many of the clinical features with MAC infections.

Pulmonary disease from rapidly growing mycobacteria is primarily seen in the southern coastal states, with the majority of isolates being due to *M. abscessus* (80%), followed by *M. fortuitum* (15%). Rapidly growing mycobacteria and MAC have been isolated from the same patients, either simultaneously or sequentially, thereby suggesting a common host susceptibility for these pathogens.

The long interval from symptom onset to isolation of rapidly growing mycobacteria is the most striking feature of disease. The average time from onset of symptoms to initial isolation of rapidly growing mycobacterium is 26 months with an upper limit of 15 years in large patient series. The typical patient is middle-aged or older, female, nonsmoking, and Caucasian, although anyone is at risk for the disease. HIV infection has not appeared to be a risk factor. Cough is invariably the presenting symptom. Sputum production and constitutional symptoms become more prominent with disease progression. Hemoptysis infrequently occurs, and patients rarely present with asymptomatic radiographic abnormalities. Associated underlying disorders include esophageal dismotility with chronic vomiting, cystic fibrosis, previous granulomatous disease, lipoid pneumonia, rheumatoid arthritis, COPD, lung cancer, and bronchiectasis. Coexisting bronchiectasis, however, may be more a result than a cause of the mycobacterial infection.

The characteristic chest radiograph shows bilateral, multilobar, patchy interstitial or alveolar infiltrates. Although all lobes may be involved, the upper lobes are the most common sites for infection. Infiltrates may resolve or progress independent of the course of the clinical symptoms. In patients with prior pulmonary disease from other mycobacterial species, infiltrates due to subsequent infections by rapidly growing mycobacteria invariably occur in previously involved lung parenchyma.

Patients who have repetitive isolation from sputum of rapidly growing mycobacteria should be considered to have lung disease. Usually all expectorated sputum cultures submitted to the laboratory before the initiation of therapy are positive. Specimens obtained from invasive procedures, such as bronchoscopy, are invariably positive in patients with positive expectorated sputum cultures. Skepticism about the diagnosis is warranted when only a single positive sputum is found in the absence of clinically apparent disease.

Recent reports recommend the following algorithm for diagnosing lung infection in patients with sputum cultures positive for *M. abscessus.* Patients with a normal chest radiograph and single positive sputum culture should be followed with repeat chest radiographs and sputum cultures if a second sputum culture is negative. If a repeat sputum culture is positive, a chest CT should be performed. Drug therapy guided by in vitro drug susceptibility testing is indicated if the CT scan demonstrates pulmonary parenchymal abnormalities. If the CT scan is negative, continued observation is warranted.

Patients with an abnormal initial chest radiograph and a sputum culture positive for *M. abscessus* should undergo repeat sputum cultures. If the repeat sputum culture is positive, the patient is a candidate for therapy, which may include symptomatic management, drug therapy, or surgery. A negative repeat sputum cutlure should be repeated again, and if still negative, the patient should undergo bronchoscopy and careful follow-up as long as sputum specimens remain negative. A positive bronchoscopy result requires considerations for therapy.

Rapidly growing mycobacteria demonstrate variable in vitro drug sensitivities. Both *M. abscessus* and *M. fortuitum* are resistant to the standard antituberculous agents used for *M. tuberculosis.* *M. fortuitum* is virtually always susceptible in vitro to sulfonamides and the new fluorinated quinolones, and some strains are susceptible to tetracycline analogues and clarithromycin. *M. abscessus* is rarely susceptible in vitro to these oral antibiotics. A few patients with *M. abscessus* have been treated successfully with prolonged oral erythromycin; however, the experience with clarithromycin has only been moderately successful. *M. abscessus* is usually susceptible to amikacin, cefoxitin, and imipenem. Unfortunately, a cure of the disease requires 4–6 months of therapy with these parenteral antibiotics and represents costly therapy that is poorly tolerated in the elderly. Cure of primary *M. abscessus* lung disease has not been reported with parenteral drug therapy alone. Periodic short intervals of therapy with parenteral agents may improve clinical symptoms without curing the patient. The best chance of cure for *M. abscessus* lung disease is surgical resection of localized disease, which represents a strong argument for early recognition of the disease.

The present patient's repeat sputums were positive for *M. abscessus*. A CT scan showed bronchiectatic changes of the lingula and anterior basilar segment of the right lower lobe. Because she was asymptomatic without pulmonary or systemic symptoms, she underwent careful follow-up without drug therapy, being watched for any evidence of radiographic or clinical progression of the disease.

Clinical Pearls

1. The rapidly growing mycobacteria *M. abscessus* and *M. fortuitum* are human lung pathogens.

2. There is usually a prolonged period from the onset of symptoms to isolation of the organism, averaging about 2 years.

3. The typical patient is middle-aged or older, non-smoking, white, and female, although considerable variability exists.

4. Diseases associated with rapidly growing mycobacterial lung disease include esophageal motility disorders with chronic vomiting, cystic fibrosis, previous granulomatous disease, and lipoid pneumonia.

5. Repeat isolation of the organism from sputum is indicative of disease and not colonization, and requires further work-up with strong consideration for therapy.

REFERENCES

1. Burke DS, Ullian RB. Megaesophagus and pneumonia associated with *Mycobacterium chelonei*. Am Rev Respir Dis 1977;116:1101–1107.
2. Swenson JM, Wallace RJ Jr, Silcox VA, et al. Antimicrobial susceptibility of five subgroups of *Mycobacterium fortuitum* and *Mycobacterium chelonei*. Antimicrob Agents Chemother 1985;28:807–811.
3. Brown BA, Wallace RJ Jr, Onyi GO, et al. Activities of four macrolides including clarithromycin, against *Mycobacterium fortuitum, Mycobacterium chelonei*, and *M. chelonei*-like organisms. Antimicrob Agents Chemother 1992;36:180–184.
4. Griffith DE, Girard WM, Wallace RJ Jr. Clinical features of pulmonary disease caused by rapidly growing mycobacteria: an analysis of 154 patients. Am Rev Respir Dis 1993;147:1271–1278.

PATIENT 95

A 74-year-old man with dyspnea and a pleural effusion

A 74-year-old man with known multiple myeloma noticed a 3-month history of progressive dyspnea and chest "heaviness." At first, his symptoms were mild, occurring only with exertion, but eventually progressed to orthopnea, paroxysmal nocturnal dyspnea, and occasional shortness of breath at rest. He denied substernal chest pain, cough, or hemoptysis. He had been treated for several years with chlorambucil for IgG multiple myeloma.

Physical Examination: Temperature 98.5°, pulse 110, respirations 22, blood pressure 125/63. Lymph nodes: none palpable. Skull: no tenderness. Chest: decreased breath sounds with dullness at the left lung base. Cardiac: grade III/VI holosystolic murmur, S3.

Laboratory Findings: Hct 33%; WBC 7,800/μl. Electrolytes: normal. BUN 32 mg/dl; creatinine 2.1 mg/dl; total protein 9.9 g/dl; albumin 3.4 g/dl. Chest radiograph: shown below.

Question: What is the most likely condition underlying the patient's respiratory complaints and chest radiographic findings?

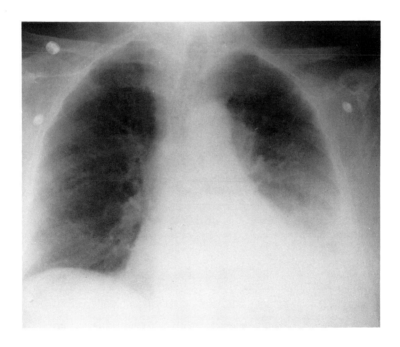

Diagnosis: Congestive heart failure with pleural effusions due to amyloid cardiomyopathy.

Discussion: Multiple myeloma, a malignant disease of plasma cells usually associated with paraproteinemia, primarily involves the bone marrow but may appear in various forms in virtually every other organ system. Thoracic involvement is particularly common, occurring in up to 46% of patients with myeloma at some time during the course of their disease.

The major manifestations of thoracic multiple myeloma include skeletal lesions, plasmacytomas, pulmonary infiltrates, and pleural effusions. Skeletal lesions are the most common thoracic form of the disease, occurring at some time in 28% of patients. Up to 15% of patients may present with thoracic skeletal lesions as the initial manifestation of their disease. Typical bony lesions include osteopenia, altered bone texture, diffuse bone destruction, "punched-out" lesions, expanding masses, osteosclerosis, and bony destruction with adjacent soft tissue masses (plasmacytomas). The ribs are the most common sites affected, followed in frequency by the vertebrae, although lesions in the sternum, clavicles, and scapulae also occur. Eight percent of patients may have generalized osteopenia as the only radiographic manifestation of the disease.

Plasmacytomas are soft tissue tumor masses that appear histologically as monotonous collections of plasma cells, which may be heterogeneous in size and shape. They occur in 12% of myeloma patients and may be the first sign of the disease in 8% of patients. Within the thorax, plasmacytomas may be "intramedullary," extending from a primary bone lesion, or "extramedullary," occurring within the soft tissues of the mediastinum, upper and lower respiratory tracts, hilar structures, or lung parenchyma unrelated to a bony site of involvement. Plasmacytomas may occur early in the course of the disease as the sole manifestation of myeloma even before the onset of paraproteinemia. Widespread disease develops in most patients within 2–3 years. Intramedullary plasmacytomas typically appear as smooth, lobulated masses that extend into the lung fields from an osteolytic rib lesion. Extramedullary plasmacytomas occur in 70% of instances at sites along the upper airways.

Pulmonary parenchymal infiltrates occur in 10% of patients with multiple myeloma and may be the presenting manifestation in 4% of patients with the disease. Most infiltrates result from infection, which is predominantly caused by *Streptococcus pneumoniae* or *Haemophilus influenzae*. Rare patients, however, may develop diffuse lung disease secondary to plasma cell infiltration into the lung.

Sometime during the course of multiple myeloma, up to 6% of patients will experience pleural effusions, one-half of which may be the sole manifestation of the disease. The effusions are only rarely a direct result of thoracic myeloma. In these patients, involvement of adjacent thoracic bony structures, tumor invasion of lung parenchyma, mediastinal lymphatic obstruction, or direct pleural extension cause the formation of pleural fluid, which may contain myeloma cells. Pleural effusions much more commonly result from congestive heart failure in patients who have developed a cardiomyopathy from myeloma-related amyloidosis. These patients interestingly have a predominance of left-sided pleural effusions.

The present patient was evaluated by thoracentesis, which demonstrated a transudative pleural effusion. The echocardiogram was compatible with amyloid cardiomyopathy with the characteristic findings of thickened ventricular walls, septum, and papillary muscles.

Clinical Pearls

1. Skeletal lesions represent the most common clinical manifestation of thoracic myeloma.

2. Thoracic plasmacytomas may be "intramedullary," arising from skeletal lesions, or "extramedullary" in location. Extramedullary lesions involve the upper airways in 70% of patients.

3. Pulmonary infiltrates in patients with multiple myeloma are more likely to represent pulmonary infections than invasion of the lung by tumor.

4. The most common cause of pleural effusions in patients with multiple myeloma is congestive heart failure related to amyloid cardiomyopathy.

REFERENCES

1. Kintzer JS, Rosenow EC, Kye RA. Thoracic and pulmonary abnormalities in multiple myeloma. Arch Intern Med 1978;138:727–730.
2. Kwan WC, Lam SC, Klimo P. Light-chain myeloma: pleural involvement. Chest 1984;86:494–496.
3. Kyle RA, Greipp PR, O'Fallon WM. Primary systemic amyloidosis: multivariate analysis for prognostic factors in 168 cases. Blood 1986;68:220–222.
4. Kravis MMJ, Hutton LC. Solitary plasma cell tumor of the pleura manifested as massive hemothorax. AJR 1993;161:543–544.

PATIENT 96

A 68-year-old woman with pleural effusions, an enlarged cardiac silhouette, and jugular venous distention

A 68-year-old woman was transferred for evaluation of persistent pleural effusions. Four months earlier, she developed fever, chills, and night sweats that resolved without treatment. Two months later, she noted the insidious onset of dyspnea with exertion and peripheral edema. Because a chest radiograph showed bilateral effusions and an enlarged silhouette and a PPD was positive with 12 mm of induration, she was started on isoniazid, rifampin, and pyrazinamide. Her sputum, gastric aspirate, and urine specimens, however, were all negative for acid-fast bacilli. The patient denied alcohol consumption but had a 30-pack-year smoking history that was discontinued 15 years earlier.

Physical Examination: Temperature 99°; pulse 96; respirations 20; blood pressure 130/65. Neck: 4-cm jugular venous distention. Chest: right dullness with decreased fremitus. Cardiac: diminished heart sounds; no gallops or murmurs. Abdomen: liver 12 cm by percussion and 3 finger-breadths below costal margin. Extremities: no cyanosis or clubbing; 1 mm pitting edema. Neurologic: normal.

Laboratory Findings: Hct 39%; WBC 7,200/μl with normal differential; erythrocyte sedimentation rate 15 mm/hr. Electrolytes and renal indices: normal. AST 24 IU/L; bilirubin 2.4 mg/dl; alkaline phosphatase 299 IU/L; LDH 89 IU/L; total protein 8.1 gm/dl. Echocardiogram: LV ejection fraction > 50%. Right thoracentesis: pleural fluid appearance: serous, nucleated cells 635/μl with 16% neutrophils; 62% lymphocytes; 18% macrophages; erythrocytes 1022/μl; total protein 3.5 gm/dl; LDH 40 IU/L; glucose: 119 gm/dl. Gram and AFB stains and cultures: negative; cytology negative. Chest radiograph: shown below left. CT scan: shown below right.

Question: What is the cause of the patient's pleural effusions?

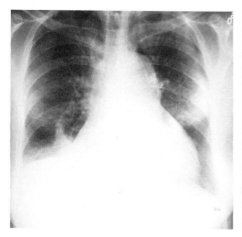 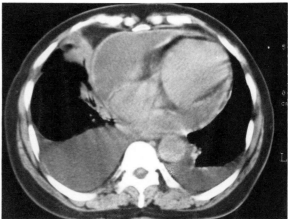

Diagnosis: Tuberculous pericarditis with effusive constriction and bilateral transudative pleural effusions.

Discussion: Constrictive pericarditis refers to a condition wherein contraction of the pericardium prevents normal diastolic filling, leading to "inflow stasis." Constrictive pericarditis may be classified as subacute (effusive) or chronic. In subacute pericarditis, fibroelastic scarring of the pericardium, often associated with a pericardial effusion in various stages of organization, constricts the heart. This constriction occurs throughout the cardiac cycle, and intrapleural pressures continue to be normally transmitted to the cardiac chambers. In chronic constrictive pericarditis, a fixed-volume, rigid shell surrounds the heart, constricting it only in diastole. Intrapleural pressures are no longer transmitted to the cardiac chambers in chronic constrictive pericarditis.

Recent series on the etiology of constrictive pericarditis note that post-cardiac surgery is the most common cause, representing about one-third of cases, followed by mediastinal radiation and uremia. Tuberculous pericarditis, bacterial pericarditis, connective tissue diseases (rheumatoid and SLE), and malignancy each represent about 5% of cases in these series. Fibrosing mediastinitis and sarcoid are rare causes. Approximately one in four instances of constrictive pericarditis is still classified as idiopathic.

Constrictive pericarditis is a relatively uncommon disorder with a varied presentation. It is often misdiagnosed as chronic liver disease, abdominal carcinomatosis, malignant pleural effusion, tuberculous pleurisy, or restrictive cardiomyopathy. Patients with subacute constrictive pericarditis have a duration of symptoms of weeks to months, history of chest pain or pericardial rub in the recent past, prominent pulsus paradoxus, and cardiomegaly. Kussmaul sign or pericardial calcification is rare. Patients with chronic constrictive pericarditis have a duration of symptoms of years, chest pain or pericardial rub in the remote past if ever, Kussmaul sign, and pericardial calcification. They do not have cardiomegaly or pulsus paradoxus.

Exertional dyspnea is the most common presenting symptom, occurring in 60–70% of patients. Mechanisms of dyspnea include restriction from bilateral pleural effusions, decreased excursion of the diaphragm from ascites, and pericardial restriction due to limited augmentation of stroke volume with exercise. Patients will often have systemic symptoms, peripheral edema, and increased abdominal girth.

The most prominent physical finding at presentation is jugular venous distention, reported in 40–95% of patients. A pleural effusion, either unilateral or bilateral, is found in approximately half of the patients at presentation. Other common physical findings include pedal edema, ascites, pericardial knock, Kussmaul sign, and pulsus paradoxus.

The chest radiograph is abnormal in most patients at the time of presentation; however, the majority of findings such as pleural effusion and increased cardiac silhouette are nonspecific. Pericardial calcification, when present, is the most specific finding.

Pleural effusions may be the primary abnormality at presentation. In the majority they are bilateral and usually symmetric. When unilateral, they have a predilection for the right, as in the patient with congestive heart failure. The effusions have been described as minimal to large, and radiographic evidence of extravascular lung water has been observed in 0–43% of patients. Pleural effusions in constrictive pericarditis are serous, transudates or exudates, with protein levels < 4.0 gm/dl, a nucleated cell count < 5000/μl, and a lymphocyte predominance. Pleural fluid glucose is similar to serum glucose, and pleural fluid acidosis has not been described. The mechanisms of pleural fluid formation in constrictive pericarditis are pulmonary venous hypertension, systemic venous hypertension, decreased oncotic pressure, and inflammatory pericardial disease.

Pericarditis should be considered in the differential diagnosis of a transudative pleural effusion. Other causes of pleural effusions that are usually exudates but may be transudates include pulmonary embolism without infarction, early malignancy, urinothorax, hypothyroidism, chylothorax, and trapped lung.

The diagnosis of constrictive pericarditis is established by clinical evaluation in conjunction with echocardiography and CT scan. Cardiac catheterization may be required to confirm the diagnosis.

Tuberculous pericarditis occurs in about 1% of patients with tuberculosis. The mortality in the pre-chemotherapy era was 90%, with a reduction in the 30–40% range following the introduction of streptomycin with about half of the deaths occurring within the first 3 months whether or not antituberculous therapy was given. The most common cause of death in some series was acute cardiac tamponade. The diagnosis must be established early; if cardiac function is impaired, appropriate drainage of the pericardial sac must be performed. Some experts recommend early use of corticosteroids with antituberculous therapy based on the drug's ability to hasten the resolution of tuberculous pleural effusions. Others suggest an aggressive surgical approach with a pericardial window. At the time of effective drainage, pericardial biopsy may be accomplished to secure the diagnosis. A general trend today is for observation on antituberculous therapy and corticosteroids as long as there is no evidence of impaired cardiac function. Pericardiectomy is recommended for those who do not respond promptly to medical therapy.

The present patient presented with radiographic evidence of bilateral pleural effusions and an abnormally thick pericardium. The transudative pleural effusion was compatible with the diagnosis. She continued to be symptomatic after 4 months of antituberculous therapy despite the addition of corticosteroids. After undergoing a pericardiectomy, she improved rapidly.

Clinical Pearls

1. Constrictive pericarditis should be included in the differential diagnosis of idiopathic pleural effusions (transudate or exudate), especially when the effusions are bilateral with a normal heart size.

2. Cardiac surgery is the most common cause of constrictive pericarditis today; mediastinal radiation remains a common etiology despite improved technology.

3. The most common presentation includes exertional dyspnea, jugular venous distention, and bilateral effusions with or without an enlarged cardiac silhouette.

4. Early antituberculous chemotherapy and possibly corticosteroids are important in preventing constriction. Patients diagnosed late and those who do not respond to medical treatment usually have a good response to pericardiectomy.

REFERENCES

1. Plumb GE, Bruwer AJ, Clagett OT. Chronic constrictive pericarditis: roentgenologic findings in 35 surgically proven cases. Mayo Clin Proc 1957;32:555–556.
2. Hancock EN. Subacute effusive-constrictive pericarditis. Circulation 1971;43:183–192.
3. Quale JM, Lipschik GY, Heurich AE. Management of tuberculous pericarditis. Ann Thorac Surg 1987;43:653–655.
4. Tomaselli G, Gamsu G, Stulbarg MS. Constrictive pericarditis presenting as a pleural effusion of unknown origin. Arch Intern Med 1989;149:201–203.

PATIENT 97

A 56-year-old woman with dyspnea and a malignant pleural effusion

A 56-year-old woman with metastatic adenocarcinoma of the breast presented with a 1-week history of increasing cough and dyspnea. One month earlier she had undergone a large volume right-sided thoracentesis for relief of dyspnea from a malignant pleural effusion. The patient denied fever, chest pain, or productive sputum.

Physical Examination: Temperature 98.7°; pulse 100; respirations 24; blood pressure 135/92. General: thin appearance. Lymph nodes: palpable right axillary. Chest: decreased breath sounds and fremitus with dullness to percussion over the right lower lung zone. Cardiac: normal.

Laboratory Findings: Hct 30%; WBC 8,700/μl with a normal differential; platelet count 200,000/μl. PT 12 sec (control 12 sec); PTT 24 sec (control 24 sec). Chest radiograph: shown below.

Question: What therapeutic options exist for the management of the patient's pleural effusion?

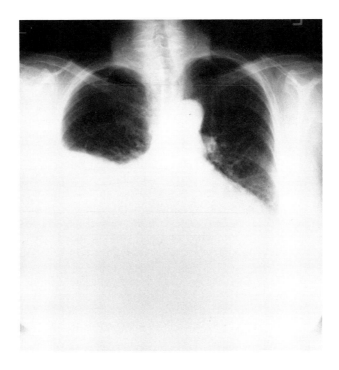

Answer: The patient is a candidate for one of the several available methods to induce pleurodesis.

Discussion: Malignant pleural effusions are a common clinical problem, representing 28–62% of pleural effusions in hospitalized patients, nearly 50% of all newly diagnosed pleural effusions, and the majority of pleural effusions in patients over 60 years of age. Unfortunately, malignant involvement of the pleura portends a poor prognosis, with a 25–54% 1-month and a 84% 6-month mortality rate. Despite advances in oncologic care, the clinical outcome in patients with malignant pleural effusions has not improved during the last 25 years.

Palliation remains the primary goal of therapy in managing pleural malignancies, with treatment options that range from simple observation to aggressive surgical decortication. Except perhaps in the instances of thoracic lymphoma, small cell lung cancer, and breast cancer, malignant pleural effusions typically do not respond to systemic chemotherapy or thoracic irradiation. Selection of a palliative plan requires individualization of care in an effort to provide relief of respiratory symptoms, prevention of fluid reaccumulation, and improvement of patient qualilty of life with the best tolerated and least interventional clinical approach necesary.

Of the available management techniques, repeated thoracentesis has not been successful because of a 97% rate of fluid reaccumulation after 30 days of observation. Draining the fluid with a chest tube for several days is equally unsuccessful. An open thoracotomy with complete or partial decortication is 100% effective, but a 23% rate of morbidity and 10% mortality limit the utility of the procedure. Decortication is presently reserved for patients with good activity levels and prognoses who have failed other palliative approaches or who present with trapped lungs unamenable to alternative techniques.

Pleurodesis by the instillation of chemical agents through a chest tube may produce pleural symphysis and thereby prevent the reaccumulation of malignant pleural fluid. Some clinicians recommend delaying the procedure until symptomatic patients reaccumulate pleural fluid after two or three therapeutic thoracenteses. Because of the risks of a trapped lung and overgrowth of the pleura with tumor that prevents a successful pleurodesis, however, other clinicians recommend early pleurodesis at the first signs of a malignant pleural effusion. Regardless of the timing of the procedure, to be successful the pleural space must be completely drained and the lung fully reexpanded before intrapleural instillation of the sclerosing agent.

Of the several sclerosing agents available, tetracycline has been the most popular in the United States since its first description in 1972 because of its safety, effectiveness, ease of use, and low cost. The mechanisms whereby tetracycline produces pleural symphysis is uncertain but may have to do with its ability to injure pleural mesothelial cells and stimulate fibroblasts to proliferate and deposit collagen adhesions between the visceral and parietal pleural surfaces. More recently, tetracycline has been shown to inhibit metalloproteinases in pleural fluid that degrade type IV collagen and gelatin deposited on mesothelial surfaces. The sclerosing action of tetracycline appears unrelated to its low pH of 2.0.

The clinical efficacy of tetracycline in controlling malignant pleural effusions ranges between 25% and 100% in reported series. The long-term success of tetracycline, however, has been variable, with pleural fluid recurrence rates up to 53% after 90 days of observation. The recent commercial unavailability of tetracycline has prompted clinical trials with the tetracycline cogeners minocycline and doxycycline. The largest clinical series to date has been with doxycycline, which in three reports appears to have an 80–90% initial success rate and 60–90% long-term efficacy.

Antineoplastic agents such as bleomycin, mitomycin, nitrogen mustard, and etoposide have been used for chemical pleurodesis, but the high cost of the drugs, systemic absorption, and interference with systemic chemotherapeutic regimens have limited their utility.

Asbestos-free talc instilled as a slurry through a chest tube is highly successful in 90–100% of patients with malignant pleural effusions and has a low rate of recurrence. Early concern regarding risks for talc-induced mesotheliomas or pulmonary restriction from thick pleural peels has not been supported by the clinical experience. Use of talc by slurry has been limited by anecdotal reports of respiratory failure with or without pneumonia in patients receiving intrapleural talc. More recent patient series using lower doses of talc, however, have not observed these complications.

Some patients with trapped lungs not treatable by other techniques may benefit from placement of a pleuroperitoneal shunt to manage their malignant pleural effusions. This catheter has a pumping chamber with two one-way valves that fits under the skin and removes 1.5 ml of pleural fluid with each compression. Although reported to have a high rate of success for relieving symptoms and excellent long-term patency, pleuroperitoneal shunts have not been prospectively compared to chemical pleurodesis.

Recently, thoracoscopy with the intrapleural insufflation of talc has regained recognition as an effective method for controlling malignant pleural effusions. First described in 1935, thoracoscopic talc insufflation under general anesthesia or local anesthesia with intravenous sedation has a 90% overall success rate with a low incidence of fluid reaccumulation. Thoracoscopy is particularly beneficial in patients with trapped lungs who may benefit from removal of visceral pleural peels to reexpand the lung and allow an effective pleurodesis. Proponents of thoracoscopic talc insufflation as a primary technique for pleurodesis in all patients with malignant pleural effusions argue that it requires a shorter duration of hospitalization and provides a high success rate compared to chemical pleurodesis. Most patients with malignant pleural effusion, however, undergo pleurodesis during hospitalizations for other indications so that the method of pleurodesis does not alter the hospital stay. Furthermore, no randomized prospective studies exist to date to clearly define the relative efficacy of thoracoscopy compared to other methods of pleurodesis.

The present patient had recurrence of a symptomatic malignant pleural effusion and underwent placement of a 24-French percutaneous chest catheter with the removal of 1.5 liters of fluid. After 48 hours, fluid drainage diminished to less that 100 ml/day, and she received intrapleural instillation of 500 mg of doxycycline. The chest tube was removed 2 days later and the fluid did not reaccumulate during the remaining 4 months of her life.

Clinical Pearls

1. The majority of patients older than 60 years of age presenting with an exudative pleural effusion have an underlying pleural malignancy.

2. Decortication is presently reserved for patients with good activity levels and prognoses who have failed other palliative approaches or who present with trapped lungs unamenable to alternative techniques.

3. Tetracylcine stimulates fibroblasts to deposit collagen and suppresses mesothelial cell growth. Both tetracycline and doxycycline inactivate metalloproteinases in pleural fluid, which are the enzymes responsible for the degradation of type IV collagen and gelatin.

4. Thoracoscopic insufflation of talc is a highly effective and well-tolerated method of pleurodesis, especially in patients with trapped lungs that can be reexpanded by removal of pleural peels. Comparative advantages to chemical pleurodesis through a chest tube, however, await confirmation by randomized prospective trials.

REFERENCES
1. Little AG, Kadowaki MH, Ferguson MK, et al. Pleuroperitoneal shunting. Ann Surg 1988;208:443–450.
2. Mänsson T. Treatment of malignant pleural effusion with doxycycline. Scand J Infect Dis 1988;53:29–34.
3. Aelony Y, King R, Boutin C. Thoracoscopic talc poudrage pleurodesis for chronic recurrent pleural effusions. Ann Intern Med 1991;115:778–782.
4. Webb WR, Ozmen V, Moulder PV, et al. Iodized talc pleurodesis for the treatment of pleural effusions. J Thorac Cardiovasc Surg 1992;103:881–888.
5. Hartman DL, Gaither JM, Kesler KA, et al: Comparison of insufflated talc under thoracoscopic guidance with standard tetracycline and bleomycin pleurodesis for control of malignant pleural effusions. J Thorac Cardiovasc Surg 1993;105:743–748.

PATIENT 98

A 70-year-old woman with exertional dyspnea, nervousness, and insomnia

A 70-year-old woman with intermittent atrial fibrillation presented with a several-year history of progressive dyspnea on exertion. She denied asthma, cough, sputum production, hemoptysis, or chest pain but did note insomnia and nervousness. The patient had a 20-pack-year smoking history but had discontinued this habit 30 years earlier. A remotely placed PPD was negative. She had a normal echocardiogram and exercise stress test and had no episodes of atrial fibrillation in the past two years. Current medications included digoxin, verapamil, and liotrix (Thyrolar) for documented hypothyroidism.

Physical Examination: Temperature 98.4°; pulse 80 and regular; respirations 18; blood pressure 145/80. HEENT: normal. Chest: normal. Cardiac: no jugular venous distention; normal heart sounds; no gallops or murmurs. Abdomen: normal. Skin: smooth. Extremities: no cyanosis, clubbing, or edema; mild tremor.

Laboratory Findings: Hct 43%; WBC 10,900/μl with a normal differential. T4 9.03 μg/dl (normal 4.5–11.5 μg/dl); TSH < 0.1 μU/ml (normal 0.4–6.0 μU/ml). FVC 2.63 L (89% of predicted); FEV$_1$ 1.90 L (90% of predicted); FEV$_1$/FVC ratio 72%; FEF 25–75% 1.17 L/sec (49% of predicted); no change with bronchodilators. RV/TLC 126% of predicted; D$_L$/VA 90% of predicted. ABG (RA): pH 7.42; PCO$_2$ 38 mmHg; PO$_2$ 85 mmHg. ECG: sinus rhythm; nonspecific ST and T wave changes. Chest radiograph: shown below.

Questions: What is the cause of the patient's dyspnea? What laboratory test would substantiate the diagnosis?

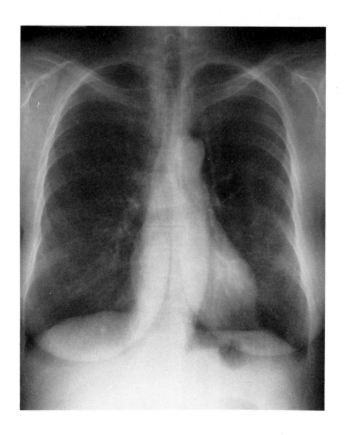

Diagnosis: Iatrogenic T3 thyrotoxicosis causing dyspnea.

Discussion: Dyspnea may occur in patients who do not have intrinsic lung disease. The most common "nonpulmonary" causes of dyspnea include congestive heart failure, anemia, obesity, pulmonary embolism, neuromuscular diseases, skeletal deformities, and hyperthyroidism. Psychogenic dyspnea should be considered as an additional cause of dyspnea when symptoms occur only at rest in patients who have organic causes of dyspnea excluded. Nonpulmonary dyspnea should be considered when the chest examination and chest radiograph are normal and pulmonary function tests cannot explain the patient's symptoms.

Dyspnea, both at rest and during exercise, is a well-recognized clinical manifestation of hyperthyroidism even in patients without overt cardiopulmonary disease. The basis for dyspnea in hyperthyroidism is not completely understood, although considerable insights have been made into its possible pathogenesis. Hyperthyroid patients have a reduced FVC, a high RV, and low maximum inspiratory and expiratory pressures. It has been postulated that these abnormalities result from respiratory muscle myopathy because the lung function impairment frequently normalizes following therapy in patients with clinical evidence of myopathy. Pulmonary function tests do not improve with therapy of the hyperthyroidism, however, in patients without underlying respiratory muscle myopathy. Generalized myopathy in thyrotoxicosis is a common clinical finding detectable by EMG in over 90% of patients. Many of these patients have associated impairment of respiratory muscles.

Other possible causes for dyspnea in hyperthyroidism include an increased hypoxic ventilatory drive, which is not abolished by beta-blockade, and increased hypercapnic ventilatory drive. Patients with hyperthyroidism also show an increased ventilatory response and often assume a rapid, shallow breathing pattern during exercise. The high respiratory rate, minute ventilation, and oxygen consumption observed in hyperthyroid patients at rest (which increase further with exercise and return to normal with treatment) suggest that a central mechanism may be involved. Hyperthyroid patients exhibit an abnormal sense of exertional dyspnea that is related to a minute ventilation out of proportion to both workload and CO_2 production. An increase in central drive during exercise may play an important role in this hyperventilation and may be related to the circulating T3 level. The observed inhibition of this response by beta-receptor antagonists suggests that the hormonal effects on the respiratory centers might be at least in part secondary to increased adrenergic stimulation.

Thyrotoxic-induced cardiac failure or airflow obstruction due to tracheal compression by a goiter are more obvious causes of dyspnea in the thyrotoxic patient. Patients with asthma who become thyrotoxic may develop further airflow obstruction that improves when euthyroidism is established.

The present patient's total T3 concentration of 368 ng/dl (normal 75–220 ng/dl), along with the normal chest radiograph and minimally abnormal PFT results, established the diagnosis of iatrogenic T3 thyrotoxicosis caused by Thyrolar, which is a mixture of the sodium salts of thyroxine and triiodothyronine in a ratio of 4:1. Because she had a known intolerance to levothyroxine (Synthroid), the patient was maintained on liotrix with a dose adjustment from 3 to 2 grains/day. Her dyspnea, insomnia, and nervousness resolved during the following several weeks. Repeat thyroid function studies showed normal total T3 and T4 concentrations.

Clinical Pearls

1. Nonpulmonary causes of dyspnea include congestive heart failure, anemia, pulmonary embolism, obesity, skeletal deformities, neuromuscular diseases, and psychiatric causes, in addition to hyperthyroidism.

2. Dyspnea, unrelated to cardiac failure or airways obstruction, is an important feature of patients with hyperthyroidism, both at rest and during exercise.

3. The dyspnea of hyperthyroidism appears to be potentially related to several causes, including respiratory muscle weakness, an inappropriate increase in ventilatory drive during rest and exercise, and inefficient rapid and shallow breathing during exercise.

REFERENCES

1. Ayres J, Rees J, Clark TJH, et al. Thyrotoxicosis and dyspnoea. Clin Endocrinol 1982;16:65–71.
2. Kendrick AH, O'Reilly JF, Laszlo G. Lung function and exercise performance in hyperthyroidism before and after treatment. Q J Med 1988;68(256):615–627.
3. Mier A, Brophy C, Wass JAH, et al. Reversible respiratory muscle weakness in hyperthyroidism. Am Rev Respir Dis 1989;139:529–533.
4. Small D, Gibbons W, Levy RD, et al. Exertional dyspnea and ventilation in hyperthyroidism. Chest 1992;101:1268–1273.

PATIENT 99

A 24-year-old man with cystic fibrosis and worsening wheezing

A 24-year-old man with a long history of cystic fibrosis and allergic rhinitis presented with a 3-month history of worsening dyspnea and cough. His sputum had not changed from its baseline appearance until the last 2 weeks when it became thick and difficult to expectorate; a chest radiograph at that time demonstrated a patchy right upper lobe infiltrate. His physician had placed him on oral antipseudomonal antibiotics, theophylline, and inhalations of beta-agonist agents every 4 hours without improvement in his symptoms, although the infiltrate resolved.

Physical Examination: Temperature 99°; respirations 20; pulse 65; blood pressure 135/75. Chest: diffuse rhonchi and wheezes. Cardiac: normal. Extremities: no clubbing.

Laboratory Findings: Hct 31%; WBC 7,500 polymorphonuclear cells 70%; eosinophils 15%. Chest radiographs: shown below.

Question: What complication of cystic fibrosis should be excluded in this patient?

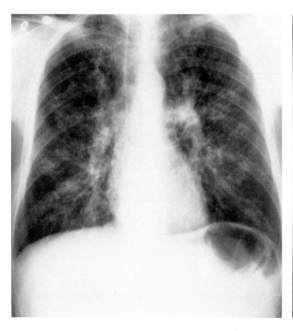 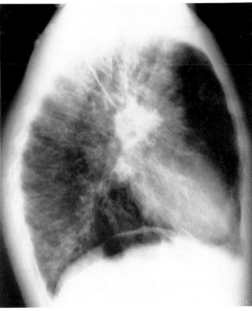

Diagnosis: Allergic bronchopulmonary aspergillosis (ABPA).

Discussion: ABPA is a hypersensitivity reaction that occurs primarily in patients with underlying asthma whose airways become colonized with the fungus *Aspergillus fumigatus*. First described in 1952, ABPA is considered to complicate lung function in as many as 22% of asthmatic patients in England and 8% of patients with asthma in the United States.

The pathogenesis of ABPA begins with the inhalation of aspergillus spores that individuals with normal lungs readily clear from their airways. In patients with asthma and abnormal bronchial secretions, however, the fungus colonizes the airways and serves as an antigen that stimulates a hypersensitivity reaction without actually invading bronchial walls. An ensuing inflammatory response releases cellular mediators and leukocyte secretory products that aggravate bronchospasm and initiate relentless airway injury that eventually results in central bronchiectasis.

Patients with asthma complicated by ABPA typically experience bronchospasm that is refractory to bronchodilators. Sputum production may increase with expectoration of tenacious secretions and plugs that may harbor fungal elements. Intermittent febrile illnesses with increased cough and evanescent radiographic pulmonary infiltrates resulting from mucus plugging may stimulate an acute bacterial pneumonia.

Cystic fibrosis (CF) has been recognized since 1965 as an additional risk factor for ABPA. Preexisting bronchiectasis, poor clearance of airway secretions, and underlying colonization of airways with *Pseudomonas aeruginosa* and *Staphylococcus aureus* related to CF create an ideal environment for aspergillus colonization. The contribution of these factors to the onset of ABPA are uncertain, however, considering that allergic rhinitis and asthma manifestations occur in 12–24% of patients with CF, and most patients with CF complicated by ABPA have underlying bronchospastic disease. In any event, it has been estimated that nearly 7% of patients with CF have coexisting ABPA. The incidence is highest in older patients with CF who have more advanced airway disease and a conducive bronchial environment for aspergillus colonization.

The chest radiograph in ABPA with or without CF shows fleeting pulmonary infiltrates, bronchiectasis, branching shadows of mucoid impaction emanating from the hila, and tramline shadows that represent thickened bronchial walls. These findings are more often observed in the upper lung zones. Most of these radiographic features are similar to those observed in advanced CF not complicated by ABPA. The laboratory features of ABPA include peripheral blood eosinophilia, sputum cultures positive for *A. fumigatus*, an elevated serum IgE, and an immediate skin reactivity to *A. fumigatus* antigen. Although these findings are sensitive indicators of ABPA, they are not specific in that many patients with underlying asthma or CF will demonstrate these laboratory results.

Diagnosing ABPA in patients with CF is complicated because the clinical, radiographic, and laboratory features of the two conditions overlap. Even identifying *A. fumigatus* in respiratory secretions may not assist diagnosis because 25–57% of patients with CF will have intermittently positive sputum cultures in the absence of aspergillus-related disease. Clinical experience demonstrates the importance of diagnosing ABPA in patients with asthma because therapy improves the course of bronchospasm and prevents the onset of bronchiectasis. Although the contribution of ABPA to the progression of cystic fibrosis lung disease is uncertain, elimination of aspergillus from the airways may improve pulmonary symptoms and the patient's short-term course in addition to preventing the acceleration of bronchiectasis. Selection of patients for therapy requires a careful clinical assessment and close observation for a response to therapy.

The therapy of ABPA is directed at eliminating fungal colonization and suppressing the hypersensitivity response with corticosteroids. Although various dosing regimens have been employed, a commonly used starting dose of prednisone is 0.5 mg/kg/day, with a taper initiated to a baseline dose as the clinical course allows over a 1–2 month period. Inhaled steroids are ineffective in controlling the clinical manifestations of ABPA. In patients with asthma, disease activity can be monitored by the serum IgE level to assist corticosteroid dose adjustments. Unfortunately, monitoring the serum IgE level in patients with CF is a less reliable gauge of the patient's clinical response. Most patients with CF tolerate corticosteroids without experiencing infectious complications. The major morbidity of prednisone in these patients is a worsening of glucose intolerance and accelerated development of cataracts.

The present patient had worsening of his bronchospasm, a fleeting upper lobe pulmonary infiltrate, and peripheral blood eosinophilia, which should always suggest the diagnosis of ABPA in the setting of CF. A subsequent sputum culture was positive for *A. fumigatus* and other laboratory findings supported the diagnosis. He was started on prednisone, which markedly improved his symptoms.

Clinical Pearls

1. Up to 7% of patients with cystic fibrosis (CF) have coexisting ABPA.

2. Most CF patients with ABPA have underlying allergic rhinitis or clinical evidence of asthma.

3. As in asthmatic patients, the presence of peripheral eosinophilia, elevated serum IgE levels, positive *A. fumigatus* precipitins, positive scratch tests for aspergillus antigens, and even positive sputum cultures for *A. fumigatus* are sensitive but nonspecific diagnostic features of ABPA.

4. Any patient with CF who has asthmatic symptoms and peripheral eosinophilia should be evaluated for ABPA.

REFERENCES

1. Hutcheson PS, Rejent AJ, Slavin RG. Variability of parameters of allergic bronchopulmonary aspergillosis in patients with cystic fibrosis. J Allergy Clin Immunol 1991;88:390–394.
2. Mroueh S, Spock A. Allergic bronchopulmonary aspergillosis in patients with cystic fibrosis. Chest 1994;105:32–36.

PATIENT 100

A 47-year-old man with left chest pain, dyspnea, and an eosinophilic pleural effusion

A 47-year-old man presented with a 4-day history of dyspnea and pleuritic chest pain. The patient reported a 30-pack-year history of smoking, long-term alcohol abuse, and an 18-year record of employment in a shipyard as a pipefitter. He took no medications and denied known HIV risk factors.

Physical Examination: Temperature 98.2°; pulse 72; respirations 20; blood pressure 110/70. General: well-nourished; no acute distress. Mouth: poor dentition. Lymph nodes: no adenopathy. Chest: diminished breath sounds and dullness to percussion, left posterior thorax; basilar rales that cleared with cough. Cardiac: normal. Abdomen: normal. Extremities: no cyanosis, clubbing, or edema.

Laboratory Findings: Hct 41%; WBC 11,000/μl. Blood chemistries: normal. Chest radiograph: shown below left. Left thoracentesis: results shown below right.

Question: What is the most likely cause of the pleural effusion?

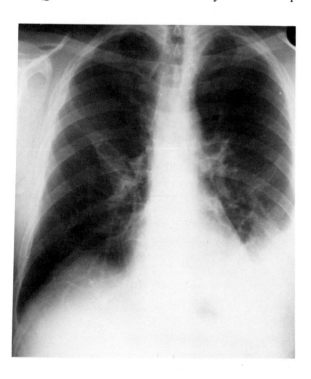

Pleural Fluid Analysis

Appearance: serosanguinous

Nucleated cells: 4800

Differential:
    1% neutrophils
    6% lymphocytes
    27% mononuclear cells
    66% eosinophils

RBC: 9250/μl

Total protein: 4.9 gm/dl
    (serum 7.2 gm/dl)

LDH: 363 IU/L (serum 150 IU/L)

Glucose: 95 mg/dl

pH: 7.33

Amylase: 28 IU/L

Gram stain and culture: negative

Cytology: negative

Diagnosis: Benign asbestos pleural effusion (BAPE).

Discussion: As early as the 1920s, pathologic descriptions of the lung in patients with asbestosis included references to abnormal pleural findings. But it was over 30 years later that the entity we know today as BAPE was first described. Subsequent reports defined that BAPE occurs in 3% of asbestos-exposed workers compared to none from a group of individuals without a history of asbestos exposure followed long-term. These observations confirmed that BAPE was a definite condition linked to asbestos exposure. By 1987, over 250 cases of BAPE had been reported in the world literature.

The clinical presentation of BAPE varies in reported series. Some reports indicate that one-half to two-thirds of patients have minimal or no symptoms. The percentage of asymptomatic patients in any series, however, depends on the number and frequency of screening chest radiographs performed. The most common symptom is chest pain. Rarely, patients have persistent, severe pain for several years after the initial episode of pleural effusion. Less than 20% of patients complain of dyspnea, cough, or fever.

The chest radiograph in BAPE usually shows a small unilateral pleural effusion; however, pleural effusions may be large and bilateral. Recurrences of effusions may occur ipsilateral or contralateral to the initial effusion and may recur years later. Parietal pleural plaques and asbestosis are seen in the minority of patients at the time of development of BAPE. Blunting of the costophrenic angle is the most common radiographic sequela, but rounded atelectasis and bilateral pleural fibrosis with or without progression also may occur.

The pleural fluid is hemorrhagic in approximately one-half of patients. The nucleated cell count is usually $< 6000/\mu l$ and may be either neutrophil or mononuclear predominant. Pleural fluid eosinophilia, which occurs in 25–50% of patients, should alert the clinician to the possibility of BAPE. Pleural fluid eosinophilia (defined as eosinophils/nucleated cells $> 10\%$) usually indicates benign disease and most commonly occurs after pneumothorax and pleural space hemorrhage. Pleural fluid from patients with BAPE also contains mesothelial cells, which in addition to eosinophilia, virtually exclude the diagnosis of tuberculous pleurisy. The effusion is always exudative with a high protein concentration. A low glucose and pleural fluid acidosis have not been described. The hyaluronic acid level is not increased and asbestos bodies have not been seen in BAPE. Asbestos bodies or fibers have been found only rarely in pleural tissue from these patients.

Criteria for the diagnosis of BAPE include exposure to asbestos, exclusion of other causes of an exudative effusion, and exclusion of malignancy for a follow-up period of 2 years. The average latency period from time of first exposure to the diagnosis of BAPE is 19 years with a range from 1–58 years. Because virtually all other asbestos-related pleuropulmonary changes or diseases have a latency period of at least 20–30 years, BAPE should be the most common manifestation in the first 20 years following exposure and may be a precursor of these other findings. Therefore, a long latency period does not necessarily indicate a malignancy. Even a minor exposure to asbestos has been reported to cause BAPE.

There is no specific treatment for BAPE. Effusions resolve within 1 month to 1 year or more (usually 3–4 months) after onset. The long-term prognosis for patients with BAPE is said to be poor. A number of malignant mesotheliomas among patients with BAPE have been reported. Whether BAPE per se is a risk factor for mesothelioma would require a large epidemiologic study.

The present patient's chest pain resolved when treated symptomatically with a nonsteroidal anti-inflamatory agent; however, he continued to complain of dyspnea with exertion.

Clinical Pearls

1. BAPE, the earliest manifestation of asbestos exposure in the chest, usually occurs within the first 20 years of initial exposure but has been reported wihtin 1 year and as late as 58 years following exposure.

2. Fifty to 70% of patients with BAPE have minimal or no symptoms at the time of diagnosis.

3. The findings of a hemorrhagic exudate with eosinophilia in a patient with asbestos exposure should suggest BAPE.

4. The most common sequela of BAPE is a blunted costophrenic angle, but rounded atelectasis and pleural fibrosis with or without progression may also occur.

REFERENCES

1. Eisenstadt HB. Asbestos pleurisy. Dis Chest 1964; 46:78–81.
2. Mattson SB. Monosymptomatic exudative pleurisy in persons exposed to asbestos dust. Scand J Respir Dis 1975;56:263–272.
3. Epler GR, McLoud TC, Gaensler EA. Prevalence and incidence of benign asbestos pleural effusion in a working population. JAMA 1982;247:617–622.
4. Hillerdal G, Ozesmi M. Benign asbestos pleural effusion: 73 exudates in 60 patients. Eur J Respir Dis 1987;71:113–121.
5. Martensson G, Hagberg S, Pettersson K, et al. Asbestos pleural effusion: a clinical entity. Thorax 1987;42:646–651.

INDEX